COMPLEMENTARY PEDIATRICS

Edited by **Öner Özdemir**

Complementary Pediatrics
Edited by Öner Özdemir

Published by InTech
Janeza Trdine 9, 51000 Rijeka, Croatia

Publishing Process Manager Irena Voric

Technical Editor Teodora Smiljanic

Cover Designer InTech Design Team

Additional hard copies can be obtained from orders@intechopen.com

Complementary Pediatrics, Edited by Öner Özdemir
p. cm.
ISBN 978-953-51-0155-0

For EU product safety concerns:
IN TECH d.o.o., Prolaz Marije Krucifikse Kozulić 3, 51000 Rijeka, Croatia,
info@intechopen.com or visit our website at intechopen.com.

Meet the editor

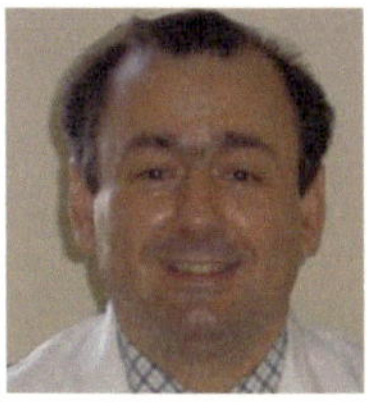

Doc. Dr. Öner Özdemir was born in Alaplı, Zonguldak, Turkey in 1965. He has graduated from İstanbul Medical School, İstanbul University and become a medical doctor in 1989. Dr. Ozdemir did his pediatric residency at Department of Pediatrics in Children's Hospital, İstanbul Medical School, İstanbul, Turkey. His clinical fellowship training was finished at Pediatric Allergy/Immunology division in Louisiana State University, Health Sciences Centre, New Orleans, LA. Dr. Ozdemir research areas are as follows: LAK-cell generation and cell-mediated cytotoxicity; human mast cell development and mast cell-mediated cytotoxicity; and apoptosis related research. He was the first place winner of Clemens Von Pirquet Award from ACAAI at ACAAI meeting in 2005 for the best research on allergy/asthma/immunology by a fellow in training. Dr. Ozdemir has more than 50 international plus 20 national publications, as well as 90 international and 30 national presentations, and more than 5 chapters related to his research areas. Currently, he works as chief at the third clinic of pediatrics associated with the division of pediatric allergy/immunology at İstanbul Medeniyet University, Göztepe Teaching and Training Hospital, Kadıköy, İstanbul, Turkey.

Contents

Preface

It is a great honor for me to be editor of the book Complementary Pediatrics. Currently; there is a lot of classical pediatric text books describing various topics. In these kinds of text books, there have always been similar topics with the same styles. In this book volume, beyond classical themes, a different approach was made to current pediatric issues and topics.

This book volume covers complementary issues of pediatric subspecialties consisting of ophthalmologic, surgical, psychosocial and administrative issues of frequently used medications. Book consists of 16 chapters which will help get us and patients enlightened with the new developments on these subspecialties' area.

First section of the book is pediatric ophthalmology, which concisely explains most common eye disorders encountered during childhood until adolescence. Pediatric Surgery section discusses very classical but unsettled approaches for issues related to circumcision and cryptorchidism. An interesting approach also has been defined for the treatment of anal fissure.

Section of special and interdisciplinary care entails pain management, snake bites, oral health, oxidative stress and a model of specialized interdisciplinary management. Oxidative stress of newborn is described in detail and therapeutic options are explained. In addition, the use of melatonin is mentioned as a useful tool to combat oxygen toxicity in newborns.

Section on psychosocial issues is usually not mentioned in old pediatric textbooks, but it is not forgotten in this book volume. This section starts with adolescent psychosocial development and continues with commonly encountered problems such as alcohol intoxication and unwanted sexual experience. Moreover, as a paramedical issue, professional liability section describes liability in detail in this book.

Frequently used medications section, lists the administration and dose of most frequently used pediatric drugs as a directory. This manual will help decrease administrative medication and calculation errors.

In conclusion; with these 16 chapters, this book volume completes knowledge on pediatric subspecialties including psychosocial and special / interdisciplinary issues.

Before I finish my last words, I feel obliged to my father Orhan and father-in-law Hasan Baş for their support during this period time.

Öner Özdemir, MD
Assoc. Prof. of Pediatrics
İstanbul Medeniyet University
Göztepe Research/Training Hospital
3rd Clinic of Pediatrics, Division of Pediatric Allergy/Immunology
Kadıköy, İstanbul,
Turkey

Part 1

Pediatric Ophtalmology

1

Pediatric Ophthalmology / Eye and Disorders

Hikmet Basmak, Nilgun Yildirim, Seyhan Topbas,
Ahmet Ozer, Nazmiye Erol, Huseyin Gursoy and Afsun Sahin
Eskisehir Osmangazi University Medical Faculty,
Department of Ophthalmology,
Turkey

1. Introduction

1.1 Growth and development of child's eye

The growth and development of eye harbors many challenging anatomical and physiological alterations starting from the intrauterine life until the early puberty. After the early puberty, the axial length of eye, which is defined as the anterior posterior diameter of the eye, remains unaltered in healthy subjects. However, the refractive status of the eye may still change in adults due to aging processes. The eye development starts in the 3-week embryo, from the optic vesicles. The eye is an organ which derives from all three of the germ layers (ectoderm, endoderm and mesoderm). The initial 3 years of life is the critical period for eye development, and rapid increase in dimensions of the organ takes place in these years. Clear vision is mandatory for the development of visual cortex in this critical period. It is accepted that normal adult visual capacity develops at 3 years of age (Fredrick, 2004).

The coordinated growth of eye's refractive components to reach a plano refraction is called emmetropization. If any failure happens in this process, refractive errors develop. The axial length is either too short, causing hypermetropia, or too long, causing myopia. Astigmatism is due to abnormal shapes in cornea. Very high degrees of hypermetropia (>5D) is not normal in newborns. The cornea and lens may flatten normally within years, but the axial length often pauses behind. This causes permanent hyperopia, which is called nanophthalmos. Generally, eyes with hyperopia of greater than 5 diopters have little chance of emmetropization (Mutti, 1992).

All anatomical alterations occur in order to achieve emmetropization. The corneal diameter at birth is about 9.5-10.5 mm. The average adult size is 12 mm. The corneal refractive power is 52 diopters at birth and 42-44 diopters in adulthood. Axial length is 17 mm at birth. It enlarges to 20 mm by the end of 12 months with continued rapid growth until 2 years old, then a slow increase to 24 mm by adulthood. The most rapid eye growth occurs within the first two years. At birth the power of the crystalline lens is 34 diopters. By 6 months of age power averages 28 diopters. By the adulthood the lens power reaches about 20 diopters. As cornea, lens, and axial length grow and change rapidly over the first months and years of life, the harmonization between these three components become crucial.

Normal infant eyes are 2 diopters hyperopic. This increases slightly to around age 7, then decreases to age 9-12 years when emmetropia is reached. Normal eyes have diminutive refractive changes after 13 years (Mutti, 1992).

2. Congenital eye anomalies

The congenital eye anomalies may appear in isolation or as part of a systemic syndrome. It may be genetically proven in some cases. Either germ line or somatic mutations can cause eye abnormalities. They may result from disruption, deformation, intrauterine infection or teratogenic exposure. Some anomalies significantly affect visual acuity. On the other hand, there are some anomalies which are noticed incidentally on routine eye check with no significance to the patient (Kherani & Robb, 2008).

2.1 Infantile hemangiomas

Infantile hemangiomas are the most common eyelid tumors in infancy. They have a bright red or purple appearance. Superficial ones typically blanch with pressure. At birth, they may be clinically undetected. However, they typically enlarge in the first 12 months followed by a slow involution during the first decade. Vision loss is related to amblyopia because of induced astigmatism or visual deprivation due to ptosis. Steroid treatment (intralesional and/or oral) is the first line of therapy (Levin, 2003).

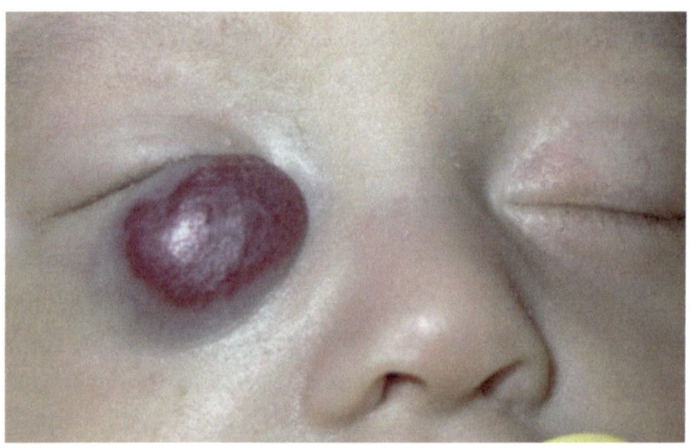

Fig. 1. Capillary hemangioma

2.2 Epibulbar dermoids

Choristomas (congenital dermoids) are masses of normal tissue found in an abnormal location. They induce astigmatism and cause refractive amblyopia. They may be excised to improve cosmetic appearance and avoid amblyopia.

2.3 Microphthalmia

A variety of disorders in which axial length is at least two standard deviations below normal is called microphthalmia. It is frequently associated with secondary orbital and ocular deformity including cataract and coloboma. It is frequently associated with various genetic conditions such as trisomy 13, Goldenhar's syndrome (Kherani & Robb, 2008).

2.4 Colobomas

It results from failure of the embryonic fissure to close along the inferonasal side of the optic cup during embryogenesis. It is frequently associated with microphthalmia. The visual prognosis is linked to the degree of optic nerve and macular involvement.

2.5 Persistant fetal vasculature (persistant hyperplastic primary vitreus)

It occurs sporadically and unilaterally in full-term health infants. The affected eye is microphthalmic with a shallow anterior chamber. A vascularized membrane behind the lens is typical. If the eye is not severely microphthalmic, surgical intervention may have a good prognosis (Levin, 2003).

3. Optic nerve disease in children

The optic nerve is approximately 50 mm long from the globe to the chiasm. It can be subdivided into four segments: Intraocular (optic disc, optic nerve head), intraorbital, intracanalicular and intracranial segment. Optic nerve is surrounded by the vascular pia, arachnoid and dura mater. The subarachnoid space is continuous with the cerebral subarachnoid space and contains the cerebrospinal fluid. The optic nerve carries approximately 1.2 million afferent nerve fibres which originate in the retinal ganglion cells (Kanski 2011).

Common congenital optic disc anomalies are present as follows: Tilted disc, optic disc pit, optic disc drusen (hyaline bodies), optic disc coloboma, morning glory anomaly, hypoplastic optic nerve and myelinated nerve fibres (Nicholson et al., 2011). Optic disc drusen is a common anomaly with a prevalence of 0.3% of the population. In buried drusen which are the most commonly encountered type, they mimic papilloedema. Exposed optic disc drusen are rare types and more easily diagnosed. They are usually innocent, but rarely may lead to visual field defects or optic disc neovascularisation. Ultrasound is important for the differential diagnosis by showing calcific deposits associated with drusen (Kanski 2011).

Optic neuritis is an inflammatory, infective or demyelinating process affecting the optic nerve. It can be classified both ophthalmoscopically and etiologically as follows. Papillitis is characterized by hyperemia and edema of the optic disc, associated with peripapillary flame-shaped hemorrhages. Neuroretinitis is characterized by papillitis in association with inflammation of the retinal nerve fibre layer and a macular star. The optic nerve head is normal in retrobulbar neuritis, because the optic nerve head is not involved. Optic neuritis may be seen due to demyelinating disease, parainfectious, infectious such as sinus-related, or associated with cat-scratch fever, syphilis, Lyme disease, cryptococcal meningitis and non-infectious such as sarcoidosis, systemic lupus erythematosus, polyarteritis nodosa and other vasculitides (Dale et al., 2009).

Papilloedema is swelling of the optic nerve head secondary to raised intracranial pressure. It is nearly always bilateral, although it may be asymmetrical. Systemic findings such as headaches, deterioration of consciousness, nausea and vomiting, may be seen in patients with papilloedema. Transient obscurations lasting a few seconds are frequent in patients with papilloedema. Horizontal diplopia due to 6th nerve palsy may accompany the clinical picture.

Optic nerve glioma is the most common primary neoplasm of the optic nerve. A low-grade form of this neoplasm, called benign optic glioma, occurs most often in the pediatric patients. On the other hand, the aggressive form of optic glioma, is most common in adults. Many children with optic nerve glioma are also known to have neurofibromatosis type 1. Another optic nerve tumor is meningioma. Meningiomas are believed to arise from arachnoid cap cells, and they are usually attached to the dura.

Optic atrophy is the final common morphologic endpoint of any disease process that causes axonal degeneration in the optic nerve. There are two types; primary and secondary. Primary optic atrophy may be caused by lesions affecting the visual pathways from the retrolaminar portion of the optic nerve to the lateral geniculate body. Secondary optic atrophy is preceded by long-standing swelling of the optic nerve head.

4. Retinitis pigmentosa

Retinitis pigmentosa (RP) is a heterogeneous group of diffuse retinal dystrophies characterized by a progressive dysfunction affecting the rod more than the cone photoreceptors (a rod-cone dystrophy). It is the most common hereditary fundus distrophy with a prevalence of approximately 1:5000. All forms of RP can present in the first or second decade of life (Kanski, 2011).

4.1 Inheritance and systemic associations

RP can be inherited as an autosomal dominant (ADRP), autosomal recessive (ARRP) or X-linked recessive (XLRP) pattern. RP can occur as an isolated sporadic disorder with no family history. The age of onset, rate of progression, eventual visual loss and associated ocular/systemic features are related to the type of inheritance (Khani, 2011). Approximately 20% of these cases are ADRP, and 6% to 9% are XLRP. The remaining 71% to 84% are either ARRP or isolated simplex cases. Up to 40% of recessive cases are associated with other systemic pathologies or syndromes and 18% have associated hearing loss. The most common forms of ADRP appear to have a later onset and less severe clinical course than XLRP. Significantly reduced visual function usually occurs at a younger age in XLRP than in other forms of RP. Most patients with XLRP are legally blind by age 30. Important systemic associations are Basen-Kornzweig syndrome (abetalipoproteinaemia), Refsum disease, Bardet- Biedl syndrome and Usher syndrome (Drack, 2006).

4.2 Symptoms and diagnosis

Typically patients present with night blindness and visual field constriction. Central vision may or may not be involved. Classical retinal signs include bone-spicule pigmentation, arteriolar narrowing and disc pallor. Cystoid macular edema may occur. The fundus may be normal in the early stages of disease and this is often the case in young children. Electroretinography (ERG) is essential in the workup of inherited retinal dystrophies. Bright flash scotopic ERGs show a reduced a-wave, indicating rod photoreceptor dysfunction with less severe photopic ERG abnormalities. Perimetry is useful in monitoring the progression of disease. Perimetry initially demonstrates small mid-peripheral scotomas that gradually coalesce to form the classical annular scooma that correlates in location and shape to the extent of fundus pathology (Kanski, 2011).

4.3 Treatment

Although the photoreceptor cell death of retinitis pigmentosa cannot at be arrested or reversed currently, some vision threatening complications (cataract and macular edema) can be successfully managed. Additional molecular and surgical therapies targeting various stages of the disease are under investigation. (gene and stem cell-based therapies, prosthetic retinal implants, germ and somatic cell gene replacement, allele-specific targeting strategies and retinal transplantation etc.)

5. Retinopathy of prematurity

Retinopathy of prematurity (ROP) is a disease of premature babies. The disease is a potentially blinding disorder affecting primarily the retinas of the premature infants. Three epidemics of ROP have been described. The first one was seen in the 1950s in the industrialized countries. The reason was uncontrolled oxygen therapy and inadequate neonatal intensive care. With developing technology in the western countries, the incidence of the surviving extremely low birth weight babies increased. This increase in survival resulted in another epidemic. This epidemic of ROP was the second epidemic, which was characterized by extremely low birth weight babies with ROP. Currently there is an ongoing epidemic in the third world countries. The characteristics of this third epidemic are the mixture of the first and second epidemics (Gilbert, 2008).

5.1 Risk factors and pathogenesis

Uncontrolled oxygen therapy and premature birth are the most important risk factors for ROP. Babies born at or before 31 weeks of gestational age, or weighing 1500 grams or less are under high risk for ROP. Systemic problems associated with prematurity may also be considered to be independent risk factors. Sepsis, anemia and growth retardation are the most significant of these systemic associations.

The retina is not completely vascularized at birth. Especially the temporal quadrant of the retina lack blood vessels in the neonates and the retinal vessels development continues until the end of the first month of age. Vascular endothelial growth factor (VEGF) is very important for the retinal vasculature development. If uncontrolled and high oxygen therapy is applied in a premature infant, the production of VEGF may increase resulting in the development of ROP. Under physiological conditions, VEGF production is stimulated by hypoxia. Therefore, it is not exactly known why high oxygen levels lead to increased VEGF levels. The possible explanation for this inconsistency is the high variations encountered during uncontrolled oxygen supply. High oxygen levels suppress VEGF initially. This is followed by an exaggerated VEGF production, after cessation of the oxygen therapy. To prevent such variations in oxygen blood levels, oxygen supply should be given in a more steady level, according to the needs of the infants.

5.2 Clinical presentation

The ROP can be categorized as active and chronic disease. Active disease is the ROP diagnosed at the early months of infancy. Most of the cases regress spontaneously. The role of an ophthalmologist is to recognize the more severe cases with the risk of progression and to apply treatment in the indicated cases. Ridge formation in the periphery of the retina is a feature of early ROP. Ridge is a fibrovascular tissue, developed as a response to hypoxia. Retinal bleeding and/or tractional retinal detachment may occur, if the disease progresses.

In 20% of the babies with active ROP, chronic sequels of the disease may evolve. Most of these are innocuous, but fibrovascular tissues leading to macular distortion or retinal detachment may also develop. These may result in visual loss or even total blindness.

5.3 Screening

Screening by an ophthalmologist is recommended for infants with a birth-weight of ≤1500 grams and/or ≤31 weeks of gestation. The time for screening is 4-7 weeks postnatally. There is inconsistency in the literature regarding the screening protocols. Protocols including more mature babies may be designed for developing countries (Basmak, 2009).

5.4 Management

Argon laser photocoagulation is performed in babies with threshold disease. Threshold disease is defined as 5 contiguous clock hours or 8 total clock hours of extraretinal neovascularisation located at or near the macula, which is the critical region of the retina for vision. Plus disease is also a feature of the threshold disease. It is defined as sausage like dilatations of the vessels around the optic disc, as a response to hypoxia. Posterior segment surgeries are indicated if retinal detachment occurs. The outcomes after laser therapy are successful in 85% of the cases, but they are not promising after surgery. Laser ablation of the avascular retina is applied to halt the progression of ROP. VEGF inhibitors alone or combined with laser therapy or surgery may be injected into the eyes to stop or slow the progression of the disease (Erol, 2011).

Pediatricians must be aware of the association between refractive disorders, amblyopia and strabismus in early or late childhood period and ROP. The risk of developing these disorders is correlated with the severity of ROP, but it still exists in regressed ROP cases with no sequel according to some literature. Therefore all ROP cases must be routinely referred to an ophthalmologist to screen for these possible associations.

6. Lacrimal system disorders in children

Unlike many insidious and asymptomatic ocular pathologies in children lacrimal system disorders alert parents immediately, because of an obvious watering eye with adherence of the lashes and with a mucoid discharge. Congenital nasolacrimal duct obstruction is the main etiology of epiphora in the pediatric age group.

6.1 Congenital nasolacrimal duct obstruction

The nasolacrimal duct is the continuation of the lacrimal sac. It opens into the nasal meatus. Its final end is partially covered by a mucosal fold called the valve of Hasner. This final lower part of the canal at the level of the valve of Hasner, is not completely developed in some of the neonates. This developmental delay present in one fifth of the neonates. Spontaneous resolution of epiphora occurs in more than 90% of the cases within a year, after completion of the lower end of the canal (Ballard, 2000).

6.2 Differential diagnosis of epiphora in children

Amniontocele (congenital dacryocele), punctual atresia or fistulae between the sac and the skin are other rare etiologies for epiphora. Amniotecele is characterized by a blue-green distention of the lacrimal sac, observed externally at the level of inner canthus. It is due to an imperforate valve of Hasner. Amniontocele is mostly self limiting within a few days of birth, especially if massage is applied (Rose, 2000).

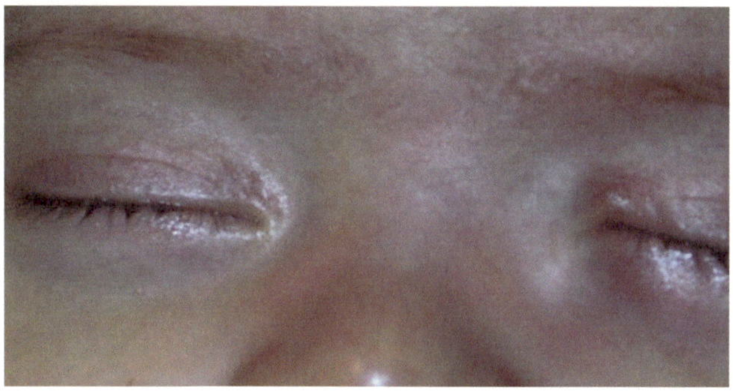

Fig. 2. Left dacryocele

6.3 Management of congenital nasolacrimal duct obstruction

Spontaneous resolution is usual, so conservative treatments including antibiotic drops and massage of the lacrimal sac region is preferred within the first year of life. The index finger is put over the inner canthal region and the massage is applied firmly downwards. Three strokes of massage, 3-4 times per day are recommended. Early intervention is indicated if recurrent dacryocystitis occur before the first year of age.

Probing of the nasolacrimal canal under general anesthesia is performed if epiphora persists beyond the first year of age. Probing is performed to disrupt the obstructive membrane at the level of valve of Hasner mechanically. The success rate of probing is very high. If it fails, the probing can be repeated once more. If epiphora persists after 2 technically satisfactory probing, more invasive procedures, including silicon tubes implantation, balloon dilatation of the nasolacrimal duct or dacryocystorhinostomy should be considered (Rose, 2000).

Dacryocystorhinostomy is an invasive surgery, which involves anastomosing the lacrimal sac to the middle meatus by the removal of the lacrimal bone, is the gold standard treatment in adults, whereas it is usually the final treatment alternative in the pediatric age group.

7. Childhood cataract

The lens is a biconvex structure that hangs behind the iris. Its diameter is about 3.5 mm at birth and it grows to about 10 mm by adulthood. There are three structural elements that constitute the lens: capsule, epithelium and fibers. The crystalline lens is a transparent structure that helps to refract light to be focused on the retina, along with the cornea. The lens is capable of changing its shape in order to modify the focal distance of the eye, so that it can focus on objects at different distances, thus allowing a clear image of the object to be formed on the retina (Kanski, 2011).

Cataract is the opacification of the crystalline lens. Cataracts result from protein denaturation, increased molecular weight of proteins, water vesicles between lens fibers, increasing proliferation and migration of the lens epithelium. Childhood cataract occurs worldwide and is an important cause of childhood blindness in many countries. Congenital cataracts occur in about 3 in 10 000 live births. Two-thirds of cases are bilateral. The cause of the cataract can be identified in about half of the cataractous eyes. Unilateral cataracts are usually isolated sporadic incidents, without a family history or systemic disease and effected infants are usually full-term and healthy. Cataract can be associated with ocular abnormalities, trauma, or an intrauterine infection such as rubella. Bilateral cataracts are often inherited and associated with other diseases. They require a full metabolic, infectious, systemic and genetic workup. The common causes are hypoglycemia, trisomy (eg, Down, Edward and Patau syndromes), myotonic dystrophy, infectious diseases (eg, toxoplasmosis, rubella, cytomegalovirus and herpes simplex [TORCH]) and prematurity. Isolated hereditary cataracts account for about 25% of the cases. The mode is most frequently autosomal dominant, but may be autosomal recessive or X-linked (Mickler, 2011).

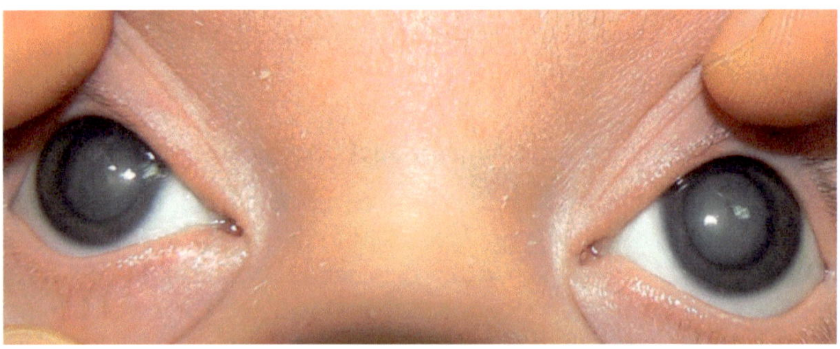

Fig. 3. Bilateral conjenital cataract

Detailed eye examination is required for the density and morphology of the any lens opacity. Potential impact on visual function of cataract is assessed on the basis of the appearance of the red reflex and the quality of the fundus view on direct and indirect ophthalmoscopy. A very dense cataract occluding the pupil will preclude any view of the fundus. In case of pediatric cataract serology should be done for intrauterine infections. Urinalysis for reducing substance after drinking milk (galactosaemia) and chromatography for amino acids (Lowe syndrome) should be performed. Other investigations include fasting blood glucose, serum calcium and phosphorus and galactokinase levels. Children who have calcium and phosphorus anomalies severe enough to cause cataracts are usually having associated severe systemic problems. Referral to a pediatrician may be warranted for dysmorphic features or suspicion of other systemic diseases. Chromosome analysis may be useful in this context. It is important to examine parents and siblings to reveal a possible etiology (Krishnamurthy & Vanderveen, 2008).

Dense cataracts require early surgery when the child is 4-6 weeks of age to prevent the development of stimulus deprivation amblyopia. If the severity is asymmetrical in bilateral cataracts, the eye with the denser cataract should be addressed first. Surgery may not require in partial cataracts if opacity is not central.

8. Childhood glaucoma

The exact definition of glaucoma is still a subject of debate. What that did not change over years is that raised intraocular pressure is the most important risk factor for glaucoma development. Glaucoma is generally the disease of adults, occurring most frequently over 40 years of age. However, it may also develop in children.

Primary congenital glaucoma (PCG) is the most common reason for raised intraocular pressure in child. It occurs in 1:10000 births and more commonly in boys. 75% of the cases are bilateral. Although autosomal recessive cases have been described, most cases of PCG are sporadic. Glaucoma develops due to the anomalous development of the anterior chamber angle. Raised intraocular pressure, cloudy cornea, large appearance of the eye (buphthalmos), optic nerve alterations due to high intraocular pressure and special biomicroscopic signs are diagnostic features of PCG.

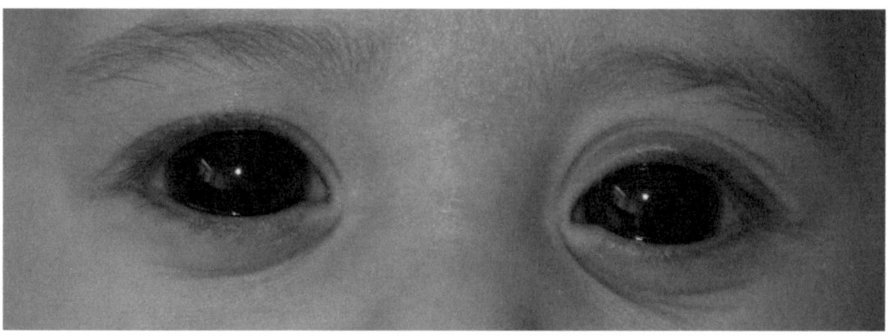

Fig. 4. Buphthalmos in PCG

PCG has 3 subtypes; true, infantile and juvenile PCG. Intraocular pressure is elevated during intrauterine life in true PCG, whereas the disease started before 3 years of age in infantile PCG. Infantile cases are the most frequently encountered ones. Treatment is surgical in all cases of PCG. Medications may also be used concomitant with the surgery. The initial evaluation must be performed under general anaesthesia. Enlargement of the eye in pediatric age group should be referred to an ophthalmologist (Idrees, 2006).

9. Pediatric eye examination

There is no consensus on when the initial eye examination in a healthy child should be performed and how often the examinations should be repeated in the presence of normal eyes. Premature infants at risk of retinopathy of prematurity must be screened by an ophthalmologist. Many congenital ocular abnormalities may be diagnosed by simple observation by a pediatrician, if they are aware of the possible congenital ocular diseases.

In developed countries, the initial eye examination by an ophthalmologist is commonly performed at 6 months of age. At this age, the alignment of the eyes and the near focussing of the infant can be checked. An infant should be able to fix and follow faces within 2-3 weeks of age (Allen, 2000). The ability of the young children to fixate and follow a small target is an important gross evaluation of vision. Consistent objection from the child to having one eye occluded suggests that the un-occluded eye is amblyopic. Refraction examination and the red reflex test should be performed. The red reflex test is a screening test for retinal abnormalities and opacities in the visual axis such as congenital cataract and corneal opacities. It is performed by focusing an ophthalmoscope light from 30 cm away from the child's eyes. If the red reflex of the 2 eyes is symmetrical, the test is normal. Dark spots in the red reflex or leukocoria (white reflex instead of red reflex) are indications for referral to an ophthalmologist.

Special tests to confirm that, an infant sees, may be performed. Optokinetic drum test and the spinning test are the most popular simple methods to confirm visual response in an infant. Forced choice preferential looking is a popular way of quantifying infant vision. Portable cards; namely Teller or Keeler cards are used to quantify infant vision. Optotype tests to quantify visual acuity may be used in children between 1-3 years of age. Cardiff acuity cards at 1-2 years of age and Sheridan Gardner optotypes at 2-3 years of age are the most commonly preferred ones. In children over 3 years of age, Snellen acuity charts may be used. Eye movements and the position of the eyes should be simply observed. Hirschberg test, which is a light reflex test, is used to exclude manifest eye deviations. If an infant with manifest deviation fixates the penlight, the corneal reflex will be eccentric in the deviating eye. The reflex will be displaced nasally in the exotropia, and temporally in the esotropia.

Pupils are smaller and poorly reacting in the newborns. Normal pupillary reactions should be documented by 3 months of age. Iris colour is permanent at 1 year of age. Colour vision assessment can be performed by the Hardy-Rand- Rittler plates in children as young as 3 years of age (Mollon et al., 1991). If the child cannot tolerate ophthalmic examination and detailed examination is indicated, sedation can be required. Routine intraocular pressure measurement in cases with congenital glaucoma is an example for such conditions.

Eye examinations after 3 years of age are more informative and more easily performed. Visual acuity assessment and the fundamental parts of eye examinations are similar with the adult patients. However, the physicians should keep in mind that, refractive status of the eye is very dynamic in preschool and school children, and preschool vision screening is recommended for all children.

10. Refractive disorders

10.1 Definitions

Ametropia, which is defined as the presence of any of the refractive disorders, is the most commonly diagnosed disorder of the human eye. Ametropia includes the hyperopia, myopia and astigmatism. The most common refractive error in the pediatric population is myopia. The World Health Organisation estimates refractive disorders to be 2-10% worldwide. The prevalence is found to be much higher in the Far East. The prevalence of astigmatism of 1 diopter or more is 50% in infancy. The prevalence decreases rapidly during the process of emmetropization. Only few children develop astigmatism greater than 1 diopter by 6 years of age (Maida et al., 2008).

10.2 Etiology

The total refractive power of the human eye is approximately 60 diopters (D). The cornea provides two thirds of this total power and the lens provides the remaining 20 D. The normal eye creates clear images by focusing the images on the retina. If the un-accommodated eye focuses the images behind the retina, hperopia (farsightedness) develops. On the other hand myopia (nearsightedness) is the state in which the un-accommodated eye focuses the images in front of the retina. The hyperopia and myopia may be due to altered total refractive power of the eye, but the axial length changes instead of that is the most common reason in most of the cases. Reduced axial length results in hyerpopia and the reverse in myopia (Riordan-Eva, 2004).

The parental history of myopia, genetic predisposition and various environmental factors are associated with the development of myopia in a child. Familial predisposition also exists in hyperopia, which is much less common in the pediatric population. The children can tolerate low amounts of hyperopia by accommodation, so most of the low amounts of hyperopia are unrecognized in this population. However, higher degrees may result in amblyopia and should be corrected promptly.

A healthy eye is able to focus all the light rays from a point source to a single point. In the presence of astigmatism, this focusing process to a single point is disrupted due to variations in the curvature of the cornea or lens at different meridians. Most of the astigmatisms are the consequences of alterations in corneal curvatures. In other words, the refractive power of some part of the cornea is higher or lower than the rest of the cornea, so the astigmatism results. If these regions of the cornea with different refractive power capacity are 90 degrees apart, the astigmatism is regular. If these regions are not 90 degrees apart, it is called irregular. Keratoconus is an important reason for irregular astigmatism.

10.3 Management

Spectacles, contact lenses, refractive surgery, intraocular lenses and clear lens extraction are the current methods of refractive correction. Refractive disorders place a significant economic and social burden on society. In USA, $4.6 billion was spent for treatment of myopia in 1990. Spectacles continue to be the safest method of correction, whereas the interventional procedures are very rarely preferred in the pediatric population. Anisometropia refers to a difference in the refractive status of the 2 eyes. If the difference is 2 diopters or more, either spherical or astigmatic, it is clinically significant. Anisometropia should be managed with caution, since it is the most important risk factor for amblyopia.

11. Amblyopia

11.1 Definition

A physician must be aware of the definition of amblyopia properly to understand the importance of early diagnosis and management of amblyopia. Amblyopia is the combination of two Greek words; amblyos - blunt and opia -vision. The parents commonly use the lazy eye terminology instead of ambloypia. Due to the suppression of the blurred vision from the diseased eye, the risk of development of unilateral amblyopia is much higher than the risk of bilateral amblyopia. However, it may also develop bilaterally, if severe visual deprivation occurs in both eyes. A same ocular pathology that develops in a child may be an important etiology for a severe amblyopia, while the same pathology in the elderly decreases the visual acuity, but does not result in an amblyopia. This is very typical for the lens pathologies. Congenital cataracts are one of the important etiologies for amblyopia, while senile cataracts are the most common treatable cause of vision loss among the elderly. Any pathology that results in abnormal visual experience in one or two eyes before the critical period of visual development may result in amblyopia. The critical period usually ends at 6-8 years of age (Morishita, & Hensch, 2008). The amblyopia is the disease of the visual cortex and it only develops in children younger than 6-8 years old. The critical period is the time of maximum neurological plasticity of the visual cortex cells. The visual acuity and binocular vision improves depending on the visual inputs until the end of the critical period. There is no consensus on which visual acuity should be adopted for the clinical definition of amblyopia. The cut-off level varies between 20/40 and 20/30 and the prevalence also varies accordingly. The prevalence of the disease may be considered approximately 2% in the general population (Webber & Wood, 2005).

11.2 Etiology

There are many treatable and untreatable causes of amblyopia. The most common etiologies are eye deviations and refractive errors. Anisometropia is a significant difference in the refractive status between the two eyes. The eye with more hypermetropia or more astigmatism is chronically blurred, so the risk of the development of amblyopia is high in that eye. Congenital cataracts, retinoblastoma, nystagmus, corneal opacities and any ocular media opacities including vitreous hemorrhages may end up with amblyopia, if they occur before the critical period of visual development (Carlton & Kaltenthaler, 2011).

11.3 Management

The severity of the amblyopia depends on the severity of the blur, the duration of the abnormal vision and the age of onset of the visual impairment. The pediatrician plays a crucial role in the early diagnosis of possible causes of amblyopia. The major determinants of success in amblyopia treatment are early recognition by the pediatrician, early referral to the pediatric ophthalmologist and prompt treatment.

The initial step in the management is the correction of the underlying etiology, if possible. Surgical treatment of the strabismus, or the congenital cataract, correction of the refractive errors by glasses or contact lenses are the main treatment modalities for the correction of the most common causes of amblyopia. In some pathologies, such as nystagmus, retinoblastoma, it is not possible to eliminate the underlying cause of blurred vision totally. Therefore, the management of amblyopia due to such untreatable diseases is very difficult.

After the correction of the underlying organic pathology, the most difficult aspect of the management starts; the occlusion of the sound eye in most cases or the alternate occlusion if the condition is bilateral. The aim of the patching the diseased eye is to improve the visual cortex which receives the inputs from the bad eye. This is possible if the neurological plasticity of the visual cortex remains. The best outcomes are achieved if the management starts before 5 years of age, but the patching may be tried up to 22 years of age (Matta et al., 2010). If children cannot tolerate patching, the penalization, which is the impairment of vision in the sound eye by eye drops, can be preferred. There is no consensus on the duration of patching per day and the total duration of the treatment. However, it is known that, it is long treatment frequently lasting more than years. Well cooperation with the parents is crucial to obtain successful outcomes. It is commonly accepted that amblyopia cannot be treated beyond a certain age. However, some trials to manage amblyopia in adults gave promising results. Perceptual visual learning and levodepo are the possible new treatment modalities for amblyopia in the elderly. These may also be tried in elder children, if conventional treatments fail (Astle et al., 2011).

12. Pediatric eye deviations

Under normal physiological conditions, the image of an object falls simultaneously on the fovea of each. This is possible if the eyes are properly aligned. This straight position of the eyes is called orthophoria. Any misalignment of the either eye is called strabismus or eye deviation in other words. There are 2 benefits of treating strabismus. The initial one is functional gain including the improvement of visual acuity and stereopsis. The second one is the cosmetic improvement.

12.1 Types of eye deviations

Tropia defines manifest deviation of eyes and phoria implies latent deviation. Phoria is detected by the simple cover-uncover test. The test is performed while the patient fixates a distant object. The physician covers one eye for 2-3 seconds and then the other eye. If orthophoria is present, no movement is detected. If latent deviation exists movement of eyes towards the opposite of the deviation is observed. For example in a patient with inward latent deviation, the uncovered eye move from inwards to outwards. Latent deviations may become manifest temporarily, when the child is tired or ill. It can also become permanently manifest during the follow-up.

Horizontal deviations are the most commonly observed types of strabismus. Esotropia is the manifest inward deviation of eyes, while esophoria is the latent inward deviation of eyes. Exotropia is the manifest outward deviation of eyes, while exophoria is the latent outward deviation of eyes. Esotropia is by far the most common form of strabismus. Infantile esotropia constitutes almost half of all cases of esotropia. Infantile esotropia is the inward deviation of eyes, which is diagnosed at 6 months of age. The angle of deviation is usually large and surgery is usually indicated. Pseudo-strabismus is the illusion of deviation in a child with orthophoria. It is most commonly in the form of pseudo-esotropia. The most common reason for this false appearance of inward deviation is broad nasal bridge with prominent epicanthal folds. This appearance usually resolves spontaneously and requires no treatment (Fredrick, & Asbury, 2004).

Paralytic strabismus in children may be in form of third, fourth or sixth cranial nerve palsy.

The most common one is the sixth cranial nerve palsy (abducens palsy), which is characterized by loss of abduction. Cranial imaging must be ordered in all forms of acquired paralytic strabismus to exclude cranial masses (Harley, 1980).

The angle of deviation in eyes with all types of deviations is measured objectively by using special prisms. The prism cover test is preferred if the child cooperates. In severe amblyopia and in very young children prism reflex test (Krimsky test) is performed. The patient fixates a light and the prism is placed in front of the deviating or bad eye to center the corneal reflex.

12.2 Management

Associated amblyopia and refractive errors must be addressed initially in all cases of strabismus. Abnormal eye movements are frequently associated with pediatric eye deviations and they can influence the management of the cases. Accommodative types of esotropias may be completely cured with spectacles. Surgical correction is decided according to the angle of deviation, if the deviation is not corrected by the spectacles during follow-up. All types of strabismus must be referred to an ophthalmologist, since early treatment by spectacles or surgery is important for normal binocular visual development.

13. Common eyelid and orbital diseases in children

The most important issue in pediatric eyelid disorders is to identify whether the lesions affect the visual development or not. If it occludes the visual axis, the pathology must be treated promptly to prevent the development of amblyopia. Entropion, ectropion, distichiasis, epicanthal folds, and telecanthus (increased distance between the medial canthus of each eye) are common congenital anomalies of the eyelids. Although they are solely cosmetic problems in most cases, they may result in corneal changes secondary to corneal irritation and exposure due to mal-position of the eyelids.

Congenital ptosis is the most important disease of the eyelids in a child. It is usually unilateral and occurs sporadically in most cases. The underlying pathology is the dysplasia of the levator palpebralis muscle. Surgical correction during the preschool years must be performed. If the disease is severe, early surgery to prevent amblyopia may be performed.

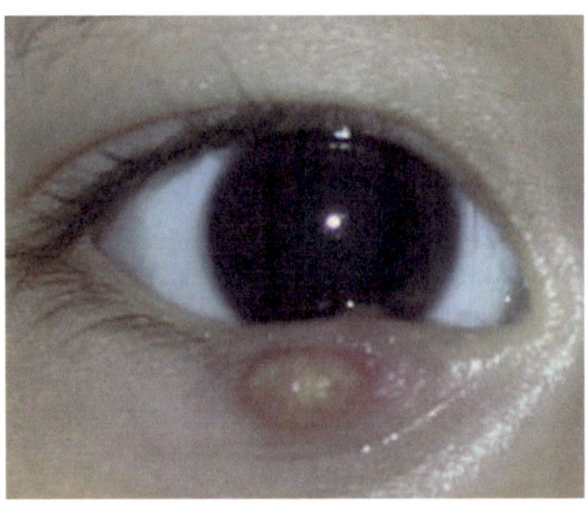

Fig. 5. Stye at lower eyelid

Chalazion (Chronic inflammation of the meibomian glands), blepharitis (effects base of the eyelashes) and acute infection of the eye lash follicle (stye) are very frequent infections of the eyelids in children. The infections are mostly innocent and respond well to conservative therapies (Hughes, 2000).

13.1 Orbital infections

The bacterial infections of the soft tissue anterior or posterior to the orbital septum are the most common diseases of the orbit in the pediatric age group. The infections occur in two clinical forms; preseptal cellulitis or orbital cellulitis. Orbital cellulitis is the most common cause of protrusion of the eyeball in children. It is a life-threatening disease of the tissues behind the orbital septum. On the other hand, preseptal cellulits involves tissues anterior to the orbital septum. Preseptal cellulitis usually responds to ampiric antibiotic treatment, whereas orbital cellulitis may be associated with serious complications requiring longer periods of treatment and surgical interventions (Kanski, 2011).

Protrusion of the eyeball, limitations of the eye movements and decreased visual acuity are signs of orbital cellulitis. Skin trauma, sinusitis, lacrimal sac infections and rarely remote infections may be the source of preseptal or orbital cellulitis. Preseptal cellulitis rarely progresses to orbital cellulitis.

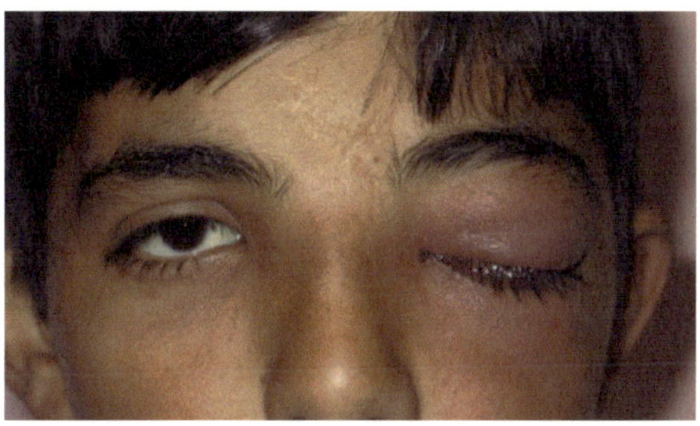

Fig. 6. Left orbital cellulitis

Subperiosteal and orbital abscesses, intracranial complications (meningitis, brain abscess) and ocular complications such as optic neuropathy and endophthalmitis may complicate orbital cellulitis. Hospitalization and aggressive medical treatment to prevent life-threatening complications is indicated in orbital cellulitis (Sullivan, 2004). Any painful periorbital edema or pain associated with eye movements should raise the suspicion of serious orbital cellulitis and referral to an ophthalmologist is indicated.

14. Conjunctival diseases in children

14.1 Ophthalmia neonatarum

Ophthalmia neonataurum means, conjunctivitis occurring in the first month of life. It is still a significant cause of blindness in underdeveloped countries. It can be bacterial, viral and chemical. The most serious form is caused by *Neisseria gonorrhoeae*. Onset is typically within the first 3-4 days of life. It causes a severe purulent discharge. Treatment includes systemic ceftriaxone and topical penicillin as well. Infection with herpes is rarer but requires prompt therapy with acyclovir. Chemical cases are caused by silver nitrate and occur within 24 hours life. Tetracyclin, erythromyicin ointments or povidone-ioidine drops can be used for prophylaxis.

14.1.1 Conjunctivitis

Conjunctivitis in children is one of the most common reasons to visit a pediatrician. Majority of these infections are self-limited and does not require therapy. This section covers a variety of infectious conjunctival diseases that might be confronted in routine pediatrics practice.

Red eye is one of the most important ophthalmological emergencies. There are several causes such as conjunctivitis, keratitis, uveitis etc. Fortunately, majority of the red eye occurs due to conjunctivitis. The underlying etiology is almost always bacterial in children. However, it can be viral or allergic. During examination there are some key points that will help to differentiate the etiology:

Symptoms: Allergic cases will always have prominent itching. Bacterial cases will always have discharge.

Presence and nature of discharge: Bacterial infections will have a purulent, yellow-green discharge. Viral cases will have a serous or mucoid discharge. Allergic cases will have serous discharge with excessive tearing.

Laterality: Bacterial cases can be either unilateral or bilateral. Viral and allergic conjunctivitis occur almost always bilateral.

Cul-de-sac: Always pull the lower eyelid away from the globe to examine the cul-de-sac. Bacterial conjunctivitis will have tarsal papillae. Viral and allergic conjunctivitis will have tarsal follicles.

Systemic associations: Viral conjunctivitis might be associated with upper respiratory infections. Allergic conjunctivitis might be seen with upper respiratory allergic symptoms.

First-line therapy for bacterial conjunctivitis is topical flouroquinolone. In many cases polysporin, erythromycin or trimethoprim/sulfa is effective. Viral conjunctivitis is self-limited. For allergic cases topical antihistaminic drops are effective.

15. Corneal diseases in children

The cornea is the anterior transparent, avascular anatomical structure of the human eye. It constitutes 2/3 of the total refractive capacity. There are many congenital and acquired corneal diseases, which may lead to blindness if left untreated. Corneal dystrophies, congenital anomalies, corneal ectasias, metabolic keratopathies and infectious diseases are the main corneal diseases that may be diagnosed in a child. Most of the corneal pathologies disturb the transparency of the organ and should be referred to an ophthalmologist immediately. Microcornea, megalocornea, anophthalmos and microphthalmos are rare congenital anomalies that affect cornea. Microphthalmos is defined as the developmental arrest of all ocular structures, while anophthalmos is the complete failure of the eye development.

Corneal involvement (corneal edema, infiltrations or erosions) may be seen in cystinosis, mucopolysaccharidoses, Wilson disease, Fabry disease and tyrosinaemia type 2. The treatment of the systemic disease is the mainstay treatment of these metabolic keratopathies.

Corneal dystrophies and corneal ectasias are frequently diagnosed during puberty or later. They are structural diseases of the cornea and mostly genetically determined, but the clinical picture rarely occurs in childhood. Keratoconus is the most common corneal ectasia of the human eye. It is typically diagnosed during puberty with unilateral impairment of vision. Corneal thinning and irregular astigmatism are the main features of the keratoconus. Hard contact lenses and corneal transplantation are treatment options based on the severity of the disease (Ciralsky & Colby, 2007).

15.1 Keratitis

Staphylococcus aeurus, staphylococcus epidermidis, and streptococcus pneumonia are the most common organisms that cause infectious keratitis. Bacterial keratitis usually occurs in patients with damaged corneal epithelial integrity. However, Neisseria gonorrhoeae, Corynebacterium diphteriae, Listeria and Haemophilus species may lead to keratitis in the presence of intact epithelium. Bacterial keratitis is characterized by oval shaped corneal infiltrations surrounded by corneal edema, conjunctival hyperemia (injection), ocular pain and photophobia.

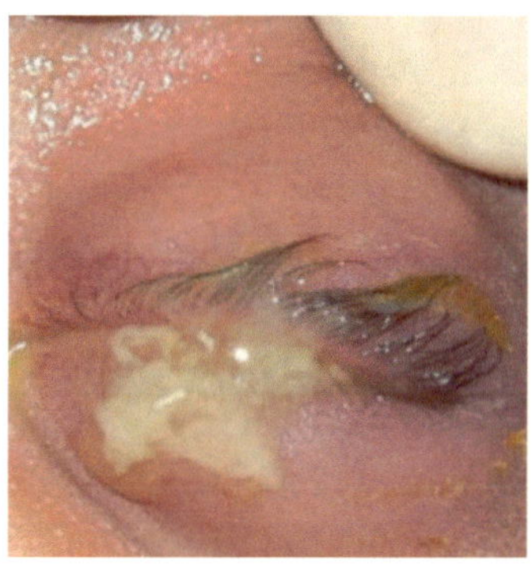

Fig. 7. Gonococcal keratoconjunctivitis

Pseudomonas aeruginosa keratitis tend be very severe and typically produces stromal necrosis with a shaggy surface and adherent mucopurulent exudates. It is an infection usually seen in contact lens users with a damaged corneal epithelial surface. The infection may progress rapidly ending with corneal perforation. In the management of keratitis, ampiric broad-spectrum therapy is recommended until the offending microorganism is identified in the culture. If the type of bacteria is identified from the stained diagnostic smear, then appropriate single drug therapy may be considered.

Herpes simplex virus (HSV) infection is more commonly acquired in adolescence than in childhood. It can be transmitted to neonates as they pass through the birth canal of a mother with genital infection that can lead to serious systemic disorders in the newborns. Primary ocular HSV infection is a form of HSV infection that typically manifests in children aged between 6 months and 5 years. It causes unilateral blepharoconjunctivitis that has signs such as cutaneous or eyelid marginal vesicles, or ulcers on the bulbar conjunctiva that can be rarely accompanied by dendritic epithelial keratitis. Primary ocular HSV infection is a self limited disease that usually resolves spontaneously. Oral antiviral therapy can speed up the resolution.

Dendritic ulcers, stromal necrotizing keratitis and disciform keratitis are forms of recurrent ocular infection of HSV. These may also occur in this age group. Topical and oral antiviral therapy can be used in the management of recurrent HSV keratitis.

Adenoviruses are the most common viral pathogens that may cause viral keratitis in a child. Pharyngoconjunctival fever (PCF) and epidemic keratoconjunctivitis (EPC) are 2 different clinical pictures that are caused by different serotypes of adenoviruses. PCF is caused by types 3, 4 and 7, while EPC is caused by types 8, 19 and 37. Corneal involvement is much more common and severe in EPC. Keratitis may persist for years in some cases. PCF is the less severe form of the disease. Keratitis is usually mild and self limiting. Mild to moderate fever may accompany PCF. The management of adenoviral keratitis is usually conservative. Topical steroids and cyclosporine may be tried to reduce inflammation. Reduction of transmission risk by avoiding contact with infected patients during the initial 7-10 days of the active disease and by good hygiene is much more important than its management. Ophthalmologists are well experienced about EKC, because unfortunately the eye clinics are usually the most common places to come in contact with the adenovirus and many ophthalmologists are infected once or more with adenoviruses. Many outbreaks occur due to improperly disinfected diagnostic instruments (Kanski, 2011).

15.2 Allergic diseases affecting the cornea

Vernal keratoconjunctivitis is an allergic eye disease that is mainly seen in male children. Symptoms include itching, photophobia, and mucoid discharge. Corneal findings consist of Horner-Trantas dots (degenerated eosinophils and epithelial cells) in the limbal area, punctate epithelial erosions and shield ulcer (an oval noninfectious epithelial ulcer). Corneal findings are generally accompanied by conjunctival ones which are hyperemia, conjunctival edema (chemosis) and papillary hypertrophy. Topical antihistamines and mast-cell stabilizers can be used in the management of vernal conjunctivitis. Severe cases may require topical corticosteroid or topical immune-modulating agents such as cyclosporine.

Atopic keratoconjunctivitis is a rare bilateral allergic eye disease that is most commonly diagnosed in young men, but also in children. Clinical picture is similar to vernal keratoconjunctivitis, but more severe. The papillary hypertrophy are less developed compared to vernal keratoconjunctivitis. The history of allergy such as allergic asthma or atopic dermatitis is commonly associated. Keratopathy leading to total corneal neovascularization may occur. Management is similar to vernalis keratoconjunctivitis, but the disease is less responsive.

15.3 Reiter syndrome

It is characterized by the ocular triad (conjunctivitis/ episcleritis, iridocyclitis, or keratitis), urethritis and arthritis. It is usually associated with gram-negative bacterial (Salmonella,

Shigella and Yersinia) dysentery. Corneal diseases usually respond to topical corticosteroids (Kanski, 2011).

16. Pediatric uveitis

The uvea is a pigmented structure that primarily lies between the retina and the sclera and constitutes the vascular portion of the eye. It comprises the iris, ciliary body and choroid. Uveitis, by strict definition implies an inflammation of the uveal tract. Uveitis is named according to the anatomical location of inflammation in the uvea. Anterior uveitis may be subdivided into: Iritis and iridocyclitis. Iritis is primarily the inflammation of the iris tissue. On the other hand, iridocyclitis involves both the iris and the pars plicata of the ciliary body. Intermediate uveitis is defined as inflammation predominantly involving the pars plana, the peripheral retina and the vitreous. Posterior uveitis involves the fundus posterior to the vitreous base. Panuveitis implies involvement of the entire uveal tract without a predominant site of inflammation (Kanski, 2011).

Pediatric uveitis may be categorized into 4 types of uveitis based on the anatomical location of the inflammatory process. These are anterior (non-granulomatous and granulomatous), intermediate and posterior uveitis. Etiologic factors associated with these uvetis in children are as follows.

Anterior non-granulomatous uveitis: Idiopathic, HLA-B27 associated, juvenile rheumatoid arthritis (JRA), ankylosing spondylitis, Reiter's disease, psoriasis, inflammatory bowel disease, nephritis, systemic lupus erythematosus, Herpes Simplex virus (HSV), Lyme disease, leukemia, drug-induced.

Anterior granulomatous uveitis: Sarcoidosis, inflammatory bowel disease, syphilis, Herpes simplex virus, tuberculosis, Behcet's disease, multiple sclerosis, fungal disease, Whipple's disease, leprosy.

Intermediate uveitis: JRA, Pars Planitis, Multiple Sclerosis, Lyme disease, Sarcoidosis.

Posterior Uveitis: Toxocariasis, Toxoplasmosis, Leukemia, Tuberculosis, Intraocular Foreign Body, Vogt-Koyanagi Harada Syndrome (VKH), Cytomegalovirus, HSV/VZV, inflammatory bowel disease, syphilis, Behcet's disease, systemic lupus erythematosus, Kawasaki's disease, sarcoidosis, polyarteritis nodosa, Wegener's granulomatosis (Kanski, 2011).

Anterior uveitis is the most common form of uveitis. Features are typically with sudden onset of unilateral pain, photophobia and redness, which may be associated with lacrimation. Occasionally patients may notice mild ocular discomfort a few days before the acute attack when clinical signs are absent. Visual acuity is usually good. The presence of vitreal cells in an active vitritis are the main signs of pars planitis. Posterior uveitis encompasses retinitis, choroiditis and retinal vasculitis. Some lesions may originate primarily in the retina or choroid but often there is involvement of both (Sauberan, 2010).

Special investigations such as skin tests, serology and radiology are indicated in posterior uveitis, granulomatous inflammation, recurrent uveitis and bilateral uveitis.

Treatment of the majority of uveitis involves predominantly the use of anti-inflammatory and immunosuppressive agents. Antibiotic therapy for infectious diseases may be necessary. Topical steroids are the mainstay treatment for anterior uveitis, while systemic steroids are indicated in most cases of intermediate and posterior uveitis. If the disease is unresponsive to systemic steroids and/or the patient cannot tolerate systemic steroids, other immunosuppressive agents including azathioprine, methotrexate and ciclosporin may be used (Jancevski ,2010).

17. Retinal detachment in children

Retinal detachment is not common in infants and children. While the incidence of retinal detachment is 12 in 100000 in all age groups, only between 1.7% and 5.7% are diagnosed during childhood. The association of retinal detachment with complex intraocular pathologies in young children often presents a challenge to treatment.

There are 3 types of retinal detachment: Rhegmatogenous retinal detachment develops when there is a hole or tear in the retina, which transmits intraocular fluid underneath the retina and subsequent separation of the retina from the underlying pigment epithelium occurs. The second most common form is tractional, where the retina is pulled away from the underlying tissues. Exudative detachment develops when subretinal fluid accumulates under the retina such as in Coat's disease or vasoproliferative disorders (Yokoyama et al., 2004).

17.1 Clinic and diagnosis

Symptoms of retinal detachment are sudden onset of floaters, light flashes, appearance of black veil and loss of visual acuity. It is important to recognize that most of the small children cannot express loss of visual acuity and often vision may already be low due to concomitant ocular pathologies. Therefore the delay in diagnosis is more common in the pediatric retinal detachments compared to that in the adult retinal detachments. In a significant proportion of the patients, the diagnosis is made by chance during a routine eye examination or by noticing leukocoria. It is important to realize that retinal detachment in children may occur in both eyes frequently.

17.2 Etiology

Trauma has been reported to be the cause in 27–51% of cases of childhood retinal detachment. Ocular trauma is an important cause of retinal abnormalities in children and it is more common in boys. Retinal dialyses may be found in the superonasal or inferotemporal quadrant. Traumatic retinal detachment is seen most commonly in older children and is usually caused by blunt trauma (Sarrazin et al., 2004). The second frequent etiological factor is high myopia in children and if it is congenital may indicate an underlying abnormality. Retinal detachment may also result from intraocular infection or inflammation. The existence of systemic or hereditary diseases such as Trisomy 13 (Patau syndrome), Walker Warburg syndrome, Meckel syndrome, Norrie disease and incontinentia pigmenti should be investigated in retinal detachments of early childhood (0-1 year). In such cases, central nervous system imaging and detailed neurological examination should be requested. Also it is important to rule out retinoblastoma. Some of these children do not live very long due to these systemic or hereditary diseases. Retinal detachment in infants and children should lead the physician to suspect a systemic disease, a syndrome, trauma, or a tumor in the eye. That should be ruled out with ultrasound or CT scan. Other causes of congenital or infantile retinal detachment should also be considered, including Stickler's syndrome, retinopathy of prematurity, persistent hyperplastic primary vitreous (PHPV), also called persistent fetal vasculature (PFV), may also present with a retinal detachment at birth; however, the associated microphthalmos and cataract often makes the diagnosis easier. Stickler's syndrome combines ocular, orthopedic and midfacial anomalies in an autosomal dominant inheritance pattern. Ocular abnormalities include high myopia, empty vitreous with membranes and bands.

17.3 Management

Prediction, prophylaxis and timely surgical treatment of retinal detachment may prevent visual loss. Retinal detachment in childhood and adolescence is different from adult cases due to higher rate of complicating predisposing factors such as trauma and high myopia and also due to the delay in the diagnosis that is mostly made after macular involvement. By appropriate surgical treatment the anatomic success rate may be as high as adult cases, however lower functional results are usually achieved because of higher rate of macular involvement (Butler et al., 2001; Topbas et al., 2003). It is important for the pediatrician to refer the children with signs and symptoms of retinal detachment, children with systemic disorders associated with retinal detachment and also children with ocular trauma history to an ophthalmologist.

18. Retinoblastoma

Retinoblastoma (RB) is the most common intraocular malignancy of the childhood, occurring in about in 1/15.000 to 20.000 live births. The tumor develops from the immature retina.

18.1 Inheritance

RB occurs in hereditary and nonhereditary forms. It can be unilateral or bilateral. The hereditary form is usually bilateral and multifocal, whereas the nonhereditary form is unilateral and unifocal. The RB gene is recognized to be a recessive suppresser gene located on chromosome 13 at the 13q14 segment and some affected children have other systemic features of the 13 q deletion syndrome. It is accepted that all bilateral and familial cases of RB will manifest a germline mutation, whereas only 10-15% of unilateral sporadic cases will show germline mutation (Shields, 2006).

18.2 Symptoms and diagnosis

RB usually diagnosed between 3 months and 3 years of age, but it can be congenital or it can occur in older children. The affected child usually presents with leukocoria and/or strabismus. More advanced tumors can cause painful secondary glaucoma or signs of orbital cellulitis. The diagnosis of RB is best made by slit lamp bio-microscopy and indirect ophthalmoscopy. Ancillary studies are ultrasonography and computed tomography. The red-reflex examination is the best way to screen for retinoblastoma.

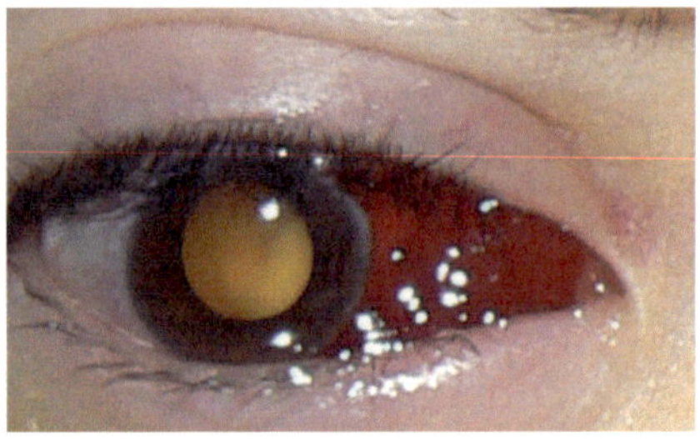

Fig. 8. Leukocoria due to RB

18.3 Metastatic spread and second primary malignancies

Metastatic spread is to regional nodes, lung, brain and bone. Second non-ocular cancers are leading cause of death in patients with the familial form of RB. Most common second tumors are soft tissue sarcoma, osteogenic sarcoma of the skull or the long bones, primitive neuroectodermal brain tumor and cutaneous melanoma. Trilateral RB refers to bilateral retinoblastoma associated with an intracranial primitive neuroectodermal tumor in the pineal or supraseller region (Murphree, 2006).

18.4 Current management of RB

Goals of treatment from most to least important ranking are: saving life, maintaining the eye and vision, and preserving cosmetic appearance. RB treatment typically requires the cooperation of an ophthalmic oncologist, pediatric oncologist and radiation therapist. Treatment varies depending on the number, size, and location of the tumors. Protocols are currently being evaluated to use chemoreduction therapy to shrink the RB in order to treat them with thermotherapy, laser therapy, cryotherapy, and local episcleral plaque radiation. More advanced tumors are managed by enucleation. External beam radiotherapy is typically reserved for eyes that fail the above methods, especially if retinoblastoma is bilateral. Lifelong monitoring is important to diagnose second primary tumor in the healthy eye as early as possible (Valenzuela, 2011).

19. Systemic disease and eye in children

19.1 Intrauterine infections

Congenital toxoplasmosis, cytomegalovirus, herpes simplex, lymphocytic choriomeningitis virus, varicella-zoster virus, West Nile virus infections are main intrauterine infections that may result in ocular pathologies. The principal ophthalmic manifestations are chorioretinal scar or an active chorioretinitis, and congenital cataract. When they are present in congenital toxoplasmosis, herpes simplex, and cytomegalovirus, they are associated with extensive eye involvement (Mets, MB. & Kumar, 2006).

19.2 Metabolic disease

Disorders of copper metabolism: Wilson's disease. The principal ophthalmic manifestations are Kayser-Fleischer ring, due to copper deposition in Descemet's membrane and sun-flower cataract.

The mucopolysaaharidoses (Hurler syndrome, Schie syndrome, Hunter's syndrome, Sanfippo's syndrome): The principal ophthalmic manifestations are progressive corneal clouding, pigmentary retinal degeneration, optic atrophy, sometimes papilloedema and in certain cases glaucoma.

The gangliosidoses: Defects in lysosomal degradation of gangliosides can result in abnormal accumulation of these lipids. (Infantile, late infantile/Juvenile GM, Tay-Sachs disease) The principal ophthalmic manifestations are macular cherry red spot, tortiosity of retinal vessels, retinal hemorrhages and optic atrophy. Strabismus, nystagmus and mild corneal cloudy can be seen.

Niemann-Pick disease: The principal ophthalmic manifestations are macular cherry red spot, mild corneal haze and fine lens opacities.

Gaucher's disease: The principal ophthalmic manifestations are ocular lesions resembling pinguecula, paralytic strabismus and corneal opacities

Albinism: Genetic disorders of melanin synthesis. The principal ophthalmic manifestations are retinal hypopigmentation, foveal hypoplasia, misrouting of optic nerve fibers at the chiasm with altered visual function, iris hypopigmentation, photophobia, nystagmus, strabismus and high refractive errors.

Galactosemia: The principal ophthalmic manifestation is cataract (Martyn, 2006).

19.3 Connective tissue disorders

Angioid streaks (blood vessel-like) and visual loss may occur in pseudoxantoma elasticum

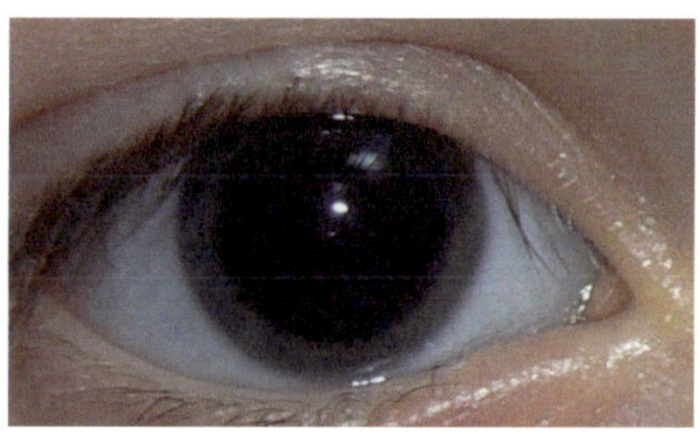

Fig. 9. Blue sclera in a case of EDS

Stretchable lids, retinal detachment and blue sclera have been reported in Ehler Danlos syndrome (EDS). Subluxation of crystalline lens, strabismus and retinal detachment may be seen in Marfan syndrome (Traboulski, 2006)

20. Ocular trauma in children

Ocular traumas in childhood are frequent and major causes of visual impairment, especially of unilateral non-congenital blindness in this age group. The frequency of eye traumas is almost double in boys especially in older age groups. This may be due to boys being more adventurous and aggressive. The 0-5 years of age group was at greatest risk regardless of gender.

20.1 Evaluation

Evaluation starts with a detailed history of the trauma, from the child if possible and also from the parents. Examination of the traumatized eye may be difficult in children. It is important to be patient and gentle. A mild sedative may sometimes be helpful. Visual function should be estimated in the beginning of the examination. Literate or illiterate Snellen charts may be used if possible. Otherwise reading any material or finger counting may help to determine the approximate level of visual acuity. Afterwards lids, conjunctivas and orbit are examined externally to reveal any lid lacerations or orbital rim fractures. The globe is examined carefully and gently. Irregular pupils, edema of the conjunctiva and blood in the anterior chamber and in the vitreous cavity are signs of severe ocular injury.

20.2 Common eye injuries and management

An external examination should be performed to look for eyelid lacerations which are seen as distortion of eyelids. A good functional and cosmetic result may only be obtained by appropriate suturing technique. Lacerations of the medial part of the lower lid may include lacrimal canaliculi. Tear drainage may be impaired leading to watering of the eye if not repaired properly.

Blunt ocular trauma may lead to traumatic hyphema, ruptured globe, retinal dialysis, retinal tears, macular hole and commosio retina. Hyphema is the collection of blood in the anterior chamber due to rupture of an iris or ciliary body vessel. Hyphema may be noticed as a red collection in the lower part of the anterior chamber or may fill the anterior chamber totally. Treatment includes bed rest, elevation of the head for approximately 45 degrees, cycloplegic and steroid eye drops. Blunt trauma may also rupture the eyeball. Conjunctival edema, soft eye and deep anterior chamber are signs of a posteriorly ruptured eye. Retinal tears and dialysis are severe consequences of blunt trauma which may lead to retinal detachment and therefore a detailed fundus examination is mandatory. Subretinal and intraocular hemorrhages may be highly associated with the shaken baby syndrome. Diffuse involvement of fundus with intravitreal and large subhyaloid hemorrhage are associated with more severe neurological injuries (MacEwen et al., 1999).

Corneal injuries may be in a spectrum from minor abrasions to serious penetrating wounds extending to the sclera. Abrasions are common and present with foreign body sensation, lacrimation and photophobia. It is important to look for a foreign body, which may be embedded at the upper tarsal conjunctiva, by everting the upper lid. Abrasions are treated by topical antibiotics and patching the eye. Irregular pupil due to iris prolapsus from the wound is a general finding of the penetrating injuries. If such an open globe injury is suspected, extreme care should be taken not to exert pressure to the globe and an eye shield should be placed over the eye. Systemic antibiotics, pain relievers and tetanus prophylaxis should be taken into consideration.

Chemical injuries may give damage to the eyelids, cornea and conjunctiva. Burns that penetrate deeper than the cornea are more serious and may lead to cataracts and glaucoma. Chemical injuries in children mostly occur at home from cleaning products or other regular household products. These injuries are dangerous and the treatment must be started immediately by irrigation with copious amounts of water as soon as possible. The type of injury, severity and the initial visual acuity are important prognostic factors for the final visual outcome. The visual prognosis is better if immediate diagnosis and treatment is provided and therefore it is important for the general physicians to recognize the severity of the trauma, provide suitable medical management and refer to the ophthalmologist as soon as possible (Moreira et al., 1988; Serrano et al., 2003).

20.3 Prevention of eye injuries

Most eye injuries can be avoided by simple measures, but still many children face serious visual impairment due to trauma. Most of the eye injuries occur at homes, in streets and roads, in schools and in other child care facilities. Adult supervision is an important factor for the prevention especially for the younger age groups. More than half of the injuries are without adult supervision at the time of event. Trauma is one of the most important preventable causes of blindness in children. Important points in prevention include parental supervision, education of children and protective eye-wears when necessary. Protective eye wears such as polycarbonate goggles should especially be recommended to functionally one eyed children (Mulvihill et al., 1997).

Recognition of eye injuries, taking immediate measures and referral to an ophthalmologist are key components in the management of eye injuries for general practitioners.

21. References

Allen, L. (2000). Pediatric eye examination, In: Pediatric Ophthalmology, Moore A,Lightman S. (eds), pp. 14-25, BMJ Books, ISBN 0-7279-1203-8, London

Astle, AT.; McGraw, PV. & Webb, BS. (2011). Can Human Amblyopia be treated in Adulthood?. *Strabismus*, vol.19, no.3, (September 2011), pp. 99-109

Ballard EA. Excessive tearing in infancy and early childhood. (1925). The role and treatment of congenital nasolacrimal duct obstruction. *Postgraduate medicine*, vol.107, no.6, (May 2000), pp. 149-54, ISSN 0032-5481

Basmak, H.; Niyaz, L. & Sahin A.; et al. (1991). Retinopathy of prematurity: screening guidelines need to be reevaluated for developing countries. *European Journal of Ophthalmology*, vol.20, no.4, (December 2009), pp. 752-55, ISSN 1120-6721

Butler, TK.; Kiel AW. & Orr GM. (1917). Anatomical and visual outcome of retinal detachment surgery in children. *Br J Ophthalmol*, vol.85, no. 12, (December 2001), pp. 1437–1439, ISSN 0007-1161

Carlton, J. & Kaltenthaler, E. (1987). Amblyopia and quality of life: a systematic review. *Eye (Lond)*, vol.25, no.4, (April 2011), pp. 403-13, ISSN 1476-5454

Ciralsky, J. & Colby, K. (1986). Congenital corneal opacities: a review with a focus on genetics. *Semin Ophthalmol*, vol.22, no.4, (October-December 2007), pp. 241-6, ISSN 0882-0538

Dale, RC.; Brilot, F. & Banwell, B. Pediatric central nervous system inflammatory demyelination: acute disseminated encephalomyelitis, clinically isolated syndromes, neuromyelitis optica, and multiple sclerosis. (1993). *Curr Opin Neurol*, vol.22, no.3, (June 2009), pp. 233-240, ISSN 1350-7540

Drack, AV. & Kimura AE. (2006). Retinitis Pigmentosa and Associated Disorders, In: *Handbook of Pediatric Retinal Disease,* Wright, KW; Spiegel PH. & Thompson LS. (Eds.), pp 135-177, Springer Science+Business Media, ISBN 10: 0-387-27932-6, USA.

Erol N. Treatment of Retinopathy of Prematurity. (2009). *Türkiye Klinikleri Journal of Ophthalmology - Special Topics,* vol.4, no.2, (July 2011), pp. 27-32, ISSN 1380-1160

Fredrick, DR. & Asbury, T. (2004). Strabismus, In: *General Ophthalmology,* Riordan-Eva P. & Whitcher JP. (eds), pp. 230-49, McGraw-Hill Companies, Inc, ISBN 0–07–137831-6, USA

Fredrick, DR. (2004). Special subjects of Pediatric Interest, In: *General Ophthalmology,*

Gilbert C. (1977). Retinopathy of prematurity: a global perspective of the epidemics, population of babies at risk and implications for control. *Early Hum Dev,* vol.84, no.2, (January 2008), pp. 77-82, ISSN 0378-3782

Goldstein, SM. & Katowitz, JA. (2008). Infections of the eye and adnexa in children, In: *Principles and Practice of Ophthalmology,* Albert, DM. & Miller, JW. (eds), pp. 4171-76, Elsevier, ISBN 978-1-4160-0016-7, Philadelphia

Harley, RD. Paralytic strabismus in children. Etiologic incidence and management of the third, fourth and sixth nerve palsies. Ophthalmology, vol.87, no.1, (January 1980), pp. 24-43, ISSN 0161-6420

Hughes, D. (2000). Eyelid disorders, In: *Pediatric Ophthalmology,* Moore, A. & Lightman, S. (eds), pp. 154-61, BMJ Books, ISBN 0-7279-1203-8, London

Idrees, F.; Vaideanu, D. & Fraser, SG.; et al. (1970).A review of anterior segment dysgeneses; Surv Ophthalmol, vol.51, no.3, (May 2006), pp. 213-31, ISSN 0039-6257

Jancevski, M. & Foster, CS. (1990). Cataracts and uveitis. *Curr Opin Ophthalmol,* vol.21, no.1, (January 2010), pp.10-14, ISSN 1040-8738

Kanski, JJ. & Bowling, B. (2011). Congenital cataract, *In Clinical Ophthalmology: A Systematic approach, pp.298-304,* Elsevier, ISBN-13:9780702040931, China

Kanski, JJ. & Bowling, B. (2011). Cornea, *In Clinical Ophthalmology: A Systematic approach, pp.* 168-238, Elsevier, ISBN-13:9780702040931, China

Kanski, JJ. & Bowling, B. (2011). Hereditary fundus dystrophies. *In Clinical Ophthalmology: A Systematic approach.* pp. 648-85, Elsevier, ISBN-13:9780702040931, China

Kanski, JJ. & Bowling, B. (2011). Neuro-ophthalmology. *In Clinical Ophthalmology: A Systematic approach.* pp.789-812, Elsevier, ISBN-13:9780702040931, China

Kanski, JJ. & Bowling, B. (2011). Orbit, *In Clinical Ophthalmology: A Systematic approach, pp.* 79-117, Elsevier, ISBN-13:9780702040931, China

Kanski, JJ. & Bowling, B. (2011). Uveitis, *In Clinical Ophthalmology: A Systematic approach, pp.* 402-474, Elsevier, ISBN-13:9780702040931, China

Khani SC. & Fasiuddin A. (2011). Generalized Inherited Retinal Dystrophies, In: *Pediatric Retina,* Reynolds, JD. & Olitsky SE. (Eds.), pp. 295-303, Springer-Verlag, ISBN 978-3-642- 12040-4, Berlin.

Kherani, F. & Robb, RM. (2008). Congenital and developmental abnormalities of the eye, orbit, and ocular adnexa, In: *Principles and Practice of Ophthalmology,* Albert, DM. & Miller, JW. (eds), pp. 4177-83, Elsevier, ISBN 978-1-4160-0016-7, Philadelphia

Krishnamurthy, R. & Vanderveen, DK. (1961). Infantile cataracts. *Int Ophthalmol Clin,* vol.48, no.2, (Spring 2008), pp. 175-192, ISSN 0020-8167

Levin, AV. (1954). Congenital eye anomalies. *Pediatr Clin North Am,* vol.50, no.1, (February 2003), pp. 56-76, ISSN 0031-3955

MacEwen, CJ.; Baines, PS. & Desai, P. (1917). Eye injuries in children; the current picture. *Br J Ophthalmol*, vol.83, no.8, (August 1999), pp. 933-936, ISSN 0007-1161

Maida, JM.; Mathers, K. & Alley, CL. (1990) Pediatric ophthalmology in the developing world. *Curr opin Ophthalmol,* vol.19, no.5, (September 2008), pp. 403-8, ISSN 1040-8738

Martyn, LJ. (2006). Metabolic disease, In : *handbook of pediatrice ye end systemic disease.* Wright, KW.; Spiegel, PH. & Thompson, LS. (eds.), pp. 350-429. Springer, ISBN 10: 0-387-27927-X, China

Matta, NS.; Singman, EL. & Silbert DI. (1951). Evidenced-based medicine: treatment for amblyopia. *Am Orthopt J, vol.*60, (November 2010), pp. 17-22, ISSN 0065-955X

Mets, MB. & Kumar, AV. (2006). Eye Manifestations of Intrauterine Infections, In: *Essentials in Ophthalmology: Pediatric Ophthalmology, Neuro-Ophthalmology, Genetics*, Lorenz, B. & Moore, AT. (Eds.), pp. 205-218. Springer-Verlag, ISSN 1612-3212, Berlin, Germany

Mickler, C.; Boden, J. & Trivedi, RH.; et al. Pediatric cataract, *Pediatr Ann, vol.*40, no.2,(February 2011), pp. 83-87, ISSN 0090-4481

Mollon, JD.; Astell, S. & Reffin, JP. (1991). A minimalist test of colour vision, In: *Colour Vision Deficiencies,* Drum B., Moreland JD. & Serra A. (eds), pp. 59-67, Kluwer Academic Publishers, Dordrecht, ISBN 0-7506-4174-6, Netherlands

Moreira, CA., Jr.; Debert-Ribeiro, M. & Belfort, R., Jr. (1960). Epidemiological study of eye injuries in Brazilian children. *Arch Ophthalmol,* vol.106, no.6, (June 1988), pp. 781-784, ISSN 0003-9950

Morishita, H. & Hensch, TK. (1991). Critical period revisited: impact on vision. *Curr Opin Neurobiol,* vol.18, no.1, (February 2008), pp. 101-7, ISSN 0959-*4388*

Mulvihill, A.; Bowell, R. & Lanigan, B.; et al. (1995). Uniocular childhood blindness: a prospective study. *J Pediatr Ophthalmol Strabismus*, vol.34, no.2, (March April 1997), pp. 111-114, ISSN 0191-3913

Murphree, AL& Christensen LE. (2006). Retinoblastoma and Other Malignant Intraocular

Mutti, DO. (1992). Hereditary and environmental contributions to emmetropization and myopia. Optom Vis Sci., vol.87, no4, (April 2010), pp.255-9, ISSN 1040-5488

Nicholson, B.; Ahmad, B. & Sears, JE. (1961). Congenital optic nerve malformations. Int Ophthalmol Clin, vol.51, no.1, (Winter 2011), pp. 49-76, ISSN 0020-8167

Riordan-Eva P. (2004). Optics & Refraction, In: *General Ophthalmology*, Riordan-Eva P. & Whitcher JP. (eds), pp. 380-96, McGraw-Hill Companies, Inc, ISBN 0-07-137831-6, USA

Riordan-Eva, P. & Whitcher, JP. (eds), pp. 353-62, McGraw-Hill Companies, Inc, ISBN 0-07-137831-6, USA

Rose, G. (2000). Pediatric lacrimal and orbital disease. In: Pediatric Ophthalmology. Moore, A. & Lightman, S. (eds), pp. 162-176, BMJ Books, ISBN 0-7279-1203-8, London

Sarrazin, L.; Averbukh, E. & Halpert, M.; et al. (1884). Traumatic pediatric retinal detachment: a comparison between open and closed globe injuries. *Am J Ophthalmol*, vol.137, no.6, (June 2004), pp. 1042-1049, ISSN 0002-9394

Sauberan, DP. (1961). Pediatric uveitis. *Int Ophthalmol Clin,* vol.50, no.4, (Fall 2010), pp.73-85,ISSN 0020-8167

Serrano, JC; Chalela, P. & Arias, JD. (1960). Epidemiology of childhood ocular trauma in a northestern Colombian region. *Arch Ophthalmol*, vol.121, no.10, (October 2003), pp. 1439-1445, ISSN 0003-9950

Shields, CL& Shields JA. (2006). Pediatric Ocular Oncology, In: *Essentials in Ophthalmology: Pediatric Ophthalmology, Neuro-Ophthalmology, Genetics*, Lorenz B. & Moore AT (Eds.), pp. 111-113. Springer-Verlag, ISSN 1612-3212, Berlin, Germany.

Sullivan, JH. (2004). Orbit, In: *General Ophthalmology*, Riordan-Eva P. & Whitcher JP. (eds), pp. 250-60, McGraw-Hill Companies, Inc, ISBN 0-07-137831-6, USA

Topbas S, Toprak A, Erol N.; et al. Results of Conventional Retinal Detachment Surgery in Paediatric Age Group. Special Topic Issue: Ophthalmologica, vol. 214, no. 3, (2000), pp. 193, ISSN 0030-3755

Traboulski, EI. & Martyn, LJ. (2006). Connective tissue, skin, and bone disorders, In : *handbook of pediatrice ye end systemic disease.* Wright, KW.; Spiegel, PH. & Thompson, LS. (eds.), pp. 227-290. Springer, ISBN 10: 0-387-27927-X, China

Tumors, In: *Handbook of Pediatric Retinal Disease,* Wright, KW; Spiegel, PH. & Thompson LS (Eds.), pp 246-283. Springer Science+Business Media, ISBN 10: 0-387-27932-6, USA .

Valenzuela, A; Chan, HSL. & Heon, E; et al. (2011). A language for retinoblastoma: Guidelines and Standard operating procedures, In: *Pediatric Retina,* Reynolds, JD & Olitsky, SE. (Eds.), pp. 205-234. Springer-Verlag, ISBN 978-3-642-12040-4, Berlin

Webber, AL. &, Wood, J. (1969). Amblyopia: prevalence, natural history, functional effects and treatment. *Clin Exp Optom,* vol.88, no.6, (November 2005), pp. 365-75, ISSN 1444-0938

Yokoyama T.; Kato, T. &, Minamoto, A.; et al. Characteristics and surgical outcomes of paediatric retinal detachment. *Eye (London)*, vol.18, no.9, (September 2004), pp. 889-892, ISSN 1476-5454

Part 2

Pediatric Surgery

2

Acquired Cryptorchidism: What Should We Know? The Results of a Systematic Review

N. Zavras[1,*], A. Charalampopoulos[1],
K. Velaoras[2] and E. Iakomidis[2]
[1]*"ATTIKO" University Hospital, Medical School of Athens,*
[2]*Penteli General Children's Hospital, Athens*
Greece

1. Introduction

Cryptorchidism or undescended testis (UDT) is the most common genital abnormality seen at term in boys (Meij-de Vries A et al 2010, Topari & Kalieva 1999). Traditionally UDT was thought to be a congenital disease, with a prevalence of about 0.8-1% by 1 year of age (Berkowitz G Set al 1993). The term acquired UDT was introduced the last few decades, after well documented clinical observations in individuals and groups of patients that many boys continue to be diagnosed and treated later in childhood (Myers NA & Officer CB 1975, Atwell JD 1985, Clarnette TD et al 1977, Schiffer KA et al 1987, Robertson JF & Azmy AF 1988, Wright JE 1989, Fenton EJM et al 1990,Mayr J et al 1995) despite the recommendations for early surgical treatment by orchidopexy (Ritzén M et al 2007). Today, acquired UDT is a recognized separate entity, and after a new clinical classification in 2003, UDT is categorized into two forms: congenital UDT and acquired UDT (Hack WW et al 2003a).

Although the pathogenesis of congenital UDT is considered multifactorial including hormonal, genetic, and environmental influences (Ghacko JK & Barthold JS 2009, Barthold JS 2008), the exact etiology of acquired UDT remains unclear (Meijer RW 2004). Furthermore, while surgical treatment is recommended for congenital UDT patients as young as 6 months (Ritzén M, 2007), to reduce the increased risks of progressive infertility, testicular malignancy, torsion, associated inguinal hernia, and because of cosmetic and psychological aspects (Ashley RA et al 2010, Lamah M et al 2001) there is much controversy in the management of acquired UDT (Hack WW et al 2010).

In this article, we present the current data of the literature of this distinct entity in a concise but comprehensive review.

2. Patients and methods

A systematic review of the literature was performed focusing on the diverse aspects of the epidemiology, pathogenesis, diagnosis and management of acquired UDT. Data were

*Corresponding Author

extracted from Medline database form inception to October 2011. A UDT was defined as a non-palpable testis inside the scrotum and for which further traction on cord traction was painful (Meij-de Vries A et al 2010). A congenital UDT was defined as a testis which had not previously descended (Meij-de Vries A et al 2010, Hack WW et al 2003b), whereas an acquired UDT was defined as an UDT in which a previous scrotal position was documented on at least one occasion (Barthold JS & González R 2003). This does not include testes identified as being cryptorchid after inguinal surgery.

3. Epidemiology

Although the incidence of congenital UDT in full term males remains constant in the last few decades (Barthold JS & González R 2003), the true incidence of acquired UDT remains unknown, because of the lack of studies documenting the prevalence of this condition (Hack et al 2010) First Villumsen et al (Villumsen AL & Zachau-Christianssen B 1966) in 1966, reported that 69/4300 boys, (84 testes), had 2%, either unilateral or bilateral ascending testes from a normal position at birth to a higher position by the age of 3 years. In 1975, Myers et al (Myers NA & Officer CB 1975) reported a study of two families in whom all nine boys had normal descended testes documented as infants, but four in one family and three in the other required surgery for UDT before their teenage years. Wyllie in 1984, (Willye GG 1984) reported a study of 100 boys with retractile testes in whom 42% had testes at a higher level after a 5-year observation. Atwell in his paper, (Atwell JD 1985) reported an incidence of 1% acquired UDTs of all orhiopexies undertaken in his unit. In a study from Oxford (John Radcliffe Hospital Cryptorchidism Study Group 1986)) was found that 40% of boys whose testicles had not descent at birth but had done so by 3 months became undescended by the age of 1 year. Since then, others have given various rates, with ascending testes comprise 16% (Fenton EJM et al 1990), 2.3% (Gracia J et al. 1997), 5% (Eardley I et al 1994), 20% (Rabinowitz R & Hulbert WC, Jr 1997), and 73% (Hack WW et al 2003b) of all orcidopexies. In a cross sectional Dutch study, Hack et al (Hack et al 2007a) found a prevalence of acquired UDT up to 2.2% among 6-13 year old boys. Acerini et al (Acerini CL et al 2009), in a UK infant cohort study observed a cumulative incidence up to 7% at the age of 24 months (0.7%, 4%, 1.3% , and 1% at ages 3 months, 12 months, 18 months , and 24 months respectively). More recently, Wohlfahrt-Veje et al (Wohlfahrt-Veje C et al 2009) reported that acquired UDTs account for 58% of all cases of cryptorchidism (congenital and acquired) at 18 months, 71% at 36 months and 69% thereafter.

Although estimates regarding the true incidence of testicular ascent vary considerably, orchidopexy rates and higher than expected mean age of orchidopexy suggest that acquired UDT is more common than indicated by the number of detailed case reports. Most authors agree that acquired UDTs is a common phenomenon outnumbering congenitalUDTs by a factor of two to three (Hack WW et al 2003b, Hack WW et al 2007a) 1, Agarwal PK et al 2006. This could mean that the pathogenesis of AUDTs, as in congenital forms, is multifactorial also.

3.1 Pathogenesis

The pathogenesis of acquired UDT is not fully clarified, since several mechanisms have been proposed to elucidate the testicular ascent. Essentially, 4 major theories have been descrived to explain the process of secondary ascent (excluding that for iatrogenic reasons). The first theory is based on surgical findings during orchidopexies. Atwell (Atwell JD 1985) noted the presence of a persistent processus vaginalis (PV) in 9/10 of his patients. He proposed that the acquired malposition of the testis is due to partial absorption of the PV into the parietal peritoneum, and this alteration in the distribution of the peritoneal lining of the abdominal cavity leads to traction of the spermatic cord and ascent of the testis. Clarnette et al (Clarnette et al 1977, Clarnette et al 1997) reported the presence of a fibrous structure extending with the cord structures, which on immunohistochemistry showed the characteristics of a remnant of the PV. Other studies found the presence of PV or hernia sac in 23%-76% of orchiopexies for acquired UDT (Robertson JF & Azmy AF 1988, Wright JE 1989, Meijer RW 2004, Gracia J et al 1997 , Eardley I et al 1994, Hack WW 2003b, Redman JF 2005). Based on these findings, it was suggested that the persistence of a patent PV or its remnants is responsible for tethering the testis in a static position during a period of somatic growth. However, recently Meij-De Vries et al (Meij-de Vries A et al 2010), studying the perioperative surgical findings in congenital UDTs and acquired UDTs, found that acquired UDTs are more likely to have a closed PV, and a normal insertion of the gubernaculum. The conflicts seems to be continued, after the current findings of Mirillas et al (Mirilas et al 2010) who studied the sonographic pattern of the PV in children with acquired UDTs and found that PV is patent in a manner similar to the inguinal hernia and hydrocele . They suggested that a scrotal testis could be retracted through the PV to a higher position with contraction of the cremaster muscle.

The second theory speculates an association between retractile testes and acquired UDTs. Agarwal et al (Agarwal PK et al 2006) reported an incidence of 32% of retractile testes which became ascending during of about 3-year follow-up period. Willie (Willye GG 1984) reported an incidence of 42% of retractile testis to become ascending. Stec et al (Stec AA et al 1987) noted an incidence of 3.2% (21 of 666 retractile testes) underwent secondary ascent and orchidopexy. They stated that the majority of retractile testes resolve without surgical intervention. Eardlay et al (Eardley I et al 1994) found that 27% of ascending testes were previously retractile. Smith et al (Smith JA et al 1989) reported an increased secondary ascent of the testes in boys with cerebral palsy, where an increased cremasteric muscle hypertonicity is noted. These findings show that about a third of ascended testes may be passing through a retractile phase through the transition from the scrotum to an extrascotal position (Hack ww et al 2003c). Natural course of acquired undescended testis in boys. *Brit J Surg*, 90, pp.728-31). The following mechanisms have been proposed to clarify the possible causes of retractile testes to become ascended: a) Smith et al (Smith JA et al 1989), speculated that cremaster muscle spasticity may be a possible cause of acquired UDT in patients with cerebral palsy. However, the proposed etiology in otherwise normal boys is not clear (Barthold JS & González R. 2003), b) The cremaster muscle is androgen sensitive and exhibits decreased activity, resulting in decreased testicular retractility, during periods of high androgen production, specifically in infancy and puberty. It has been shown, that target disruption of estrogen receptors in mice produces cremasteric hypertrophy and testicular retraction (Bartlett JE et al 2008). Theoretically, environmental chemicals that influence sex steroid production or action could exaggerate the physiological hyperactivity of the cremaster muscle in young boys and increase the risk o testicular ascent (Gray LE & Osthy 2001). However, reproductive hormone activity is low during mid childhood, and the association between ascent testis and these substances is theoretical, and c) Robertson et al (Robertson JF & Azmy AF 1988) suggested that peri-testicular adhesions might be responsible for retaining the retractile testis in an inguinal position but this association has not been proved yet.

A third hypothesis proposed by Rusnack et al (Rusnack SL et al 2002) who found that primary undescended testes, ascending testes and the contralateral descended testes share the same histopathology concerning the total and differential germ cell counts per tubule. These findings suggest that an endocrine defect could be the cause of acquired UDT, since no thermal effect can be blamed for the decreased germ cell count in the descent testes. A further implication of an endocrine defect in the pathogenesis of acquired UDT is derived from recent reports which found an increased risk of AUDTs with proximal hypospadias (Tasian GE et al 2010, Itesako T et al 2011). The authors suggest that the role of prenatal and postnatal androgen disruption may link these conditions.

Finally, the fourth theory speculates the role of genitofemoral nerve (GFN) as a factor in testicular ascent. Hutson et al (Hutson JM & Hasthorpe S 2005) found that the GFN acts as second messenger for androgen by release calcitonin gene related peptide (CGRP) to control descent of the testis. They proposed the following mechanism by which the influence of the GFN is implicated: at birth the spermatic cord is 4 to 5 cm in length, but by the 10th year, it is 8-10 cm. This doubling in length is inhibited if there is a residual fibrous remnant of the PV, which may caused by deficient CGRP release from the GFN postnatally. Shono et al (Shono T et al 1999) reported that the proximal division of the GFN in neonatal rats causes testicular maldescent and may also induce testicular ascent in adulthood. They proposed that some intrauterine disorders of the GFN may cause testicular ascent.

The perception of acquired UDT has not been widely accepted. Rabinowitz et al (Rabinowitz R & Hulbert WC, Jr. et al 1997) studied 21 patients (23 undescended testis) and found that the gubernaculum attachment in half of the cases was abnormal. They stated that "this condition is ought to a missed diagnosis at a younger age. The testis is undescended, bur almost completely descended. With somatic growth the distance between the terminal portion of the gubernaculum and the scrotum increases, making the diagnosis more obvious". Furthermore, Redman in his paper (Redman JF 2005) challenged the concept of acquired UDT, arguing for "abandoning the concept and diagnosis of the ascending testis and embracing the phenomenon that the examination of the testis in infants and boys is an inexact process".

3.2 Natural history

The assessment of the natural history of acquired UDT is complicated by the difficulty in differentiating between "high retractile" testes and testes that have ascended from a normal descended position in the scrotum (Taghizadeh AK & Thomas DF 2008). However, some conclusions concerning the natural history are extracted by three long-term prospective studies performed by Eisjbouts et al, Sijstermans et al, and Hack et al. Eisjbouts et al (Eijsbouts SW et al 2007) evaluated prospectively 107 patients (132 acquired UDT) with a mean age 8.9±2.9 years. The mean follow-up was 4.5 years (range 0.3-12.1 years). The results showed that 75/132 (56.8%) testes descended spontaneously at puberty. Orchidopexy was performed in 57/132 (43.2%) testes. They noted that acquired UDT showed an increasing chance of descending spontaneously with increasing age, and an appropriate for the age testicle volume. Sijsterman et al (Sijsterman K et al 2006) reported that among 129 acquired UDTs, (mean follow-up 2.5 years, range: 0.2-8.5 years), 98 (76%) descended spontaneously at puberty with appropriate testicular growth; in the remaining 31 (24%) orchidopexy was performed at puberty, due to non-descent. Hack et al (Hack WW et al 2010) assessed prospectively the natural history and long-term testicular growth of acquired UDT after spontaneous descent or pubertal orchidopexy in case of non-descent, in 391 boys with 464 acquired UDT. At the time of referral the median age was 7.1 years. The mean follow-up was 4.7 years (range 0.1-12.0 years). They found that a 77.7% has a tendency of spontaneous descent at puberty, and in nearly all cases, after spontaneous descent or after pubertal orchidopexy, with long-term testicular volumes appropriate for age. Pubertal surges in luteinizing hormone and testosterone, as also is seen in the first 3 months after birth (Hamza AF et al 2001) when spontaneous descent of congenital UDT can still occur, are hypothesized to be responsible for pubertal spontaneous descent (Sijsterman K et al 2006).

3.3 Acquired UDT and fertility

There is limited evidence from the available data of the literature about the impact of acquired UDT in the fertility. As mentioned above, biopsies taken from ascending testes showed comparable histological findings to biopsies taken from the contra lateral descended testes and primary undescended testes (Rusnack SL et al 2002). Gracia et al (Gracia J et al. 1997) reported an impaired spermatogenic potential in 25/ 35 (71.4%) biopsied ascending testes. Meijer et al (Meijer RW et al 2004) reported that 24 / 30 acquired UDTs (80%) were small for the children's age and 1 (3%) was atrophic. These findings imply that acquired UDTs might influence fertility.

3.4 Acquired UDT and cancer

It is generally accepted that UDT is a risk factor for testicular cancer (Pettersson A et al 2007). Among men who have had UDTs the risk of cancer is increased two to eight times, and among all men with testicular cancer have a history of cryptorchidism (Topari J & Kalieva M 1999, Dieckemman KP et al 2004). However, orchidopexy does not reduce the risk of cancer but renders the retained testis amenable to self-estimation later in adulthood (Hack WW et al 2010). It remains unknown whether the risk of malignancy in acquired UDT and congenital UDT is the same. Nevertheless, the risk of cancer in acquired UDT might be lower than in congenital UDT, since neonatal gonocytes have transformed normally before the abnormality develops (Hutson JM &Clarke MC 2007).

4. Diagnosis

Past history and clinical examination are essential for the correct diagnosis of an acquired UDT. Commonly, acquired UDT is seen after the age of 4-5 years ((Myers NA & Officer CB 1975), and peaks around age 8 (Wohlfahrt-Veje C et al 2009). Clinically, acquired UDTs may be distinguished from retractile testis because they have a smaller size, immediate retraction out of the scrotum and pain after manipulation (Agarwal PK et al 2006).

However, early forms, even in boys less than 1 year, have also been recognized (Hack WW 2007b). Wright (Wright JE 1989) proposed the following criteria that have to be satisfied for the diagnosis of acquired UDT: a) it must be recorded by an experienced observer that the testis once had reached the bottom of the scrotum, b) the same or an equally experienced observer must later be unable to manipulate it into the scrotum, and the testis must remain above the scrotum when the child squats or sits bolt upright with the thighs abducted. c) there must have been no surgery or inflammatory episode to have caused the ascent, and d) the testis must remain above the scrotum when the child is anesthetized.

Potential impediments that may interfere in the correct diagnosis an ascending testis include: a) obesity, b) a small contracted scrotum, and c) an uncooperative or fretful patient (Redman JF 2005). The contractions of the cramasteric muscles, hydroceles, thick walled hernia sacs, and long looping vasa are further possible factors to a correct diagnosis (Redman JF 2005)

5. Management

The proper management of acquired UDT remains controversial mainly due to a lack of longitudinal follow up data ((Hack WW et al 2010). Currently two main polices have been proposed : a) the policy of prompt surgical correction (Taghizadeh AK & Thomas DF 2008, Bonney T et al 2008) and b) consrvative policy either of "wait and see"(Meij-de Vries A et al 2010) or hormonal treatment (Meijer RW et al 2001). The target of the first policy is to achieve normal or at least improved fertility, and to prevent malignancy (Hack WW et al 2010). However, it is still unknown whether the risks of infertility and cancer migh benefit at all from surgery as in congenital UDT (Hack WW et al 2010). In addition, it must be noted that there is no evidence that the ascended testis has a higher malignancy rate compared with the normal descended testis (Ong C et al 2005). The second policy is based on studies which showed a spontaneous descent of acquired UDTs at the beginning of puberty in 57% to 77.5% of the cases, with normal testicular growth (Hack WW et al 2010, Acerini CL et al 2009). This policy is supported by the following: 1) surgery itself can lead to complications such as direct injury to the vas deferens or testicular vessels (Mouriquand PDE 2008), 2) Meijer et al (Meijer RW et al 2001) treated successfully with human chorionic gonadotropin (HCG) 14/ 15 acquired UDTs (93.3%) (54). In addition, Hutson et al (Hutson JM & Basley SW 1991) predicted acquired UDTs to respond well to HCG therapy. These findings suggest that surgery should be reserved for those testes which fail to respond to hormonal therapy and those with anatomical abnormalities; 3) there is no strong evidence that early operation in boys 4-14 years has any effect on subsequent fertility (Chilvers C et al 1986). Although these results seem promising of a conservative approach to acquired UDTs, more long term follow-up studies are necessary to determine the consequences in fertility potential of boys with a history of acquired UDTs.

6. Conclusions

This study showed, that there is an ongoing interest for the exact pathogenesis and the optimal mode of treatment of acquired UDTs. However, the data are inconclusive, as there are no available studies reaching a worldwide consensus. Large series, randomized-controlled studies and close follow-up beyond the puberty are recommended to further elucidate acquired UDT.

7. References

Acerini CL, Miles HL,Dunker DB, Ong KK, Hughes IA. (2009). The descriptive epidemiology of congenital and acquired cryptorchidism in a UK infant cohort. *Arch Dis Child*,94,pp. 368-72

Agarwal PK, Diaz M, Elder JS . (2006). Retractile testis-is it a normal variant? *J Urol*, 175,pp. 1496-99

Ashley RA, Barthold JS, Kolon F.(2010) Cryptorchidism: pathogenesis, diagnosis, treatment and prognosis. *Urol Clin North Am*,37, pp.183-93

Atwell JD.(1985).Ascent of the testis: fact or fiction. Br J Urol, 57, pp.474-7

Barthold JS, González R. (2003).The epidemiology of congenital cryptorchidism, testicular ascent and orchiopexy. *J Urol*, 170pp. 2396-401

Barthold JS.(2008) Undescended testis: current theories of etiology. *Curr Opin Urol*;18pp.395-400

Bartlett JE, Washburn T, Eddy EM, Korach KS, Temelcos C, Hutson JM .(2001). Early development of the gubernaculums and cremaster sac in estrogen receptor knock-out mice. *Urol Res*, 29,pp.163-7

Berkowitz GS, Lapinski RH, et al.(1993). Prevalence and natural history of cryptorchidism. *Pediatrics* , 92, pp. 44-9

Bonney T, Hutson J, Southwell B, Newgreen D.(2008). Update on congenital versus acquired undescended testis: incidence, diagnosis and management. *ANZ J Surg*,102,pp. 1010-3

Chilvers C, Dadley NE, Gough MH, Jackson MB, Pike MC. (1986). Undescended testis: the effect of treatment on subsequent risk of fertility and malignancy. *J Pediatr Surg*, 21, pp.691-6

Clarnette TD, Rowe D, Hashorpe S, Hutson JM.(1977). Incomplete disappearance of the processus vaginalis as a cause of ascending testis. *J Urol*;157, pp. 1889-91

Clarnette TD, Rowe D, Hasthorpe S, Hutson JM et al.(1997). Incomplete disappearance of the processus vaginalis as a cause of ascending testis. *J Urol*, 157,pp.1889-91

Dieckemman KP, Pichlmeier U.(2004). Clinical epidemiology of testicular germ tumors. *World J Urol*,22,pp.2-14

Eardley I, Saw KC, Whitaker RH . (1994). Surgical outcome of orchiopexy. II. Trapped and ascending testis. *Br J Urol*, 73pp.204-6

Eijsbouts SW, de Muinck Keizer- Scharma SM, Hazebroek FW . (2007). Further evidence for spontaneous descent of acquired undescended testis. *J Urol*, 178,pp. 1726-9

Fenton EJM, Woodward AA, Hutson IL, Marschner I.(1990). The ascending testis. *Pediatr Surg Int*5, pp. 6-9

Ghacko JK, Barthold JS. (2009). Genetic and environment contributors to cryptorchidism. Pediatr Endocrinol Rev,6, pp.476-80

Gracia J, Navarro E, Guirado F, Pueyo C, Ferrández A .(1997). Spontaneous ascent of the testis. *Br J Urol*, 79, pp. 113-5

Gray LE, Osthy J.(2001). Effects of environmental antiandrogens on reproductive development in experimental animals. *Hum Reprod Update*,7,pp.248-64

Hack WW, Meijer RW, Bos SD, Haasnoot K.(2003a). A new clinical classification for undescended testis. *Scand J Urol Nephr*, 37 43-7

Hack WW, Meijer RW, van der Voort- Doedens LM, Bos SD, De Kok ME.(2003b). Previous testicular position in boys referred for an undescended testis: further explanation of the late orchidopexy enigma? *BJU Int*, 92,pp. 293-96

Hack WW, Sijstermans K, van Dijk J, van der Voort-Doedens LM, de Kok ME, Hobbelt-Stoker MJ .(2007) Prevalence of acquired undescended testis in 6-year, 9-year. And 13-year-old Dutch boys. *Arch Dis Child*, 92,pp. 17-20

Hack WW, van der Voort-Doedens LM, Goede J, van Dijk JM, Meijer RW, Sijstermans K .(2010). Natural history and long-term testicular growth of acquired undescended testis after spontaneous descent or pubertal orchidopexy. *BJU Int*, 106,pp.1052-59

Hack WW, van der Voort-Doedens LM, Sijtermans K, Plerik FH .(2007). Reduction in the number of orchidopexies for cryptorchidism after recognition of acquired undescended testis and implementation of expectative policy. *Acta Pediatr*, 96, pp. 915-8

Hack WW, Meijer RW, van der Voort-Doedens LM, Bos SD, Haasnoot K . (2003c).Natural course of acquired undescended testis in boys. *Brit J Surg*, 90, pp.728-31

Hamza AF, Elrahim M, Elnagar, Maaty SA, Bassiouny E, Jehannin B.(2001). Testicular descent: when to interfere? Eur J Pediatr Surg 11,pp.173-6

Hutson JM, Basley SW. (1992). Descent of the testis. Chapter 4: Classification and causes of undescended testes in humans. Edward Arnold (Ed). London Melbourne Auckland; pp 57-59

Hutson JM, Clarke MC. Current management of the undescended testicle.(2007). *Semin Pediatr Surg* ,16,pp. 64-70

Hutson JM, Hasthorpe S.(2005). Testicular descent and cryptorchidism: the state of the art in 2004. J Pediatr Surg, 40,pp. 297-302

Itesako T, Nara K, Matsui F, Matsumoto F, Shimada K.(2011). Acquired undescended testis in boys with hypospadias. *J Urol*, 185,pp. 2440-3

John Radcliffe Hospital Cryptorchidism Study Group.(1986). Boys with late descending testis: the source of patients with "rectractile" testes undergoing undergoing orchidopexy. *BMJ*, 293, pp.789-90

Lamah M, McCaughey ES, Finley FO,Burge DM. (2001). The ascending testis: is late orchidopexy due to failure of screening or late ascent? *Pediatr Surg Int*,17,pp.421-3

Mayr J, Rune GM, Holas A, Schimpl G Schmidt B,Haberlik A. (1995). Ascent of the testis. *Eur J Pediatr*, 154, pp. 893-5

Meij-de Vries A, Hack WW, Heij HA, Meijer RW (2010).Perioperative surgical findings in congenital and acquired undescended testis. *J Pediatr Surg*, 45, pp. 1874-81

Meijer RW, Hack WW, van der Voort-Doedens LM, Haasnoot K, Bos SD. (2004). Surgical findings in acquired undescended testis. *J Pediatr Surg*, 39, pp. 1242-44

Meijer RW, Hack WW,Haasnoot K. (2001). Successful treatment of acquired undescended testes with human gonadotropin. *Eur J Pediatr*, 160, pp 66-7

Mirilas P, Menetssidou A, Kontis E, Argyris I, Tsitouridis I, Petropoulos A .(2010). Sonographic evidence for patency of the processus vaginalis in children with acquired undescended testis. *Int J Andr*, 34,pp. 49-54

Mouriquand PDE.(2008). Undescended testes in children: the paediatric urologist's point of view. *Eur J Endocrinol*, (Suppl 1),pp. S83-6

Myers NA, Officer CB.(1975). Undescended testis: congenital or acquired? *Aust J Paediatr* , 11, pp.76-80

Ong C, Hasthorpe S, Hutson JM. (2005). Germ cell development in the descended and cryptorchid testis and the effect of hormonal population. *Pediatr Surg Int*, 21,pp, 240-254

Pettersson A, Richiardi L, Nordenskjold A, Kaijser M, Akre O . (2007). Age at surgery for undescended testis and risk of testicular cancer. *N Engl J Med*;356,pp.1835-41

Rabinowitz R, Hulbert WC, Jr. (1997). Late presentation of cryptorchidism: the etiology of testicular re-ascent. *J Urol*,157, pp. 1892-94

Redman JF. (2005).The ascending (acquired undescended) testis: a phenomenon? *BJU Int*,95,pp. 1165-7

Redman JF.(2005). The ascending (acquired) testis: a phenomenon? *BJU Int*, 95,pp.1165-67

Ritzén EM, Bergh A, Bjerknes R, Christiansen P, Cortes D, Haugen SE, Jörgensen N, Kollin C, Lindahl S, Läckgren G, Main KM, Nordenskjöld A, Rajpert-De Meyts E, Söder O, Taskinen S, Thorsson A, Thorup J, Toppari J, Virtanen H..(2007). Nordic consensus on treatment of undescended testes. *Acta Pediatr*, 96,pp. 638-43

Robertson JF, Azmy AF.(1988). Assent to assent of the testis. *Br J Urol*, 61,pp. 146-47

Rusnack SL, Wu HY, Huff DS, Snyder HM 3rd, Zderic SA, Carr MC, Canning DA. (2002). The ascending testis and the testis undescended since birth share the same histopathology. J Urol, 168,pp.2590-1

Schiffer KA, Kogan SJ, Reda EF, Levitt SB (1987). Acquired undescended testis. *Am J Dis Child* 141,pp, 106-7

Shono T, Zakaria O, Imajima T, Suita S .(1999). Does proximal genitofemoral nerve division induce testicular maldescent or ascent in the rat. *BJU Int*, 83,pp.323-26

Sijsterman K, Hack WW, van der Voort-Doedens LM, Meijer RW, Haasnoot K .(2006). Puberty stage and spontaneous descent of acquired undescended testis: implication for therapy? *Int J Androl*, 29,pp. 597-602

Smith JA, Hutson JM, Beasley SW, Reddihough DS.(1989). The relationship between cerebral palsy and cryptorchidism. *J Pediatr Surg*; 24,pp.1303-5

Stec AA, Thomas JC, DeMarco RT, Pope JC 4th, Brock JW 3rd, Adams MC . (2007). Incidence of testicular ascent in boys with retractile testes. *J Urol*, 178,pp. 1722-5

Taghizadeh AK, Thomas DF. (2008).Ascent of the testis revisited: fact not fiction. Br J Urol Int,102,pp. 676-78

Tasian GE, Zaid H, Cabana MD, Baskin LS .(2010). Proximal hypospadias and risk of acquired cryporchidism. *J Urol*, 184,pp. 715-20

Topari J, Kalieva M. Maldescendus testis.(1999). Horm Res, 51, pp.261-9

Villumsen AL, Zachau-Christianssen B.(1966). Spontaneous alterations in positions of the testis. *Arch Dis Child*, 41,pp. 198-200

Willye GG. (1984).The retractile testis. *Med J Aust*,140,pp.403-5

Wohlfahrt-Veje C, Boisen KA, Boas M, Damgaard IN, Kai CM, Schmidt IM, Chellakooty M, Suomi AM, Toppari J, Skakkebaek NE, Main KM .(2009). Acquired cryptorchidism is frequent in infancy and childhood. *Int J Andrology*,32,pp. 423-28

Wright JE. Testes do ascent. (1989). *Pediatr Surg Int*, 4,pp. 269-72

Zorgniotti AW (ed). Temperature and Environmental Effects on the Testis. Mew York: Plenum Press, 1991

3

Merits and Arguments Related to Circumcision

Hosni Khairy Salem
Kasr Al Ainy Hospital,
Cairo University, Cairo,
Egypt

1. Introduction

Christians and no believers perform Circumcision for health and hygienic reasons especially in U.S.A. and some countries of the Middle East. It is uncommon in Northern Europe, Central and South America and Asia (Leitch, 1970). It is one of the" oldest operations but it has not received enough consideration or progress in the Middle East. It is always regarded as a minor outpatient procedure often performed by primitive clamps by barbers, Mohels, medical students and house officers (Kaplan, 1977).In hospitals, male circumcision is performed by junior gynecologists, urologists, or surgeons. The objective of this article is to perform a review of the literature regarding the different aspects of male circumcision and discussing the following points; history of circumcision, urgent indications of circumcision, merits and arguments related to circumcision, religious factors, contraindications of circumcision, timing of circumcision, different techniques of circumcision , complications after circumcision and relation to STDs or UTI.

2. History of circumcision

Circumcision is one of the oldest operation in the history and the first unequivocal description of circumcision is found in the forth dynasty Egyptian toombs (3000 BC). According to Herodotus, it was practiced at puberty. It is carved on portraits in the Karnak temple of Mount Saini Statues of Pharaohs. Its technique is seen in a bas brief on Mastaba of Sakkarah in the fifty dynasty (Bistschai& Brodnay, 1956; Arnaout et al., 1962 and Badr, 1963). Whether it had a religious or hygienic in purpose in Ancient Egypt, it is unknown. According to Herodotus, the Egyptians taught the procedure to Jews, Syrians and Phoenicians. Later, the custom spread to Ethiopians but Herodotus did not know that Columbus would find the natives of the West Indias circumcised. Captain Cook found the practice used by natives of Australia, Fijt, New Caledonia, New Hebrides and Madagascar (Blandy, 1968).It is a religious ritual practiced by Jews and Muslims. Jews practice it on the eighth day after birth. From Jews, it passes to the Christians who performed it for hygienic purposes then passed to Muslims as an important ritual of cleanliness for males. It was introduced to the western cultures by Biblical injunctions (Arnaout et al., 1962).Circumcision has also been practiced in other locations and for various reasons throughout the world e.g., in the-one continent of Africa, only certain tribes circumcise e.g., Zulo, Xahsa, Bechuana and Falasha while among its many Christian communities; circumcision has a religious significance only in Ethiopia (Blandy et al., 1968).

3. The prepuce (what is removed during circumcision?)

The glans is covered by the prepuce which is formed of two layers of skin reflected at the neck of the penis behind the corona glandis; the inner layer of the prepuce is confluent along the line of the neck with thin skin-which covers and adheres firmy to the glans on the undersurface of the glans penis, a small median fold passes to the deep surface of the prepuce (frenulurn). The prepuce is separated from the glans by a potential space (preputial sac) which presents two shallow fossae on either side of the frenulum. On the corona glandis and on the neck of the penis, there are numerous small preputial sebaceous glands which secrete smegma beneath the foreskin (a mixture of sebaceous material and shed keratin). It has a peculiar odor, and may be seen exiting from the foreskin tip or accumulate in clumps beneath the foreskin (Gray's Anatomy, 1950).

4. Indications of circumcision

4.1 Phimosis

It is a condition in which the contracted foreskin cannot be retracted over the glans and the commonest cause is chronic infection from poor local hygiene. In diabetic older men, balanoposthitis may lead to phimosis (Eiger, 1972). Congenital narrowing of the preputial orifice associated with long foreskin leads to ballooning out of the prepuce on micturition with a thin weak stream of urine leading to difficult micturition with residual urine, hydroureter and hydronephrosis but more often occurs as a result of atresia meati which may lie hidden by phimosis (Blandy et al, 1968, Bailey & Love's, 1992). It is reported that most cases of phimosis occur in uncircumcised males although excessive skin left, which may become stenotic lead to phimosis.

Circumcision has been the traditional treatment for phimosis but not the only management option; the best of which appears to be gentle physical retraction combined with topical steroid treatment of the unretractable foreskin (Dewan et al., 1996).

Circumcision for phimosis in infant and young boys is done due to a request by the patients (religious and personal), or due to recurrent balanitis with inability to retract the prepuce and rarely due to a very long prepuce. In adults, it is done due to inability to retract for intercourse, tight frenum, balanitis and sometimes, prior to radiotherapy for penile carcinoma.(Bailey& Love's, 1992).

4.2 Paraphimosis

Tight prepuce has been retracted and cannot be returned to its normal position. This is due to chronic infection under the redundant foreskin which leads to contracture of the preputial opening (phimosis) and formation of a tight ring of skin when the foreskin is retracted over the glans. The skin ring leads to venous congestion which leads to engorged oedematous glans making the condition worse. As the condition progresses, arterial occlusion and necrosis of the glans may occur. Treatment can be done by firm squeezing of the glans for five minutes to reduce tissue oedema and to decrease the glans size then the skin can be drawn forwards over the glans. If this is unsuccessful, general anaesthesia must be given and the constricting band is incised and circumcision is done to trim the redundant skin later on and antibiotics should be given (Bailey & Love's, 1992).

4.3 Trauma

It is a rare indication for circumcision (Blandy et al., 1968).

4.4 Balanoposthitis

Inflammation of the glans penis is known as balanitis while the inflammation of the prepuce is known as posthitis. Frequently, the opposing surfaces of the prepuce and glans are implicated in the inflammation process (Balanoposthitis).

The immediate cause of acute balanoposthitis is the multiplication within the preputial sac of pyogenic organisms as Streptococcal pneumococci and coliform bacilli. A contributing cause of balanoposthitis is diabetes (Manson, 1966 and Ross, 1941).

4.5 Prophylactic neonatal circumcision

Circumcision is done as prophylactic reasons to reduce the incidence of: urinary tract infection, penile carcinoma and carcinoma of the cervix "and sexually transmitted diseases.

4.6 Religious reasons

Circumcision is a religious rite among Muslims and Jews (Arnaout et al., 1962).

5. Circumcision/sexually transmitted diseases (STDs) &HIV

Donovan et al. in 1994,stated that the uncircumcised penis is hypothetically at increased risk of STDs especially-genital herpes, gonorrhea, syphilis, immunodeficiency virus type 1 (HIV-1) infection, candidiasis and chancroid due to larger surface area, thinner epidermal barrier, more liability for epithelial microtrauma and the moist warm neck under the foreskin favoring the persistence of fastidious microorganisms. However, none of these hypotheses has been proven. Moses et al. in 1994, in eighteen cross sectional studies from six countries reported a statistically significant association between male circumcision and the risk for HIV infection. Male circumcision should be considered as an essential strategy for AIDs-control (Tyndall et al., 1996). Caldwell in 1996 reported that in parts of subsaharan Africa, nearly 25% of the population is HIV positive as a result of heterosexual transmission of the virus. Lack of circumcision makes men in this region particularly susceptible. Taylor and Rodin in 1975, reported that there was a positive relationship between lack of circumcision and genital herpes simplex virus infection (HSV). Simonsen et al. in 1988, reported that in a controlled study of Human Immunodeficiency Disease (HIV), they found that men who were uncircumcised were 2.5 times more likely to have HIV infection.

6. Circumcision/urinary tract infections

Winberg's study in Scandinavia 1975, where circumcision is uncommon showed that in male infants with pyelonephritis, the prepuce is colonized with the offending organism. This only occurs during the first months of life where boys have a urinary tract infection more frequently than girls.

Ginsburg and McCracken in 1982, like Winberg found that early in life, the number of boys with acute pyelonephritis was greater than girls and 95% of all boys with urinary tract infection were uncircumcised. The association between circumcision and infection has since been confirmed by Wiswell and Roscelle in two epidemiologic studies, the latest involving over 400,000 infants. That study showed that the incidence of urinary tract infection was only 0.1% when circumcision was performed. Finally, taking into consideration the fact that most males in these Scandinavian studies are uncircumcised, it may consider the prepuce as a risk factor. Wiswell and Roscelle in 1986 and Horzog 1989, stated that the infection rate in uncircumcised infants was ten times greater than in circumcised males. So, prophylactic neonatal circumcision is mandatory to reduce the incidence of UTI.

7. Circumcision/carcinoma of the penis

KuroviUa et al. in 1971 Stated that, Jews do not have cancers of the penis because they perform ritualistic circumcision upon their male children on the 8th day of life. Muslims also perform ritualistic circumcision. Compared with Hindus, who live in a similar environment but who do not circumcise, Muslims are relatively free from penile cancers while those who delay circumcision till boys are about 10 years of age; by that time, occult cancerous changes have become so well established beneath the prepuce that the disease can not be prevented. Study of men with cancers of the penis shows a high proportion with conditions of the prepuce that make its retraction difficult or impossible. Difficulty in retracting the prepuce especially in a man careless of hygiene is likely to result in accumulation and retention of the smegma, probably the exciting agent in the production of penile cancer. It is evident that the complete prophylaxis conferred by a well performed circumcision early in infancy is not produced by the circumcision of adults. When an infant is circumcised and the glans is no longer protected by the prepuce, a dense, thicker epidermis develops that-resists formation of cancer by chronic irritation. An association has been reported between cancer of the cervix and penis (Smith et al., 1980) . It has long been known that carcinoma of the cervix is rare in nuns and that the incidence of such cancer is low in populations in whom most males are circumcised (Blandy et al., 1968).

8. Contraindications of circumcision

Any penile abnormality in which the foreskin may be used in later reconstruction e.g., Hypospadias or Epispadias. Epispadius is a contraindicatios for circumcision.

1. In doubtful sex as male and female pseudo-hermaphrodism or true hermaphrodism where both ovaries and testes are present.
2. In anemic, marasmic or weak children as well as in the presence of acute disease or active infections.
3. Unfavorable general conditions, e.g., prematurity, uncorrected bleeding diathesis (Grimes, 1978).

9. The optimum age for circumcision

The third week is the best time for circumcision because pain is minimal, bleeding is minimal, wound healing is perfect, and the risk of infection and psychological effects are minimal because the blood is still loaded with maternal antibodies with the near sterility of the skin of the neonate.

Circumcision can be done at any later healthy period preferably before school age.

If it is confirmed that the uncircumcised male neonate is at a higher risk of serious urinary tract infection than the circumcised one and therefore, the operation should be done shortly after birth.

Jewish ritual of circumcision on the eighth day is known to be more effective prophylaxis than procedures performed at the age between 4-14 years (Blandy, 1968).

However, operations performed at adolescence or later in life are completely attended with undesirable erections, protracted healing and infection (Arnaout et al., 1962).

In Muslim areas, circumcision is usually performed in the first few months of life. In Uganda and similarly in Kenya, circumcision age is 12-20 years.

Also, circumcision can be done in the first day of life provided no hypospadius, bleeding tendency or intersex is present.

10. Different opinions & arguments in neonatal circumcision

It is a custom: The most important, arguments are those of custom and tradition.

It confers beauty: It is difficult to evaluate the consideration of beauty since these are subjective. In cultures where circumcision is norm, young women find the uncircumcised penis radiculously ugly. Young ladies refuse intercourse without wearing an appropriate brooch through his penis.

It promotes health: through the prevention of venereal diseases, cancer of the penis and cervix uteri. Hutchinsons in 1891, the greatest syphilologist suggested that, the presence of the foreskin constitutes a constant source of irritation leading to high risk of syphilis in early life and cancer in the aged. Penile cancer is never seen in a Jew and chancres are rare.

In some countries, insurance excluded infants under the age of 15 years. The reason was that the money used to pay for the possible unnecessary circumcisions would cover much of the cost of emerging neonatal and premature intensive care units. Circumcision is done when the boy is more than one day old and after he has been checked for bleeding tendency (Blandy et al, in 1968).

There are children who are brought in by their parents for circumcision for ethnic or social reasons (Shanon et al., 1979).

On the other hand, the risk cost- effectiveness and medical resources should probably be allocated to health measures of demonstrated value. Laumann et al. in 1997, in The National Health and Social life survey, indicated that there are no significant differences between circumcised and uncircumcised men in contracting sexually transmitted diseases.

Also, uncircumcised men appear slightly more likely to experience sexual dysfunction especially later in life. Their results support the view that physicians and parents must be informed about potential benefits and risks of circumcision.

Tran and Giacomantanio in 1996, reported that the increased rate of penile cancer among uncircumcised men appears to justify the procedure but that alone is not sufficient justification. The final decision in neonatal circumcision should be made by parents with balanced counsel from the attending physicians. The Infectious Disease Committee of the Canadian of Society in 1996, stated that circumcision of newborns should not be routinely performed.

11. Anaesthetic techniques during circumcision

Circumcision may be conducted using a wide variety of general, regional and local anaesthetic techniques. The choice of an ideal anaesthetic technique depends upon surgical and patients factors. In addition, sedation is commonly used to supplement local anaesthetic based techniques as part of a so-called monitored anaesthesia care (MAC) technique.

12. Methods of circumcision

Circumcision is one of the oldest and commonest operations in medicine. There are several, methods aiming for completely exposure of the glans and complete excision of the prepuce.

In infants and neonates:

Primitive methods: Bamboo - Lazem - shield (Ritual Jewish Circumcision).

Standard methods: Bone forceps, surgical dissection - circumcision by the use of special instruments (Gomco clamp- plastibell device- Mogen clamp) (Holman et al,1990).

In older children and adults:

Dorsal slit and dissection technique-sleeve resection method.

In Sudan, Bamboo size of the glans is applied over the glans down to the corona to protect the glans inside it while the prepuce is pulled out over the outer surface of the bamboo and cut off at the appropriate level.

Blunt circumcision on clamps (lazem or kalloba) (Arnaout et al., 1962), made of non-cutting blades articulating at one end are widely used by village barbers in rural areas.

Ritual Jewish Circumcision: The Jewish ritual operation is usually done by a professional circumciser who is trained to do the operation as well as to observe the rituals. Circumcision is usually done in a Synagogue but now is done in hospitals.

13. Complications of circumcision

The common complications due to circumcision are not usually serious. These include:

1. Asymmetrical removal of the foreskin which may require recircumcision for cosmetic purposes.

2. The suture line may become infected specially by Staphylococcal infection. (Annunziato and Goldbum in 1978).
3. Meatal stenosis is probably the most common potentially adverse result of neonatal circumcision. Lacking of the foreskin coverage leads to irritation and inflammation of the meatal tissues by the very alkaline urine formed after meals. This leads to stenosis or meatal adhesions. Formal meatotomy is required when the stream is very fine in calibre (Blandy et al., 1968).
4. Bleeding from an artery or vein. Shulman et al. in 1964, reported that the most common complication in 800 infants undergoing ritual circumcision by Mohels on the 8th day of life in Jews is haemorrhage which occurs in ten patients.
5. Removal of excessive skin of the penile shaft along with the prepuce. On healing of the wound, the penis sets buried in the scrotum. This results in a concealed or denuded penis. Repair is complicated by the lack of the available skin to cover the shaft of the penis. (Radhakrishnan & Reges, 1984).
6. If the urethra is grapsed in the circumcision clamp or from stitches placed in the urethra, the injury is usually a fistula at the corona (Shulman et al., 1964).
7. Penile glans amputation during circumcision. Sherman et al. in 1996, reported seven cases of traumatic amputation of the glans penis and/or urethra during circumcision due to errors in the circumcision technique. The excised glandular tissue remains viable up to eight hours after injury. Reanastomosis of the glans and/or urethra following distal amputation even when there is a delay in the surgical repair of up to eight hours is usually successful.
8. Gangrene of the penis and scrotum (Du-Toit & Villet in 1979).
9. Complete avulsion of the skin of the penis and scrotum (Malherbe, 1975). Shulman et al. in 1964, reported that 1:800 would develop complications requiring admission to the hospital, e.g., necrosis of the glans, laceration of the scrotum and removal of the entire penile skin.

14. Laser circumcision

The laser beam cuts as well as controls bleeding from the skin, resulting in a very tidy wound. This technique allows exact proportions of skin and mucous membrane to be removed. Laser circumcision is the technique of choice for children circumcision and can also be applied to adult patients. Clinical comparative studies between the Neodymium:yttriumaluminum-garnet (Nd:YAG) laser and conventional circumcision in boys are very few. Vaos compared the clinical effects of the Nd:YAG laser contact technique with those of a conventional technique on the grounds of certain perioperative parameters, including operative time, length of hospital stay, postoperative complications and morbidity. Seventy-five patients undergoing circumcision were reviewed retrospectively. Operative time, length of hospital stay, and postoperative morbidity were analyzed. The study concluded the Nd:YAG laser contact technique is an effective laser-assisted procedure alternative to the conventional technique in circumcision with virtually no significant postoperative morbidity (Vaos,2004).

Similar study using Carbon dioxide laser circumcision found this technique to reduce operative time translating into cost effectiveness. Morbidity rates of laser circumcision compared favorably to those of conventional circumcision (How et al 2003).

15. Psychological effect of circumcision

An early operation minimizes the potential psychological damage caused by genital surgery (Manley, 1982). Also, avoids sensitive phases of psychosocial development (maternal bonding, separation anxiety, development of genital body image, gender identity, and phallic awareness), the disruption of which is thought to predispose to psychological problems in later life. The age at which surgery took place was not associated with abnormal psychological adjustment later in life (Freud 1955).

16. Conclusions

The advantages of male circumcision are much more than the disadvantages and this explains the increased number of parents asking for circumcision for their male infants.

17. References

[1] Leitch I.O.W. Circumcision, A continuing engima Aust. ped. J.G. 59-1970.
[2] Kaplan G.W.: Circumcision. An overview current problemsi in ped. 7: 1; 1977.
[3] Bistschai J. and Brodney, ML: A History of urology in Egypt Cambridge, Mass-Riveside press; 1956.
[4] Arnaout H.; Elfiky G.F. and Sherif M.: Circumcision. Kasr-ElAini J Surg. 3:169; 1962.
[5] Badr M.M.: The History of urology in Ancient Egypt. L Intern. Coll. surgeons 39:404; 1963.
[6] Blandy J.P.: Circumcision Hospital Mediane. 3:551; 1968.
[7] Gray's Anatomy D.: D.Davis 4th ed. (254-585-1561- Langrnans green and co. 1950).
[8] Eiger MS.: The case for circumcision. Today's Health. (50)4: p. 14; 1972.
[9] Bailey and Love's, short practice of surgery. Urethra and penis, vol II, 21Ist ed; 1992.
[10] Dewan PA; Tieu HC and ChTeng BS.: Phimosis is a circumicsion necessary. J. Ped. Child. - Health. Aug.; 32(4):285; 1996.
[11] Manson-Bakr; PH.: Manson's 16th. ed; page 677 London 1966.
[12] Ross J.C.: Brit. J. Surg., 42,29,194; 1941.
[13] Donovan B; Bassett I and Bodsvorth NJ.: Male circumcision and common sexua, transmissible diseases in a developed nationsetting: Genitourim Med. Oct.; 70(5):317; 1994.
[14] Moses S; Plummer FA; Bradley JE; Ndinya-Acloal-Jo; Nagelkerke NJ and Roland- AR.: The association between lack of male circum. and risk for HIV. infection: A review of the epidemiological data: sex- Transm. Dis. Jul- Aug: 21(4): 201; 1994.
[15] Tyndall MVV; Ronald AR; Agoki E; iMalisa \V; Bvvayo JJ; Nadinya Achola Jo; Moses S and Plummer FA.: Increased risk of infeciion with human immunodeficency virus type 1 among uncircumcised men presenting with genital ulcer dis. in Kenya: clin. Infect. Dis. Sep; 23(3) 449; 1996.
[16] Caldwell JC and Caldwell P.: African AIDS, epidemic. Sci. Am. Mats; .274(3) 62; 1996.
[17] Taylor P.K.; Rodin P.: Herpes genitalis and circumcision. British Journal of veneral diseases, 51:274; 1975.

[18] Simenson J; et al.: Human Immunodeficiency virus infection among men. Africa. Engl. J. Med. 319(5): p. 274; 1988.
[19] Winberg J; Bergstrom T and Jacobsson B.: Morbidity, age and sex distribution, recurrences and renal scarring in symptomatic UTI. In children. Kidney Int. 4(suppl.) 3:8-101-8-106; 1975.
[20] Ginsburg CM; MC Cracken GH Jr.: UTI. in young infants ped. 69:409; 1982.
[21] Wiswell TE and Roscelle JD.: Corroborative evidence for the decreased incidence of UTI. incircumcis. Male infants-ped. 78; 1986.
[22] Herozog L.W.: Urinary tract infection and circumcision: Acase Control, A, J, Did Child 143(3): pp 348-50; 1989.
[23] Kurovilla J.T.; Garlick R.H. and Nammon K.E.: Results of surgical treatment of penile'carcinoma: Aust. N.Z.J. surgery 41:157, 1971.
[24] Smith PG., Knlen IJ. White GC, et al.: Mortality of wives of men dying of cancer of penis. British Journal of Cancer. 41:422; 1980.
[25] Grimes DA.: Routine circumcision of the newborn infant: a reappraisal. Am. J. Obst. Gynecol. Jan. ID; ou (2): 125; 1978.
[26] Hutchinson J.: A plea for circumcision. Archives of surgery "" 2:15; 1891.
[27] Shannon FT; Horvvood LJ and Fergusson DM.: Infant circumcision. N-Z-Med.-J. Oct. 10; 90 (645):283; 1979.
[28] Laumann EO; Masi CM and Zuckerman EW.: Circumcision in the United States prevalance, nrophylaclic effect? And sexual practice, JAMA.. April 2; 277(13): 1052; 1997.
[29] Tran PT and Giacomantonio M.: Routine neonatal circumcision. Can- Fam-Physician. Nov.; 42:2201; 1996.
[30] Holloman JR; Lewis EL and Ringler RL.: Neonatal circumcision techniques. Am. Fain. Physician. Aug., 52(2):511; 1995.
[31] Annunnziato D. and Goldbum L.M.: Staphylococcal scalded skin syndnome. A complication of circumcision. AM. J. Dis. Child. Dec; 132(12): 1187, 1978.
[32] Shuliman J.; Ben Hur N. and Neuman Z.: Surgical Complications of circumcision 9Am- J. Dis. Child 107: 149, 1964.
[33] Radhakrishnan, J. and Reges, H.M.: Penoplasty for buried penis secondary to radical circumcision, J. ped. surg., 199:6p 629; 1984.
[34] Sherman J; Borer, JG; Horowitz M; Glassberg KL: Circumcision successful glandular reconstruction and survival following traumatic amputation. J-uroi. Aug; 156 (2pt2); 842; 1996.
[35] Du Toit DF and Villet WT.: Gangrene of the penis after circumcision S- Afr. Med- J. Mar. 24; 55(B) :521; 1979.
[36] Malherbe WD.: Injuries to the skin of the male external genitalia in southern Africa S- Afr. Med-J. Feb. 1; 49(5): 147; 1975.
[37] Vaos. G. Photomedicine and Laser Surgery. August 2004, 22(4): 318-322 doi:10.1089/pho.2004.22.318.
[38] How A.,Ong C.,Jacobsen A.,Joseph V. Carbon dioxide laser circumcisions for children,Pediatric Surgery International,2003-04-0,Springer Berlin / Heidelberg SN - 0179-0358.

[39] Manley C. Elective general surgery at one year of age: psychological and surgical considerations. Surg Clinics North Am 1982; 62: 941–53.

[40] Freud S. A Case of Hysteria: Three Essays on Sexuality and Other Works. London: Hogarth Press, 1955.

4

Nifedipine Gel with Lidocaine in the Treatment of Anal Fissure in Children: A Pilot Study and Review of the Literature

Baruch Klin[1], Ibrahim Abu-Kishk[2],
Yigal Efrati[1] and Gad Lotan[1]
[1]Department of Pediatric Surgery &
[2]Pediatric Intensive Care Unit, Assaf Harofeh Medical Center,
Zerifin, Affiliated to the Sackler School of Medicine,
Tel-Aviv University, Tel-Aviv,
Israel

1. Introduction

Anal fissures are common in infancy and represent the most common cause of bright rectal bleeding at any age. Delayed diagnosis and treatment can lead to a disturbing cycle of constipation, repeat rectal bleeding, and crying, due to increasing pain during and after defecation. In spite of its high frequency, the problem remains underrated by most clinicians, with only a paucity of data on the management of anal fissures in children being found in the literature. The objective of this work is to bring this common and distressing problem into a more positive light, based on our good results achieved by the nifedipine gel with lidocaine treatment.

2. History

The first description of anal sphincterotomy in the world literature is found in Alexis Boyer's 11-volume Traite des Maladies Chirurgicales published between 1818 and 1826 (DeMoulin, 1977). His descriptions of the condition are dramatic, detailing the severe suffering patients endured. Louis Lemmonier, in 1869, gave the world the first anatomic description of an anal fissure. Boyer established the relationship between anal sphincter spasm and no healing of anal fissures, as well as the association between constipation and anal fissure. He was the first to divide the sphincter to cure the problem. This procedure, routine and quite safe today, caused deaths and pelvic abscesses in four patients, as reported by Velpeau in 1832. During the 1950s, fissure excision, anal sphincter stretching, injection therapy (local anesthetic and sclerotherapy) and sphincterotomy were performed for chronic anal fissures. Later, in the late 1960s and early 1970s, cutaneous island advancement flaps were added to this group (Ruiz-Moreno, 1968; Samson & Stewart, 1970). The modern reintroduction of sphincterotomy for anal fissure can be attributed to Eisenhammer (1951). In 1953, Inburg published his technique of partial internal sphincterotomy, cutting the sphincter through the bed of the fissure. It was not until the mid to late 1970s that lateral internal sphincterotomy became accepted as the standard of care to treat anal fissures surgically (J. Nelson, 2006).

3. Definition

An anal fissure is a linear, longitudinal split in the lining of the distal anal canal, extending from below the dentate line to the anal verge. They are usually very painful because of their somatic innervations, the pain resulting from spasm of the anal sphincter in response to stretching and tearing during passage of stool. A well developed anal fissure rests directly over the internal sphincter and the circular fibers of this sphincter are visible on the floor of the fissure on naked eye inspection.

4. Anatomy

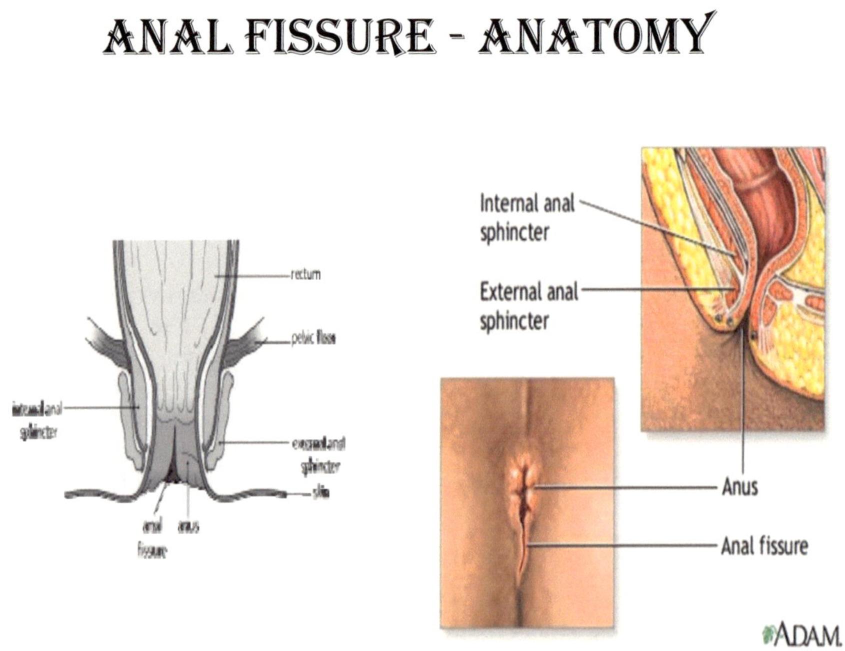

Fig. 1. Anal fissure anatomy.

5. Incidence and etiology

Anal fissures presents mostly in children aged 6-24 months. The overall incidence in children is not well described. Anal fissures are located in the posterior midline in 90% of the cases, although 10-20% in women and 1-10% in men are located in the anterior midline (Notaras, 1988). The posterior commissure of the anoderm is less well perfused than other anodermal regions (Schouten et al., 1994). Pressure over the branches of the inferior rectal artery (increased tone at the internal sphincter and high canal pressures) causes relative ischemia (Klosterhalfen et al., 1989). First described as a disease entity in 1934, the cause of anal fissures is still unknown. Constipation and passage of hard stool were traditionally blamed and believed to be the causative factor of anal fissure, but a history of constipation is elicited in only approximately 20% of the patients (McCallion & Gardiner, 2001). Trauma, usually because of passage of a large or hard stool, is believed to be a common initiating factor. Ball suggested that passage of hard stool tore down the anal valve, leaving the coiled-up skin at the anal verge as the "sentinel pile" (Lund & Scholefield, 1996). The remaining fissures are associated with chronic diarrhea, food allergy, Crohn's disease, syphilis, human immunodeficiency virus (HIV), or tuberculosis.

6. Pathophysiology

The pathophysiology is fairly complex and multifactorial, with anodermal ischemia, infection, chronic constipation, hypertonicity of the smooth muscle of the internal anal sphincter (IAS) and elevated maximal anal resting pressure (MARP) being involved (Gillet & Padias, 2006; Schouten et al., 1996). The exact mechanism surrounding the pathophysiology of anal fissures has not been clearly established, but current theories involve the tonicity of the anal sphincter and anal blood flow. A relative lack of nitrate oxide synthase, as found in other spasmodic states of the gastrointestinal tract, has been suggested as a possible mechanism for IAS hypertonia (Lund, 2006). As fissures are most commonly seen in the posterior midline, inadequate blood flow to this region has been hypothesized to play a role in the development of fissures. End arterioles from the inferior rectal artery pierce both sphincters to reach the submucosa of the anal canal and travel cephalad in this plane. Klosterhalfen et al. (1989) suggested that hypertonic sphincter decreases blood flow in these terminal vessels as they pass through the IAS fibers. Recognized features common to most chronic anal fissures are a high resting anal canal pressure due to hypertonicity of the internal anal sphincter, reduced vascular perfusion index at the site of the fissure, and the presence of "ultraslow" pressure wave activity in the internal anal sphincter (Hancok, 1977, Schouten & Blankensteijn, 1992).

7. Classification

Anal fissures may be classified as acute or chronic and typical or atypical. Acute fissures cause bright red bleeding with bowel movements and anal pain or spasm that can last for hours after the bowel movement. They have the appearance of a simple tear, superficial or deep in the anoderm. Chronic anal fissures present with induration at the edges, a sentinel pile, visible fibers of the internal anal sphincter, chronic granulation tissue in the base of the fissure and a hypertrophied anal papilla. They are acute fissures that fail to heal following 6 to 8 weeks of intensive treatment. Typical fissures are usually in the posterior or anterior midline, and are not associated with other diseases. Atypical fissures can occur anywhere in the anal canal, and tend to be associated with other diseases.

8. Differential diagnosis

Pruritus ani, inflammatory bowel disease (mostly Crohn's disease), tuberculosis, immune system diseases, acquired immunodeficiency syndrome (AIDS), Chlamydia, venereal diseases, neoplasm, and sexual abuse.

9. Innervation and pharmacology of the internal sphincter

The enteric nervous system consists of two major plexuses of interconnecting ganglia, the myenteric (Auerbach's) plexus and the submucous (Meissner's) plexus. The enteric nervous system contains entire reflex pathways that permit peristaltic contractions independent of extrinsic innervations. The internal anal sphincter receives its sympathetic innervations from the hypogastric pelvic plexuses. Parasympathetic innervation is from the first, second, and third sacral segments via the pelvic plexus. Internal anal smooth muscle relaxation can be inhibited by stimulation of nonadrenergic noncholinergic enteric neurons, parasympathetic muscarinic receptors, or sympathetic beta adrenoceptors, and by inhibition of calcium entry into the cell. Sphincter contraction depends on an increase in cytoplasmic calcium and is enhanced by sympathetic alpha adrenergic stimulation (Bhardwaj et al., 2000). A number of putative nonadrenergic transmitters have been suggested, the work being concentrated on the function of adenosine triphosphate (ATP), vasoactive intestinal peptide (VIP), and nitric oxide (NO) and their role in mediating the rectoanal inhibitory reflex (RAIR), as they are known to act together in mediating enteric inhibitory cotransmission in other areas of the gut. NO activates soluble guanylate monophosphate (cGMP) and relaxation of smooth muscle. NO has been widely demonstrated to be the main chemical neurotransmitting agent in the nonadrenergic neurons mediating relaxation of the internal anal sphincter. Working on the opposum internal anal sphincter, Rattan and Chakder suggested that NO was a nonadrenergic noncholinergic inhibitory neurotransmitter (Rattan & Chakder, 1992). NO caused tetrodotoxin-resistant relaxations of internal anal sphincter strips. The internal anal sphincter generates a high degree of tone in the resting state and is responsible for 50-85% of overall resting anal tone. This is due to both intrinsic myogenic activity and extrinsic adrenergic innervations. The effects of adrenergic agonists are well documented. Parks et al demonstrated that internal anal sphincter strips contracted to noradrenaline, had a variable response to adrenaline and relaxed in response to isoprenaline (Parks et al., 1969). Analysis of these responses using appropriate adrenoceptor antagonists has shown that contractions were mediated via alpha-receptors and relaxations via beta-receptors. Contractions to noradrenaline and adrenaline can be converted to relaxations by the addition of an alpha-receptor antagonist. Burleigh et al. (1979) have shown that acetylcholine has a predominantly inhibitory effect on internal anal sphincter smooth muscle acting through muscarinic receptors. Furthermore, electrical field stimulation of internal anal sphincter strips resulted in relaxation of the smooth muscle. These relaxations are abolished by tetrodotoxin, indicating that they are nerve mediated. Transient internal anal sphincter relaxation in response to rectal distension was first described by Gowers in 1877. O'Kelly et al. (1994) suggested that NO might be important in mediating the rectoanal inhibitory reflex. A review on the pharmacology of the internal anal sphincter was reported by Cook et al. (2001).

10. Clinical picture

The clinical picture involves a history of constipation in 20% of the cases, intense crying with bowel movements, streaks of bright red blood on the surface of hard stool, on the diaper, or on the toilet paper, following bowel movements, discharge and pruritus. The clinical hallmark of anal fissure is pain during, and especially some time after defecation. Inspection of the anal region reveals a posterior midline laceration, a sentinel skin tag, and signs of inflammation.

11. Medical treatment

Acute fissures often resolve within 10-14 days of conservative management. However, as long as 6-8 weeks may be necessary for the fissure to heal. Recurrence after conservative management can be observed in 27% of the cases. Dietary modification (increased fluid and fiber intake), stool softeners (lactulose) and warm baths are all part of the conservative treatment (Shafik, 1993). Conservative treatment is safe, has few side effects, and should usually be the first step in therapy. Shub et al. (1978) reported that 44% of fissure patients healed with sitz baths, a psyllium fiber supplement, and emollient suppositories. In 27% of these "healed" patients, the fissures recurred over a 5-year follow-up period.

The optimal treatment for an anal fissure is to induce a temporary reduction of anal canal resting pressure to allow healing of the fissure without permanently disrupting normal sphincter function. Internal anal smooth muscle relaxation can be inhibited by stimulation of non-adrenergic non-cholinergic enteric neurons, parasympathetic muscarinic receptors, or sympathetic beta adrenoceptors, and by inhibition of calcium entry into the cell.

11.1 Glyceryl trinitrate

Glyceryl trinitrate (GTN) is a vasodilator and causes relaxation of smooth muscle. Relaxation of the internal sphincter tone is achieved by the reduction of intracellular calcium in the smooth muscle cells by nitric oxide donation. Topical GTN heals anal fissures better than a placebo, irrespective of dose, but is associated with headache in around 25% of the patients. During the late 90's, GTN ointment was the best one could offer for a child with anal fissure. Exogenous nitrates release nitric oxide in vivo and have been used clinically as nitric oxide donors. Loder et al. (1994) demonstrated that topical application of 0.2% GTN led to decreased resting anal pressure. Chemical sphincterotomy using GTN with adjunctive stool softeners has been demonstrated to be quite effective at relieving symptoms and promoting healing. They significantly decrease pain during the therapy period. A study of 80 patients reported in the Lancet in 1997 showed healing in 26/38 (68%) after GTN, compared with 3/30 (8%) after placebo (Lund & Scholefield, 1997). Another study comparing GTN, lidocaine and placebo, was reported in the Journal of Pediatric Surgery in 1999. Complete healing was observed in 26/31 (83.9%) after GTN, 7/14 (50%) after lidocaine, and 6/11 (35.3%) after placebo (Tander et al., 1999). Kenny et al. (2001) questioned the healing power of GTN, reporting 31 children with an overall fissure healing rate of 84%, but with no differences being observed between GTN and placebo. Bacher et al. (1997) conducted a randomized trial of 0.2% GTN vs. 2% lidocaine gel, each applied 3 times daily, in a mixed group of acute and chronic fissure patients. After 1 month, healing rates were higher with GTN in both the acute (91.6%, GTN vs. 50%, lidocaine) and chronic (62.5%, GTN vs. 20%, lidocaine) fissure groups. A randomized, placebo-controlled treatment of anal fissure by lidocaine, EMLA, and GTN in 102 children, showed faster response rates by GTN application, and similar and high success rates by 8 weeks of EMLA treatment (Sönmez et al., 2002). The average age of patients was 3 years (range, 2.5 months to 15 years). Symptoms at admission consisted of hard stools in 90% of patients, pain or crying during defecation in 87%, bleeding in 84%, excessive straining at defecation in 35%, and mucosal prolapse in 9%. Despite the encouraging results reported with topical nitrates, severe headaches and noted relapse rates are major drawbacks. Dorfman et al. (1999) reported a 27% symptomatic relapse rate (median follow-up, 6 months). Associated side-effects were observed in 78% of patients, including headaches in 63% and light-headedness in 52%. Carapeti et al. (1999) noted relapse rates of 33% with 0.2% GNT and 25% with escalating-dose GTN (mean follow-up, 9 months). Headaches were observed in 72% of the patients. More recent studies have shown lower healing rates with GTN than were initially reported. Patient non-compliance and tachyphylaxis are also major drawnbacks to this treatment. Local application of another precursor of nitric oxide, L-arginine, has been reported as effective in promoting fissure healing without headache as a side effect (Gosselink et al., 2005).

11.2 Calcium channel blockers

They improve fissure healing by inhibiting calcium ion entry through voltage-sensitive areas of vascular smooth muscle, causing muscle relaxation and vascular dilatation. Topical diltiazem (Cardizem) has similar efficacy to GNT, with fewer side effects, but the experience with children is small.

11.3 Nifedipine

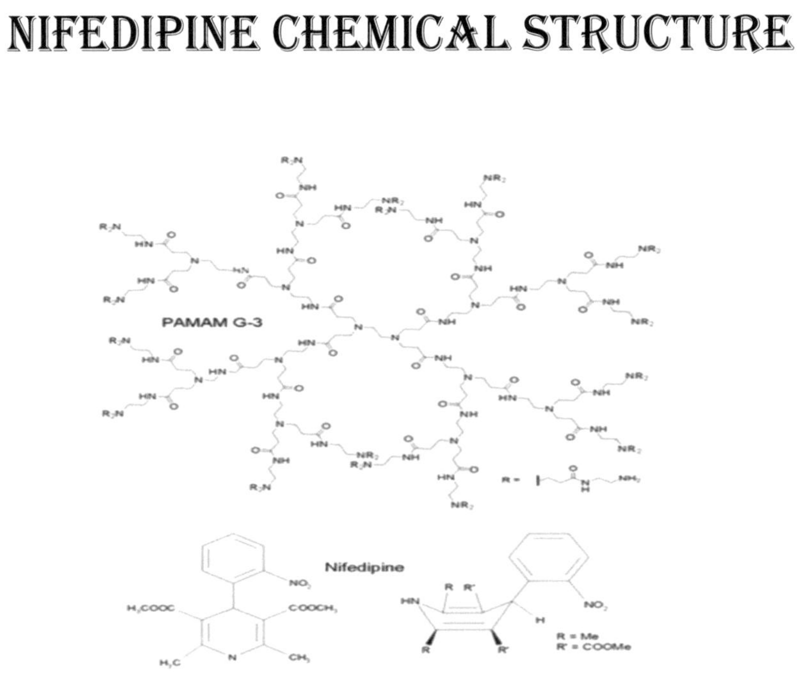

Fig. 2. Nifedipine chemical structure.

Nifedipine (Adalat) has a modulating effect on the microcirculation (Oshiro et al., 1995). The advent of this calcium channel blocker as nifedipine gel was a turning point and a major contribution to the healing of posterior anal fissures. Used to treat hypertension, angina pectoris, Raynaud's syndrome, congestive heart failure, and cardiomyopathies, it may cause side effects like headache, upset stomach, dizziness, tiredness, flushing, heartburn, tachycardia, muscle cramps, enlargement of gum tissue around teeth, constipation, nasal congestion, and cough. The first clinical study on the effects of calcium antagonists on resting anal pressure showed that pressures were reduced with sublingual nifedipine in both healthy volunteers and patients with hypertonic sphincters (Chrysos et al., 1996). A medline database literature search concerning the non-surgical treatment of chronic anal fissures, including 282 patients, called the attention to nifedipine gel. The study compared nifedipine with lidocaine with hydrocortisone acetate, showing 98% complete healing after nifedipine and 61% complete healing in the control group. Nifedipine reduced MRAP by 30% and maximum squeeze pressure by 16.8% (McCallion & Gardiner, 2001). Another large study by Perroti et al. (2002) comparing nifedipine and lidocaine with hydrocortisone and lidocaine, showed complete healing in 94.5% of the nifedipine treated patients and only 16.4% of the control patients.

Preliminary results of a multicenter study on nifedipine for local use in conservative treatment of anal fissures was reported by Antropoli in 1999. Total remission from acute anal fissure was achieved after 21 days of therapy in 95% of the nifedipine-treated patients, with a mean reduction of 30% in maximum resting anal pressures. A randomized controlled double-blind trial comparing nifedipine gel plus lidocaine, topical lidocaine alone and hydrocortisone acetate ointment, showed topical nifedipine plus lidocaine gel to be effective and well tolerated in the treatment of chronic anal fissures (Perroti et al., 2002). In other studies reported by Merenstein & Rosenbaum (2003) and Slawson (2003), remarkable improvement in healing was observed when 1.5% lidocaine and 0.3% nifedipine were applied twice daily for 6 weeks. Ezra & Susmalliam (2003) showed a better healing rate with topical nifedipine than with GTN. Katsinelos et al. (2006) reported that aggressive treatment of acute anal fissure with 0.5% nifedipine gel ointment prevents its evolution to chronicity. Twenty-seven of their 31 patients achieved complete remission and healing of the anal fissure following an 8-week treatment course (85.2%). Recurrence was observed in 16% of their patients. A systematic review of medical therapy for anal fissure including 31 trials from 1966 to 2002 returned the black shadow of pessimism to most physicians' minds. Nine agents were studied: GTN, isosorbide dinitrate, botulinum toxin, diltiazem, nifedipine, hydrocortisone, lidocaine, bran, and placebo. The results were only marginally better than placebo (R. Nelson, 2004)! A Cochrane Collaboration Review from 2009, by the same author, showed no better results. GNT was found to be marginally, but significantly, better than placebo in healing anal fissure (48.6% vs. 37%, $p < 0.004$), but late recurrence of the fissure was common, in the range of 50% of those initially cured! Botox and calcium channel blockers were equivalent to GNT in efficacy, with fewer adverse effects. No medical therapy was found to come close to the efficacy of surgical sphincterotomy (R.L. Nelson, 2006). Combined treatments have also been reported. The combination of nifedipine and botulinum toxin was superior to nitroglycerin and pneumatic dilatation with respect to both healing (94% v. 71%) and recurrence rate (2% v. 27%) (Tranqui et al., 2006). Headache is the most common complication of administering topical nifedipine in adults, but not in children. Nifedipine gel in the treatment of anal fissure has now been accepted even in China, with good results (Hong-yu et al., 2004). Reversible chemical sphincterotomy with nifedipine gel looks now as the most promising development in the treatment of anal fissures in children. The outcome is extremely good and side effects almost nonexistent.

11.4 Botulinum toxin (Botox)

Botulinum neurotoxin is a lethal biological substance produced by the anaerobic bacterium Clostridium botulinum. Serotype A is commercially available and has proven to be of therapeutic value in a variety of clinical conditions such as strabismus, torticollis, hyperhidrosis, achalasia and chronic anal fissure (Jankovic & Brin, 1991). Botulinum toxin (Botox) is associated with a similar rate of healing of anal fissure as GTN, but is more expensive. The technique, dose and site of injection do not affect the rate of healing. The experience in children is very small. Jost & Schimrig (1993) first reported the use of botulin toxin (BT) for anal fissure in 1933. The commercially available agent prevents neural transmission by preventing acetylcholine release from presynaptic nerve terminals. BT exerts its effects on the acetylcholine releasing parasympathetic peripheral nerve endings as well as the ganglionic nerve endings, leading to flaccid paralysis of the internal anal sphincter (IAS). This effect stays for about 3 months, a period sufficient for most non-complicated anal fissures to heal. Jost (1997) subsequently reported on a series of 100 patients treated with BT injection. In all, 78 patients became pain-free within 3 days, and healing rates at 3 and 6 months were 82% and 79%. BT injection was compared with topical GTN (0.2% twice daily) in a randomized trial of 50 chronic anal fissure patients (Brisinda et al., 1999). Resting anal pressure decreased in both groups, but did so to a greater extent in the BT group (29% with BT vs. 14% with GTN at 2 months). Healing rates were 96% in the BT group and 60% in the GTN group. No adverse effects were seen in the BT group.

11.5 Hyperbaric oxygen

Hyperbaric oxygen therapy provides a significant increase in tissue oxygenation in hypoperfused wounds. This increase in oxygen tension induces positive changes in the wound repair process by enhancing fibroblast replication, collagen synthesis and neovascularization. Cundall et al. (2003) reported a small series of adult patients with chronic anal fissure treated by hyperbaric oxygen. They found the procedure safe and appropriate in patients who have failed medical treatment, in those at risk of fecal incontinence, and in patients who are unfit for operation or in whom surgery has failed (Cundall et al., 2003).

11.6 Naturopathic treatment

Homeopathic medicines are excellent to alleviate the pain and spasm. Some of the more often indicated medicines are Chamomilla, Graphites, Nitric acid, Ratanhia, Sepia, Silicea and Thuja. Aesculus and Paeonia may be indicated if keynote symptoms are present. Homeopathic medicines often work faster and provide greater pain relief than analgesics and narcotics. In order to facilitate healing of the fissure, a topical cream consisting of Vitamins A and E, panthenol, calendula, goldenseal and Emu oil , can be used (Kruzel, 2006).

11.7 Iontophoresis

Iontophoresis using a zinc or copper electrode and applying a positive current will help to facilitate healing by hardening the underlying fissure, decreasing bleeding and affording pain relief.

11.8 Nd:YAG or CO2 laser

Contact Nd:YAG laser therapy appears to be efficient and safe in the treatment of anorectal lesions, including anal fissures (Sankar & Joffe, 1988; Walfisch et al., 1994). With the advent of the CO2 laser, a laser sphincterotomy and fissurectomy have proved to be very effective, with good results, prompt rehabilitation, reduced amount of complications and fewer recurrences (Ali, 1988; Skobelkin et al., 1989). It involves laser vaporization of the fissure locally. Patient acceptance is remarkable, and the treatment can be carried out at a fraction of the cost of hospital surgical treatment. There are no reports of laser treatment for anal fissures in children.

11.9 Wonder remedies

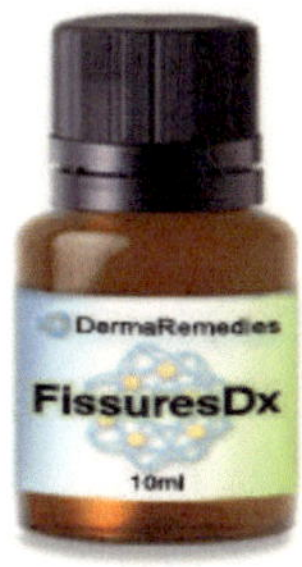

Fig. 3a. Anal Fissures DX: a unique formula with anti-inflammatory properties, providing immediate soothing relief.

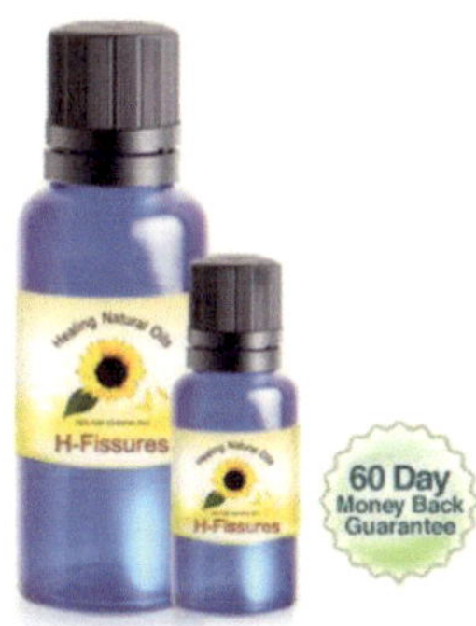

Fig. 3b. H-Fissures: healing natural oil with anti-inflammatory properties, specially formulated to provide instant relief from the pain and discomfort of fissures, reducing the swelling without skin irritation.

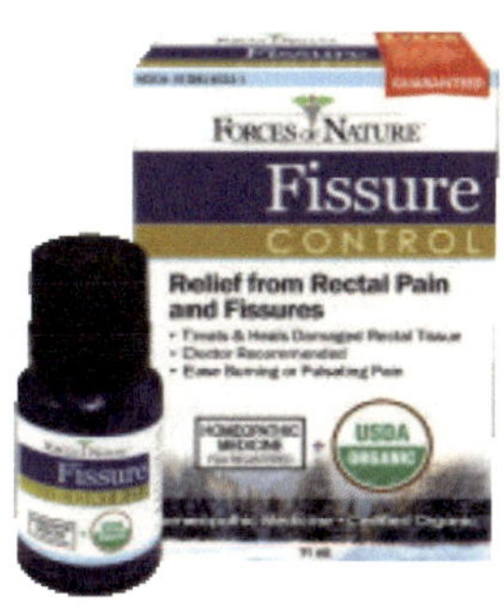

Fig. 3c. Fissure Control: a breakthrough topical homeopathic treatment made of a blend of herbs (Chamomile, Lavandula Angustifolia, Helichrysum, and Hamamelis Virginiana).

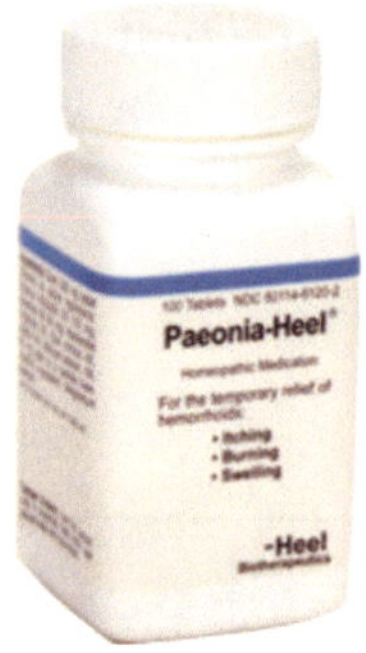

Fig. 3d. Paeonia-Heel: a homeopathic medicine containing Paeonia officinalis (Peony), Graphites (graphite), Nux vomica (vomit nut), Sulfur (sulphur), Acidum nitricum (nitric acid), and Hamamelis (witch-hazel).

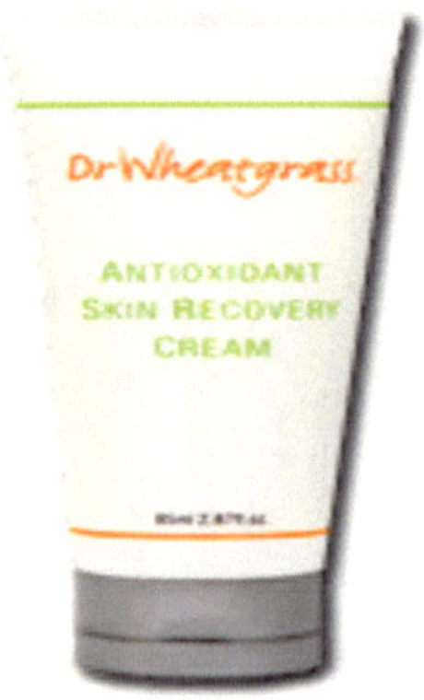

Fig. 3e. Dr Wheatgrass's cream: enriched with highly bioactive wheatgrass-derived antioxidants, containing vitamins A,C and E, phytosterols, aminoacids and minerals. The Figure shows Dr Wheatgrass's antioxidant skin recovery cream.

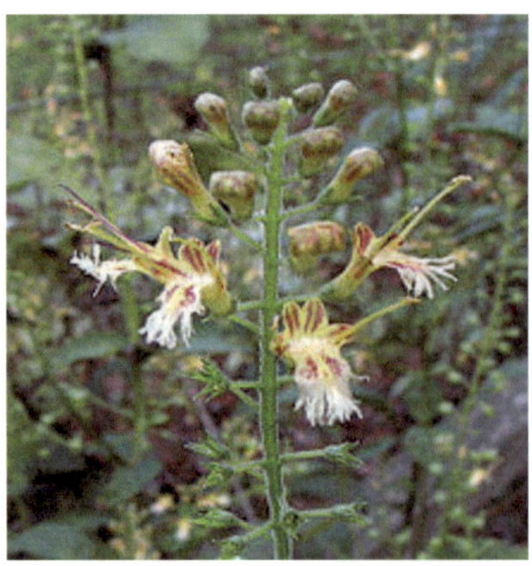

Fig. 3f. Nature's Wonderland Stone Root Herbal Supplement: Collinsonia Canadensis, sour and spicy in taste, and warming in action. It relaxes constriction and clears venous congestion and inflammation. The Figure shows the Collinsonia Canadensis flowers.

12. Surgical treatment

Surgical treatment is rarely needed for infants and children. Open or closed lateral internal sphincterotomy (healing rates of 93% to 100%, recurrence rates of 0% to 25%), internal sphincterotomy (for chronic anal fissures), and posterior midline sphincterotomy are all part of the surgical arsenal. The open lateral sphincterotomy is the procedure of choice for children. Relative contraindications to operative treatment include inflammatory bowel disease and profound immunosupression.

12.1 Anal dilatation

First described in 1829 by Recamier and popularized by Lord in the treatment of hemorrhoids, anal stretching has been used in the past based on the concept of loosening the sphincter muscle and increasing the blood flow to the anoderm. Anal dilatation was reintroduced for anal fissure therapy in 1964, with success rates of 87% to 100% (Watts et al., 1964), but are not recommended in children because of the very high rate of recurrence (10% - 30%) , risk of sphincter damage and incontinence after excessive stretching.

12.2 Fissurectomy

Fissurectomy as a treatment for anal fissures in children was found successful only when combined with postoperative laxative therapy (Lambe et al., 2000a). An important part of their technique was the use of stay sutures to avoid the need for an anal retractor, thereby preventing stretching of the internal anal sphincter. A triangular part of the anoderm is excised along with the fissure itself. A good and reliable operation, but leaves behind a large and uncomfortable external wound, which takes a long time to heal. Application of a split thickness graft to the wound has been advocated, in order to improve healing.

12.3 Internal anal sphincterotomy

Internal anal sphincterotomy (IAS) was popularized for the treatment of anal fissure during the 1950s by Eisenhammer (1951). Lateral internal sphincterotomy (LIS) has been found to be the preferred operation. LIS can be performed using either the open or closed technique , the method of Notaras, dividing the IAS via a small stab wound (Notaras, 1971). Equal success has been reported with open or closed lateral sphincterotomy for acute and chronic anal fissures in children. A systematic review on the treatment of anal fissure was published by Steele & Madoff in 2006. Current concepts in anal fissures were reported by Ayantude et al. (2006) in the same year, involving a literature search from 1970 to 2004.

Chronic anal fissures tend to be refractory and are usually reluctant to heal with conservative treatment. Chronicity is defined by chronology (6-8 weeks) and morphologic features (visible transverse internal anal sphincter fibers, chronic granulation tissue, indurated edge, a sentinel pile, and a hypertrophic anal papilla). A very large series of adult patients was published by Lysy et al. in 2006. Prolonged periods of treatment were necessary and 384 patients were healed (84.4%) by the end of four months. Older age and longer time interval between symptom appearance and treatment negatively affected fissure healing. The explanation for the latter was that longer time exposure of the fissure area to inflammation and ischemia and subsequent fibrosis may compromise the healing process. After recurrence, patient education for self and prompt retreatment was found to improve outcome. Chronic anal fissures are caused by internal sphincter hypertonia, which leads to reduced blood flow and tissue hypoxia, with consequent healing failure. A cautious surgical approach is required to treat those who do not respond to medical treatment, and should include excision of the fissure along with its sentinel tag and internal sphincterotomy at the base of the ulcer (Cohen & Dehn, 1995; Lambe et al., 2000b). The wound is left open and should heal in 7-14 days without scarring. Local reconstruction with advancement flaps is a relatively new and effective adjunct to chronic fissure excision. Practice parameters for the management of anal fissures from the American Society of Colon and Rectal Surgeons were reported by Orsay et al. (2004) and a very extensive review on the diagnosis and care of patients with anal fissure was reported by the American Gastroenterological Association (Madoff & Fleshman, 2003).

13. Our experience: Nifedipine gel 0.2% with lidocaine

13.1 Subjects

Seventy children suffering from acute and chronic anal fissures treated by us between 2004 and 2010 comprised the study population. They were all treated topically with nifedipine gel 0.2% with lidocaine for 4 weeks and followed up for as long as possible in our outpatient clinic (a maximum of 5 years).

13.2 Methods

Because anal fissure has such a distinctive appearance, its healing is the most objective measure of treatment efficacy available that can be standardized. Combining all analyses in which a placebo was used as the comparison group, the healing rate in the placebo group is 35.5 percent, a level of response that is fairly uniform across studies (standard deviation, 11.8 percent). For these reasons we did not find necessary to use a control group in the present pilot study.

13.3 Results

There were 28 males and 42 females. Their clinical presentation consisted of constipation, rectal bleeding, anal and abdominal pain, perianal itching and rectal prolapse (58, 50, 33, 6, 4, and 1 cases, respectively). Posterior, anterior, multiple, both posterior and anterior, and both posterior and lateral fissures were the main physical findings (44, 16, 5, 4, and 1 cases, respectively). Fifty eight patients completed the 4-week treatment course, with another 7 patients requiring a second 4-week treatment course in order to achieve complete remission, indicated by resolution of symptoms and complete healing of the fissure (65 patients altogether). The remaining 5 patients had recurrence of symptoms in 2, 4, 11, 18 and 19 months, respectively, treated successfully by an additional 4-week course of nifedipine. The recurrence rate observed was very low (7.14%). All the 70 patients had a mean follow-up of 1.88 years, ranging from 6 months to 5.2 years. Problems with compliance were not observed, one of the main reasons for treatment failure in adults. No side effects of nifedipine were observed.

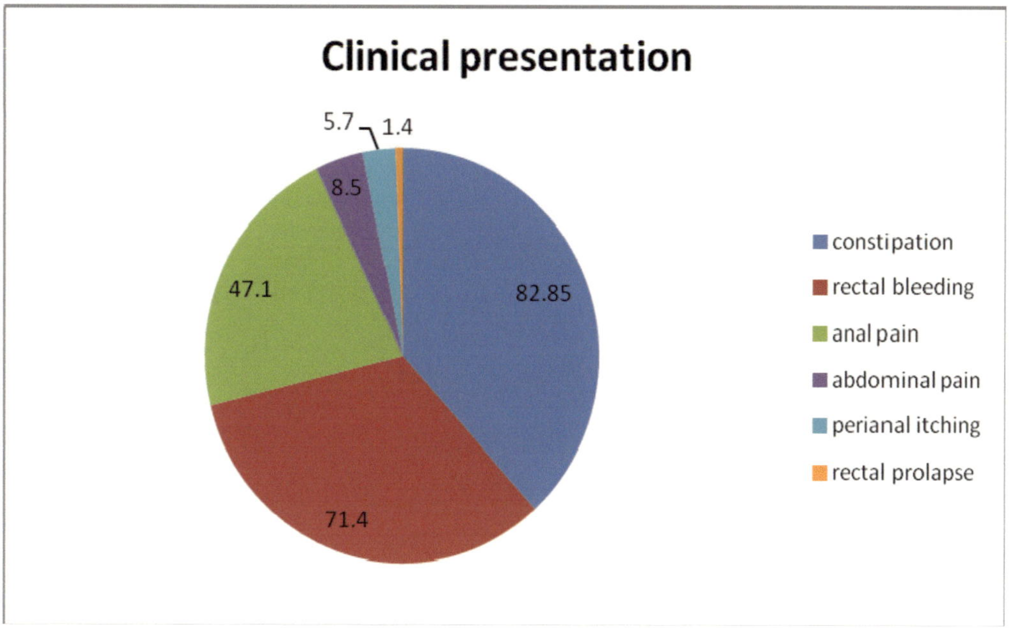

Fig. 4. Clinical presentation (percentage)

14. Special situations

1. Crohn's disease: Platell et al. (1996) noted symptomatic anal pathology in 42.4% of Crohn's disease patients, 27.6% of them presenting anal fissures. Frequently, they are multiple or off the midline, and often coexist with other pathology (Sangwan et al., 1996). They can be locally aggressive, progressing to form deep ulcers with granulating bases and overlapping skin edges.
2. HIV/AIDS: Anal fissures maintain their typical appearance, but have poor wound healing (Lord, 1997). Barrett et al. (1998) reported their experience with perianal disease in 260 HIV-positive patients, 32% of them with anal fissures (Barrett et al., 1998). Eighteen patients underwent sphincterotomies. Viamonte et al. (1993) reviewed the treatment of 33 HIV-positive fissure patients. Thirteen underwent LIS, with excellent results (12 improved).

15. Conclusions

Topical 0.2% nifedipine with lidocaine appears today as the most efficient mode of treatment for anal fissures in children, with a significant healing rate and no side effects. It is safe and effective, prevents the evolution of acute anal fissures in children to chronicity, avoids surgical procedures in the great majority of cases, avoids complications and does not require hospitalization.

Efficacy of medical treatment (number of patients)

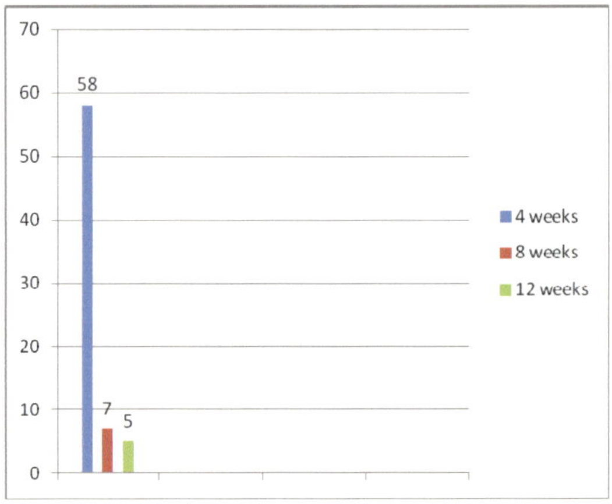

Fig. 5. Efficacy of medical treatment.

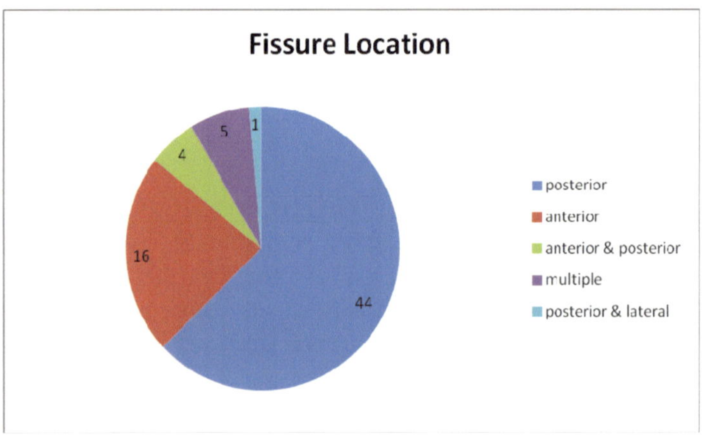

Fig. 6. Fissure location

16. Acknowledgment

The authors wish to express their gratitude to Mrs. Fredrica Gendler for her continuous help, highly professional and invaluable assistance.

17. References

Ali, M.M. (1988). Treatment of chronic anal fissure utilizing CO2 Laser. *Laser Medicine and Surgery News and Advances*, Vol.6, No.1, (February 1988), pp. 39–40

Antropoli, C., Perrotti, P., Rubino, M., Martino, A., De Stefano, G., Migliore, G., Antropoli, M., & Piazza, P. (1999). Nifedipine for local use in conservative treatment of anal fissures: preliminary results of a multicenter study. *Diseases of the Colon and Rectum*, Vol.42, No.8, (August 1999), pp. 1011-1015

Ayantude, A.A., & Debrah, S.A. (2006). Current concepts in anal fissures. *World Journal of Surgery*, Vol.30, No.12, (December 2006), pp. 2246-2260

Bacher, H., Mischinger, H.J., Werkgartner, G., Cerwenka, H., El-Shabrawi, A., Pfeifer, J., & Schweiger, W. (1997). Local nitroglycerin for treatment of anal fissures: an alternative to lateral sphincterotomy? *Diseases of the Colon & Rectum*, Vol.40, No.7, (July 1997), pp. 840-845

Barrett, W.L., Callahan, T.D., & Orkin, B.A. (1998). Perianal manifestations of human immunodeficiency virus infection: experience with 260 patients. *Diseases of the Colon and Rectum*, Vol.41, No.5, (May 1998), pp. 606-611

Bhardwaj, R., Vaizey, C.J., Boulos, P.B., & Hoyle C.H. (2000). Neuromyogenic properties of the internal anal sphincter: therapeutic rationale for anal fissures. *Gut*, Vol.46, No.6, (June 2000), pp. 861-868

Brisinda, G., Maria, G., Bentivoglio, A.R., Cassetta, E., Gui, D., & Albanese, A. (1999). A comparison of injections of botulinum toxin and topical nitroglycerin ointment for the treatment of chronic anal fissure. *The New England Journal of Medicine*, Vol.341, No.2, (July 1999), pp. 65-69

Burleigh, D. E., D'Mello, A., & Parks, A. G. (1979). Responses of isolated human internal anal sphincter to drugs and electrical field stimulation. *Gastroenterology*, Vol.77, No.3, (September 1979), pp. 484-490

Carapeti, E.A., Kamm, M.A., McDonald, P.J., Chadwick, S.J., Melville, D., & Phillips, R.K. (1999). Randomised controlled trial shows that glyceryl trinitrate heals anal fissures, higher doses are not more effective, and there is a high recurrence rate. *Gut*, Vol.44, No.5, (May 1999), pp. 727-730

Chrysos, E., Xynos, E., Tzovaras, G., Zoras, O.J., Tsiaoussis, J., & Vassilakis, S.J. (1996). Effect of nifedipine on rectoanal motility. *Diseases of the Colon and Rectum*, Vol.39, No.2, (February 1996), pp. 212-216

Cohen, A., & Dehn, T.C. (1995). Lateral subcutaneous sphincterotomy for treatment of anal fissure in children. *The British Journal of Surgery*, Vol.82, No.10, (October 1995), pp. 1341-1342

Cook, T.A., Brading, A.F., & Mortensen, N.J. (2001). The pharmacology of the internal anal sphincter and new treatments of ano-rectal disorders. *Alimentary Pharmacology & Therapeutics*, Vol.15, No.7, (July 2001), pp. 887-898

Cundall, J.D., Gardiner, A., Laden, G., Grout, P., & Duthie, G.S. (2003). Use of hyperbaric oxygen to treat chronic anal fissure. *The British Journal of Surgery*, Vol.90, No. 4, pp. 452-453

DeMoulin, D. (1977). A fundamental affair - a short history of anal fissure. *Archivum Chirurgicum Neerlandicum*, Vol.29, No.3, (1977), pp. 163-166

Dorfman, G., Levitt, M., & Platell, C. (1999). Treatment of chronic anal fissure with topical glyceryl trinitrate. *Diseases of the Colon and Rectum*, Vol.42, No.8, (August 1999), pp. 1007-1010

Eisenhammer, S. (1951). The surgical correction of chronic internal anal sphincteric contracture. *South African Medical Journal*, Vol.25, No.28, (July 1951), pp. 486-489

Ezri, T., & Susmallian. S. (2003). Topical nifedipine vs. topical glyceril trinitrate on chronic anal fissure. *Diseases of the Colon and Rectum*, Vol.46, No.6, (June 2003), pp. 805-808

Gillett, B.P., & Paidas, C.N. (2006), Anal fissure, In: *eMedicine*, Accessed 4th August, 2011, Available from: www.emedicine.medscape.com/article/934952-print

Gosselink, M.P., Darby, M., Zimmerman, D.E., Gruss, H.J., & Schouten, W.R. (2005). Treatment of chronic anal fissure by application of L-arginine gel : a phase II study in 15 patients. *Diseases of the Colon and Rectum*, Vol.48, No.4, (April 2005), pp. 832-837

Gowers, W.R. (1877). The automatic action of the sphincter ani. *Proceedings of the Royal Society of London*, Vol.26, pp. 77–84

Hancock, B.D. (1977). The internal sphincter and anal fissure. *The British Journal of Surgery*, Vol.64, No.2, (February 1977), pp. 92–95

Hong-yu, T., Jia-he, X.U., Mei-fu, S., & Yu-miao. H. (2004). Nifedipine gel in the treatment of anal fissure. *Chinese Journal of New Drugs and Clinical Remedies*, Vol.01, ISSN 1007–7669

Jankovic, J., Brin, M.F. (1991). Therapeutic uses of botulinum toxin. *The New England Journal of Medicine*, Vol.324, No.17, (April 25), pp. 1186–1194

Jost, W.H., & Schimrig, K. (1993). Use of botulinum toxin in anal fissure. *Diseases of the Colon and Rectum*, Vol.36, No.10, (October 1993), pp. 974

Jost, W.H. (1997). One hundred cases of anal fissure treated with botulin toxin: early and long-term results. *Diseases of the Colon and Rectum*, Vol.40, No.9, (September 1997), pp. 1029–1032

Inburg, K.R. (1953). Partial internal sphincterotomy compared with some other methods in the treatment of anal fissure. *Acta Chirurgica Scandinavica*, Vol.183, pp. 1–40

Katsinelos, P., Kountouras, J., Paroutoglou, G., Beltsis, A., Chatzimavroudis, G., Zavos, C., Katsinelos, T., & Papaziogas, B. (2006). Aggressive treatment of acute anal fissure with 0.5% nifedipine ointment prevents its evolution to chronicity. *World Journal of Gastroenterology*, Vol.12, No.38, (October 2006), pp. 6203–6206

Kenny, S.E., Irvine, T., Driver, C.P., Nunn, A.T., Losty, P.D., Jones, M.O., Turnock, R.R., Lamont, G.L., & Lloyd, D.A. (2001). Double blind randomised controlled trial of topical glyceryl nitrate in anal fissure. *Archives of Disease in Childhood*, Vol.85, No.5, (November 2001), pp. 404–407

Klosterhalfen, B., Vogel, P., Rixen, H., & Mittermayer, C. (1989). Topography of the inferior rectal artery: a possible cause of chronic, primary anal fissure. *Diseases of the Colon & Rectum*, Vol.32, No.1, (January 1989), pp. 43–45

Kruzel, T.A. (2006). Naturopathic treatment of anal fissure. *Naturopathic Doctor News & Review*, (March 2006).

Lambe, G.F., Driver, C.P., Morton, S., & Turnock, R.R. (2000a). Fissurectomy as a treatment for anal fissures in children. *Annals of the Royal College of Surgeons of England*, Vol.82, No.4, (July 2000), pp. 254–257

Lambe, G.F., Driver, C.P., Morton, S., & Turnock, R.R. (2000b). Fissurectomy as a treatment for anal fissures in children. *Annals of the Royal College of Surgeons of England*, Vol.82, No. 4, (July 2000), pp. 254–257

Loder, P.B., Kamm, M.A., Nicholls, R.J., & Phillips, R.K. (1994). Reversible chemical sphincterotomy by local application of glyceryl trinitrate. *The British Journal of Surgery*, Vol.81, No.9, (September 1994), 1386–1389

Lord, R.V. (1997). Anorectal surgery in patients infected with human immunodeficiency virus: factors associated with delayed wound healing. *Annals of Surgery*, Vol.226, No.1, (July 1997), pp. 92–99

Lund, J.N., Scholefield, J.H. (1996). Aetiology and treatment of anal fissure. *The British Journal of Surgery*, Vol.83, No.10, (October 1996), pp. 1335–1344

Lund, J.N., & Scholefield, J.H. (1997). A randomized, prospective, double-blind, placebo-controlled trial of glyceryl trinitrate ointment in treatment of anal fissure. *Lancet*, Vol.9044, No.349, (January 1997), pp. 11–14

Lund, J.N. (2006). Nitric oxide deficiency in the internal anal sphincter of patients with chronic anal fissure. *International Journal of Colorectal Disease*, Vol.21, pp. No 7, (October 21), pp. 673–675

Lysy, J., Israeli, E., Levy, S., Rozentzweig, G., Strauss-Liviatan, N., & Goldin, E. (2006). Long-term results of "chemical sphincterotomy" for chronic anal fissure: a prospective study. *Diseases of the Colon and Rectum*, Vol.49, No.6, (June 2006), pp. 858–864

Madoff, R.D., & Fleshman, J.W. (2003). AGA technical review on the diagnosis and care of patients with anal fissure. *Gastroenterology*, Vol.124, No.1, (January 2003), pp. 235–245

McCallion, K., & Gardiner, K.R. (2001). Progress in the understanding and treatment of chronic anal fissure. *Postgraduate Medical Journal*, Vol.77, No.914, (December 2001), pp. 753–758

Merenstein, D., & Rosenbaum, D. (2003). Is topical nifedipine effective for chronic anal fissures? *The Journal of Family Practice*, Vol.52, No.3, (March 2003), pp. 190–192

Nelson, J. (2006). History of anal fissure treatment. *Seminars in Colon & Rectal Surgery*, Vol.17, No.3, (March 2006), pp. 104–105

Nelson, R. (2004). A systematic review of medical therapy for anal fissure. *Diseases of the Colon and Rectum*, Vol.47, No.4, (April 2004), pp. 422–431

Nelson, R.L. Non surgical therapy for anal fissure. (2006). *Cochrane Database of Systematic Reviews*, Issue 4, Art. No.CD003431, DOI: 10.1002/14651858.CD003431.pub2

Notaras, M.J. (1988). Anal fissure and stenosis. *The Surgical Clinics of North America*, Vol.68, No.6, (December 1988), pp. 1427–1440

Notaras, M.J. (1971). The treatment of anal fissure by lateral subcutaneous internal sphincterotomy - a technique and results. *The British Journal of Surgery*, Vol.58, No.2, (February 1971), pp. 96–100

O'Kelly, T.J., Davies, J.R., Brading, A.F., & Mortensen, N.J. (1994). Distribution of nitric oxide synthase containing neurons in the rectal myenteric plexus and anal canal. Morphologic evidence that nitric oxide mediates the rectonal inhibitory reflex. *Diseases of the Colon and Rectum*, Vol.37, No.4, (April 1994), pp. 350–357

Orsay, C., Rakinic, J., Perry, W.B., Hyman, N., Buie, D., Cataldo, P., et al. (2004). Practice parameters for the management of anal fissures (revised). *Diseases of the Colon and Rectum*, Vol.47, No.12, (December 2004), pp. 2003–2007

Oshiro, H., Kobayashi, I., Kim, D., Takenaka, H., Hobson, R.W. 2nd, & Durán, W.N. (1995). L-type calcium channel block the microvascular hyperpermeability induced by platelet-activating factor in vivo. *Journal of Vascular Surgery*, Vol.22, No.6, (December 1995), pp. 732–739; discussion 739–741

Parks, A.G., Fishlock, D.J., Cameron, J.D., & May, H. (1969). Preliminary investigation of the pharmacology of the human internal anal sphincter. *Gut*, Vol.10, No.8, (August 1969), pp. 674-677

Perrotti, P., Bove, A., Antropoli, C., Molino, D., Antropoli, M., Balzano, A., De Stefano, G., & Attena, F. (2002). Topical nifedipine with lidocaine ointment vs. active control for treatment of chronic anal fissure: results of a prospective, randomized, double-blind study. *Diseases of the Colon and Rectum*, Vol.45, No.11, (November 2002), pp. 1468–1475

Platell, C., Mackay, J., Collopy, B., Fink, R., Ryan, P., & Woods, R. (1996). Anal pathology in patients with Crohn's disease. *The Australian and New Zealand Journal of Surgery*, Vol.66, No.1, (January 1996), pp. 5–9

Rattan, S., & Chakder, S. (1992). Role of nitric oxide as a mediator of internal anal sphincter relaxation. *The American Journal of Physiology*, Vol.262, No.1 Pt 1, (January 1992), pp. G107–G112

Ruiz-Moreno, F. (1968). Sliding mucocutaneous flap for the treatment of anal ulcer. *Diseases of the Colon & Rectum*, Vol.11, No.4, (July–August 1968), pp. 285–288

Samson, R., & Stewart, W. (1970). Sliding skin grafts in the treatment of anal fissures. *Diseases of the Colon & Rectum*, Vol.13, No.5, (Setember–October 1970), pp. 372–375

Sangwan, Y.P., Schoetz, D.J. Jr,, Murray, J.J., Roberts, P.L., & Coller, JA. (1996). Perianal Crohn's disease. Results of local surgical treatment. *Diseases of the Colon and Rectum*, Vol.39, No.5, pp. 529–535

Sankar, M.Y., & Joffe, S.N. (1988). Laser surgery in colonic and anorectal lesions. *The Surgical Clinics of North America*, Vol.68, No.6, (December 1988), pp. 1447–1469

Schouten, W.R., & Blankensteijn, J.D. (1992). Ultra slow wave pressure variations in the anal canal before and after lateral internal sphincterotomy. *International Journal of Colorectal Disease*, Vol.7, No.3, (September 1992), pp. 115–118

Schouten, W.R., Briel, J.W., & Auwerda, J.J. (1994). Relationship between anal pressure and anodermal blood flow. The vascular pathogenesis of anal fissures. *Diseases of the Colon & Rectum*, Vol.37, No.7, (July 1994), pp. 664–669

Schouten, W.R., Briel, J.W., Aurwerda, J.J., & Boerma, M.O. (1996). Anal fissure: new concepts in pathogenesis and treatment. *Scandinavian Journal of Gastroenterology. Supplement*, Vol.218, pp. 78–81

Shafik, A. (1993). Role of warm-water bath in anorectal conditions: The "thermosphincteric reflex". *Journal of Clinical Gastroenterology*, Vol.16, No.4, (June 1993), pp. 304–308

Shub, H.A., Salvati, E.P., & Rubin, R.J. (1978). Conservative treatment of anal fissure: an unselected, retrospective and continuous study. *Diseases of the Colon and Rectum*, Vol.21, No.8, (December 1978), pp. 582–583

Skobelkin, O.K., Tolstykh, P.I., Derbenev, V.A., Ste'nko, V.G., & Kochurkov, N.V. (1989). [Carbon dioxide laser in the surgical treatment of proctologic diseases]. *Vestnik Khirurgii Imeni I. I. Grekova*, Vol.143, No.9, (September 1989), pp. 3–5 [Article in Russian]

Slawson, D. (2003). Topical nifedipine plus lidocaine gel effective for anal fissures. *American Family Physician*, Vol.67, No.8, (April 2003) pp. 1781

Sönmez, K., Demiroğullari, B., Ekingen, G., Türkyilmaz, Z., Karabulut, R., Başaklar, A.C., & Kale, N. (2002). Randomized, placebo-controlled treatment of anal fissure by lidocaine, EMLA, and GNT in children. *Journal of Pediatric Surgery*, Vol.37, No.9, (September 2002), pp. 1313–1316

Steele, S.R., & Madoff, R.D. (2006). Systematic review: the treatment of anal fissure. *Alimentary Pharmacology & Therapeutics*, Vol.24, No.2, (July 2006), pp. 247–257

Tander, B., Güven, A., Demirbağ, S., Ozkan, Y., Oztürk, H., & Cetinkurşun, S. (1999). A prospective, randomized, double-blind, placebo-controlled trial of glyceryl nitrate ointment in the treatment of children with anal fissure. *Journal of Pediatric Surgery*, Vol.34, No.12, (December 1999), pp. 1810–1812

Tranqui, P., Trottier, D.C., Victor, C., & Freeman J.B. (2006). Nonsurgical treatment of chronic anal fissure: nitroglycerin and dilatation versus nifedipine and botulinum toxin. *Canadian Journal of Surgery*, Vol.49, No.1, (February 2006), pp. 41–45

Viamonte, M., Dailey, T.H., & Gottesman, L. (1993). Ulcerative disease of the anorectum in the HIV+ patient. *Diseases of the Colon and Rectum*, Vol.36, No.9, (September 1993), pp. 801–805

Walfisch, S., Ohana, N., & Charuzi, E. (1994). Nd:YAG laser for anorectal surgery: initial experience in Israel. *Harefuah*, Vol.126, No.1, (January 1994), pp. 1–4, 56 [Article in Hebrew]

Watts, J.M., Bennett, R.C., & Goligher, J.C. (1964). Stretching of anal sphincters in treatment of fissure-in-ano. *British Medical Journal*, Vol.8, No.2, (August 1964), pp 342–343

Part 3

Special or Interdisciplinary Care

5

Oxidative Stress of Newborn

Eloisa Gitto[1], Gabriella D'Angelo[1],
Erika Cusumano[1] and Russel J. Reiter[2]
*[1]Institute of Medical Pediatrics, Neonatal Intensive Care Unit,
University of Messina,
[2]Department of Cellular and Structural Biology,
The University of Texas,
[1]Italy
[2]USA*

1. Introduction

Free radicals are highly reactive molecules containing one or more unpaired electrons. They donate or abstract electrons from other molecules in an attempt to pair their electrons and generate a more stable species. Oxygen-derived reactants collectively termed reactive oxygen species (ROS) as well as reactive nitrogen species (RNS) are normally produced in living organisms. When produced in excess, they are important mediators of cell and tissue injury [Halliwell, B. (1999), Fridovich, I. (1998), Gitto, E. et al. (2002)]. The resulting damage is referred to as oxidative stress. Free radicals are highly unstable and several enzymes and small-molecular-weight molecules with antioxidant capabilities protect against them [Halliwell, B. (1992)]; these protective molecules are part of the antioxidative defence system. There is a critical balance between free radical generation and antioxidant defences. Free radical reactions lead to the oxidation of lipids, proteins, polysaccharides and to DNA damage (fragmentation, base modifications and strand breaks); as a consequence, radicals have a wide range of biologically toxic effects [Saugstad, OD. (1996), Sarker, AH. et al. (1995)]. The generation of both ROS and RNS are summarised in figure 1.

Newborns and especially pre-term infants are probably more prone to oxidative stress than are children and young adults. There are some special reasons for this. These infants very often 1) are exposed to high oxygen concentrations, 2) have infections or inflammation, 3) have reduced antioxidant defence, and 4) have free iron which enhances the Fenton reaction leading to production of highly toxic hydroxyl radicals [Saugstad, OD. (2003, 2005)]. The Fenton reaction describes the interaction of hydrogen peroxide with a transition metal resulting in the generation of the highly toxic hydroxyl radical. Oxidative stress has been postulated to be implicated in several newborn conditions and, in 1988, SAUGSTAD [Saugstad, OD. (1988)] coined the phrase "oxygen radical diseases of neonatology". The idea contends that oxidative stress affects different organs, often simultaneously, giving rise to different signs according to the organ most affected. He included bronchopulmonary dysplasia/chronic lung disease, retinopathy of prematurity and necrotising enterocolitis in this category. Later, it became clear that free radicals are also involved in periventricular leukomalacia [Haynes, RL. et al. (2003)] as well as in regulating the ductus arteriosus and pulmonary circulation [Clyman, RI. et al. (1989), Archer, SL. et al. (1989), Sanderud, J. et al. (1993)]. If the concept of "oxygen radical diseases in neonatology" is correct, it means that the conditions mentioned are not different diseases but belong to the same frequently have higher plasma levels of non-transferrin-bound iron and higher erythrocyte free iron than adults [Ogihara, T. et al. (1996)].

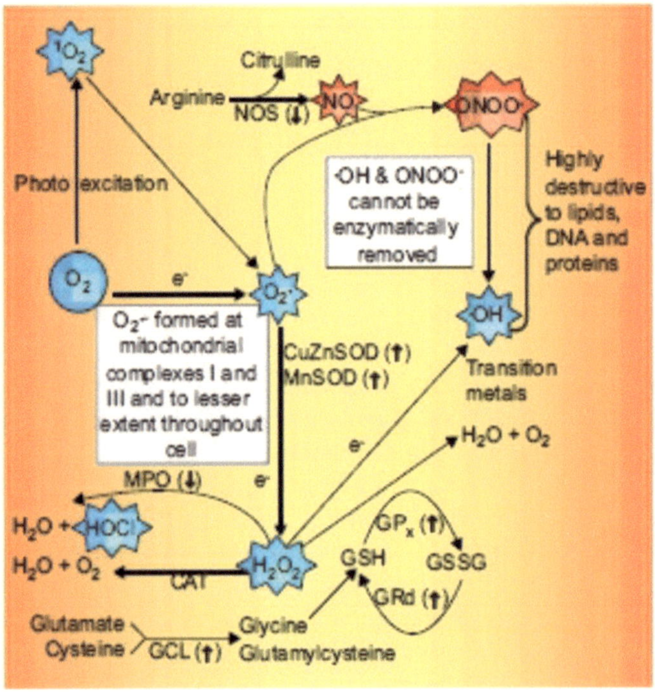

Fig. 1. Summary of the production of reactive oxygen species (ROS) and reactive nitrogen species (RNS).

2. Oxidative stress in pregnancy, in pre-eclampsia and at parturition

Pregnancy is a physiological state accompanied by a high metabolic demand and elevated requirements for tissue oxygen. This increased oxygen demand augments the rate of production of ROS and even women with normal pregnancies experience increased oxidative stress and lipid peroxidation relative to age-matched, non pregnant women. Several studies have shown that the antioxidative defense system is altered during pregnancy. Circulating levels of lipid peroxides increase significantly in the maternal circulation when a woman becomes pregnant. Various antioxidants, however, including vitamin E, ceruloplasmin, erythrocyte thiols and iron-binding capacity also increase. Several of these elevate progressively with advancing gestation, while serum iron concentrations progressively decrease. While there is a gradual favoring of antioxidant activity over oxidation during normal pregnancy, there is an insufficient increase in antioxidants to offset the rise in free radical generation. In contrast to the low-molecular weight antioxidants, the activity of an important family of antioxidative enzymes, the superoxide dismutases (SOD), are depressed in the blood of pregnant women [Wisdom, SJ. et al. (1991)]. In addition, Walsh and Wang [Walsh, SW. & Wang, Y. (1993)] reported a deficiency in another antioxidative enzyme, glutathione peroxidase (GPx), during pregnancy. GPx is an important antioxidant enzyme present in virtually all tissues. The enzyme limits the accumulation of lipid peroxides and utilizes reduced glutathione (GSH) as its cofactor to convert lipid peroxides into relatively harmless hydroxylated fatty acids, water and glutathione disulfide. Given these actions, it might be expected that a deficiency in this enzyme may lead to elevated oxidative stress during pregnancy. The placenta is a major source of oxidative stress during pregnancy. It is rich in polyunsaturated fatty acids, and the placenta is an abundant source of lipid peroxides which are secreted into the maternal circulation. In normal pregnancy, placental lipid production is believed to be kept under control by placental antioxidant enzymes [Walsh, SW. et al. (1993)]. Major antioxidant enzymes such as SOD, catalase (CAT), GPx, glutathione reductase, glutathione S-transferase and glucose-6-phosphate dehydrogenase are all present in the placenta. In the normal placenta, the activities of SOD and CAT increase as gestation progresses, while the activity of GPx is diminished. On the other hand, placental production of lipid peroxides progressively drop as normal gestation advances, most likely because of the elevated activities of SOD and CAT. Thus, in normal pregnancy, placental antioxidant defenses are considered sufficient to control lipid peroxidation. Pre-eclampsia is a multisystem disorder unique to human pregnancy. It is a complication in 5–10% of pregnancies and remains a leading cause of maternal and neonatal mortality and morbidity. This human disorder is a leading cause of premature delivery and intrauterine fetal growth retardation (IUGR). Pre-eclampsia is usually diagnosed in late pregnancy because of increased blood pressure and proteinuria with the symptoms of pre-eclampsia typically disappearing shortly after delivery of the placenta. A significant rise in lipid peroxidation levels in the placenta of pre-eclampsia has been suggested [Walsh, SW. et al. (2000), Hubel, CA. (1999), Gupta, S. et al. (2005), Vanderlelie, J. et al. (2005), Atamer, Y. et al. (2005)]. Several lines of evidence support this assumption, including increased lipid peroxidation products, elevated nitrotyrosine immunostaining and reduced antioxidant enzyme activities in preeclamptic placentas. In a case control study, Vanderlelie et al. [Vanderlelie, J. et al. (2005)] measured tissue levels of SOD, GPx and lipid peroxidation in placental samples from women with normal pregnancies (18 women) and with pre-eclampsia (20 women). Placental tissue homogenates from pre-eclamptic patients contained significantly higher levels of lipid peroxides [malondialdehyde (MDA) and 4-hydroxy-2 (E)- nonenal; 20.68 versus 5.33 mm/mg protein], whereas there were significantly lower levels of SOD (2.02 versus 2.48 U/ mg protein) and of GPx (11.50 versus 17.33 mmol/min/mg) than in control placentas. These finding are consistent with a limited enzymatic antioxidant capacity and elevated breakdown of lipids in placental tissue of women suffering from pre-eclampsia. Increased levels of thromboxane and lipid peroxides associated with a loss of GPx activity was also reported in placentas from pre-eclamptic patients compared with those from normal pregnancies [Walsh, SW. & Wang, Y. (1993)]. In parallel, the in vitro production of lipid peroxides and thromboxane is augmented in both trophoblast cells and villous tissues from women with pre-eclampsia [Walsh, SW. & Wang, Y. (1995)]. Furthermore, production of 8-iso-PGF2a and MDA (a lipid peroxide metabolite), as measured by levels in the medium, is higher for pre-eclamptic placental tissue explants than for normal placental explants [Walsh, SW. et al. (2000)]. Collectively, the data provide convincing evidence that oxidative stress and especially lipid peroxidation are abnormally increased in the placentas of pre eclamptic women. Many et al. [Many, A. et al. (2000)] found particularly intensive immunoreactivity for nitrotyrosine in invasive cytotrophoblasts in placental biopsies and vascular endothelium in the floating villi obtained from women with pre-eclampsia. The presence of nitrotyrosine is suggestive of damage caused by peroxynitrite, a potent nitrosative agent [Beckman, JS. & Koppenol, WH. (1996)]. Overall, the findings of nitrotyrosine residues in the cellular components of pre-eclamptic placentas may reflect increased production of the superoxide anion radical, as it couples with nitric oxide to generate peroxynitrite. Placental generation of ROS and reactive nitrogen species (RNS) in pre-eclampsia might be facilitated by a reduction in local antioxidant defense, although it is not clear whether this reduced antioxidant defense is part of the problem or secondary to free radical damage. The activities of placental SOD and glucose 6 phosphate-dehydrogenase are reduced in pre-eclampsia compared to placentas from normal pregnancy [Poranen, AK. et al. (1996)]. Moreover, the activities and mRNA expression of Cu/ZnSOD and GPx, and tissue levels of vitamin E are significantly lower in placental tissues from pre-eclampsia than from normal pregnancy [Wang, Y. & Walsh, SW. (1996)]. In summary, there appears to be an increment in ROS generation in the placenta of pre-eclamptic women. There is also evidence for increased nitrotyrosine residue formation in the pre eclamptic placenta suggestive of peroxynitrite formation, perhaps arising from local NO production coupled with increased generation of superoxide anion radical and either regionally decreased or inadequate SOD. The transition from fetal to neonatal life at birth includes acute and complex physiologic changes. The delivery of the fetus from an intrauterine relatively hypoxic environment with a PO2 of 20–25 mmHg to an extrauterine normoxic environment with a PO2 of 100 mmHg increases oxidative stress. This four to fivefold rise in oxygen tension is believed to induce a greater production of ROS [Shoji, H. & Koletzko, B. (2007)]. In addition, labor and childbirth may be associated with periods of both hypoxia and oxidative stress for the newborn, while neonatal plasma is relatively deficient in antioxidants. Several investigators studied the relationship between the oxidative state of the mother and the newborn at the moment of birth. Arguelles et al. [Auguelles, S. et al. (2006)] measured oxidative stress markers [carbonyl groups, lipid peroxides and total antioxidant capacity (TAC)] and found a good correlation between the oxidative status of the mother and of the neonate, with higher oxidative stress correlating with an even higher oxidative stress of the newborn based on measurements in umbilical cord blood. They also report that smoking mothers and their newborns had a higher concentration of the carbonyl groups, lipid peroxides and a lower TAC. Term labor is typically associated with oxidative stress for the neonate, but there is no difference between the degree of fetal oxidative stress in vaginal delivery and cesarean section [Fogel, I. et al. (2005), Hracsko, Z. et al. (2007)]. It is unclear, however, whether oxidative stress is related to the delivery itself or whether it reflects a pre-existing fetal oxidative status. Lauries et al. [Laurie, S. et al. (2007)] demonstrated that distressed fetuses delivered by emergency cesarean exhibited increased MDA concentrations, a parameter indicative of oxidative damage, and an enhanced GPx activity in amniotic fluid and umbilical cord blood compared to non distressed fetuses delivered by elective cesarean section. This is probably an indication of higher fetal oxidative stress.

2.1. Oxidative stress in neonatal diseases

Perinatal asphyxia is an insult to the fetus or newborn resulting from a lack of oxygen (hypoxia) or a reduced perfusion (ischemia) in various organs. While virtually every organ of the body is affected by asphyxia leading to multiorgan failure, the most severe insult occurs in the central nervous system, which also lacks many repair processes [Scher, M. (2001)]. The mechanism of cellular injury after hypoxia or ischemia is poorly understood, but is probably mediated by an excess release of neurotransmitters, generation of ROS/RNS and the initiation of lipid peroxidation which, in turn, leads to a cascade of damaging events [Harris, ED. (1992)].

At the cellular level, cerebral hypoxia–ischemia sets in motion a series of biochemical events commencing in a shift from oxidative to anaerobic metabolism; this leads to an accumulation of NADH, FADH, lactic acid and H+ ions [Palmer, C. et al. (1990)]. If the asphyxic insult persists, the fetus is unable to maintain circulatory centralization, cardiac output and cerebral perfusion falls. Owing to the acute reduction in its oxygen supply, oxidative phosphorylation and ATP production in the brain are diminished [Yager, JY. et al. (1992), Berger, R. et al. (1994)]. As a result, the Na+/K+ pump in cell membranes are deprived of the required energy to maintain ionic gradients. With a reduced membrane potential, increased numbers of calcium ions flow through voltage-dependent ion channels, down an extreme extra-intracellular concentration gradient, into the cell. Intracellular accumulation of Na+ and Cl) ions leads to swelling of the cells as water enters by osmosis (cytotoxic cell edema) [Vannucci, RC. et al. (1993)]. This damage is thought to be caused by the post ischemic production of oxygen radicals, synthesis of NO, inflammatory reactions and an imbalance between excitatory and inhibitory neurotransmitter systems. Part of the secondary neuronal cell damage may be caused by induction of a well-known cellular suicide program referred to as apoptosis [Berger, R. & Garnier, J. (2000)]. Production of reactive species in the early reperfusion phase plays a substantial role in the resulting brain cell damage. Among the toxicants generated are the superoxide anion radical (O2 •)) and hydrogen peroxide (H2O2). The latter agent can be converted to the highly reactive hydroxyl radical by transition metals, in particular free iron, ultimately leading to lipid peroxidation of the brain cell membranes as well as damage to other macromolecules [Halliwell, B. & Gutteridge, JC. (1990)].

Recent studies reported increased intra-erythrocyte free iron levels in infants with asphyxia [Buonocore, G. et al. (1998)]. Iron may be released from hemoglobin in erythrocytes as result of oxidative stress [Ferrali, M. et al. (1992)]. As the erythrocyte is a target of extracellular free radicals, free iron release may be followed by extracellular oxidative stress caused by O2 •) generation because of phagocyte activation [Buonocore, G. et al. (1994)]. Intra-erythrocyte free iron concentrations appear to be a reliable marker of cell oxidative stress and an indicator of the risk of oxidative injury in other tissues. Increased production of free radicals including the O2 •) and NO induces oxidative stress in the placenta by formation of the pro-oxidant ONOO); this reactant is formed when O2 •) couples with NO• [Crow, JP. & Beckman, JS. (1996), Szabo, C. & Oshima, H. (1997)]. ONOO) is cytotoxic due to a number of independent mechanisms including the initiation of lipid peroxidation, the inactivation of a variety of enzymes (most notably, mitochondrial respiratory enzymes) and membrane pumps [Crow, JP. & Beckman, JS. (1995)] and depletion of GSH [Phelps, DT. et al. (1995)]. Moreover, ONOO) causes DNA damage [Inoue, S. & Kawanishi, S. (1995), Salgo, MG. et al. (1995)] resulting in the activation of the nuclear enzyme poly (ADP-ribose) synthetase, depletion of NAD and ATP, and ultimately leading to cell death [Szabo, C. et al. (1997)]. The higher levels of free radical production associated with repetitive ischemia likely reflect differences in oxygen availability during these events. During repetitive ischemia, the availability of oxygen to the fetus for intermittent periods of reperfusion facilitates free radical production. With the increased availability of oxygen, oxidative reactions rather than reductive reactions are favored. Hyperoxic exposure itself, although essential for promoting survival of infants with RDS, induces excessive production of ROS in the respiratory system. There exist, however, several potential causes of intracellular and extracellular oxidant stress in the preterm newborns with RDS. The high inspiratory concentrations of oxygen required to achieve adequate arterial oxygenation, pro-oxidant drugs and infections or extrapulmonary inflammation can all promote ROS accumulation and the utilization and depletion of antioxidative agents [Kothecha, S. (2000)].

In experimental models of respiratory distress, the specific targets of a hyperoxic insult to the lung are the vascular endothelial cells and the epithelial cells of the alveoli. ROS induce ultrastructural changes in the cytoplasm of pulmonary capillary endothelial cells and cause focal hypertrophy and altered metabolic activity. Thus, increased oxidative stress accompanied by reduced endogenous antioxidant defenses may play a role in the pathogenesis of a number of inflammatory pulmonary diseases including respiratory distress in the newborn [Bhandari, V. et al. (2000), Ikegami, M. et al. (2000)]. A deficit in the precise balance between exposure to oxidants and endogenous antioxidants obviously leads to elevated oxidative damage. The molecular damage caused by free radicals and related reactants appear to be involved in the pathogenesis of a growing number of diseases, including RDS of the newborn [Lamb, NJ. et al. (1999), Huertas, JR. et al. (1998)]. When phagocytes such as neutrophils are stimulated by microorganisms or other means, they are activated and increase their oxidative metabolism; as a result, toxic oxygen derivatives, i.e. ROS, are formed. If these oxygen based products are not inactivated, their high chemical reactivity leads to damage to a variety of cellular macromolecules including proteins, carbohydrates, lipids and nucleic acid. This results in cell injury and may induce respiratory cell death [Esteban, J. et al. (1999)]. Under these conditions, a surfactant deficiency may be aggravated by the inactivation of the small amount of endogenous surfactant that is produced [Boda, D. et al. (1998)]. Furthermore, if exogenous surfactant is given, it may also be destroyed [Ikegami, M. et al. (2000), Huertas, JR. et al. (1998)]. Reactive oxygen species also have been implicated in the molecular damage seen in the bronchoalveolar lavage (BAL) fluid of patients with RDS [Banks, BA. et al. (1998), Dellinger, RP. (1999)]. This assertion is supported by several findings; H2O2 is detected in the expired air of RDS patients, and myeloperoxidase (MPO) and oxidized-1-antitrypsin have been found in BAL fluid. Moreover, increased plasma lipid peroxidation products have been measured in critically ill patients and in patients with sepsis and at risk of developing RDS. Also, evidence of augmented levels of oxidized lipids and proteins have been found in the plasma of patients with RDS. Elevated levels of ROS also have been implicated in the molecular damage seen in the BAL fluid of patients with RDS. BAL fluid normally contains a large amount of the antioxidant GSH; however, in patients with RDS this is mostly in the oxidized form [Janssen, YMW. et al. (1998)]. Consistent with this, oxidative inactivation of 1-antiprotease also has been observed in RDS. Elevated concentrations of xanthine and hypoxanthine are present in the plasma and BAL fluid of patients with RDS and are a potential source of ROS in the presence of exogenously added xanthine oxidase. Also, elevated concentrations of orthotyrosine and metatyrosine in BAL fluid protein imply the formation of the damaging •OH in the lungs of these patients, as orthotyrosine and metatyrosine are isomers of tyrosine thought to be formed exclusively by aromatic hydroxylation of phenylalanine by •OH [Kim, K. et al. (1999)]. Chlorotyrosine and nitrotyrosine also have been found in BAL fluid from patients with RDS. Increased concentrations of chlorotyrosine residues in BAL fluid proteins from patients with RDS indicate hypochlorous acid (HClO) production by the activated inflammatory cells in the lungs of these patients. Chlorotyrosine is formed by HClO-dependent chlorination of paratyrosine. HClO is a damaging oxidant formed from H2O2 and chloride ions by the enzyme MPO, present in activated inflammatory cells. HClO has been implicated as the major damaging species produced by activated neutrophils. While HClO itself is a destructive oxidant, it also may interact with low molecular mass iron or O2 •) to produce the •OH. Nitrotyrosine concentrations also are significantly elevated in the BAL fluid protein of patients with RDS [Ogihara, T. et al. (1999)]. Nitration of tyrosine residues is an in vivo marker of the formation of ONOO). Earlier studies reported increased nitrotyrosine concentrations in the lungs of patients with RDS. Additionally, under acidic conditions ONOO) decomposes to form a powerful oxidant with properties similar to •OH. There is, however, another possible explanation for the formation of nitrotyrosine. Recent work shows that nitrotyrosine can arise from the reaction of tyrosine with nitroxyl chloride, an intermediate formed by the interaction of nitrite (the auto-oxidation product of nitric oxide) with HClO. Interestingly, nitrotyrosine concentrations in BAL fluid protein from patients with RDS treated with NO were elevated compared with those found in lung-injured patients not receiving this therapy [Metnitz, PGH. et al. (1999)]. Increased nitrotyrosine concentrations may reflect augmented ONOO) formation in patients receiving NO. As the patients receiving inhaled NO are no sicker, in terms of Acute Physiology and Chronic Health Evaluation II score or FIO2 requirements, than those patients not receiving this therapy, it implies that inhaled NO may react with O2 •) in these circumstances to form the nitrating agent [Vento, G. et al. (2000)]. Finally, MPO concentrations are significantly elevated in the BAL fluid from patients with RDS, suggesting lung neutrophil recruitment and activation [Yitig, S. et al. (1998)]. Collectively, the data are compelling that RDS is associated with elevated ROS/RNS generation and the consequential increased oxidative damage to the respiratory tree.

Sepsis represents a serious problem in newborns with an incidence of one to 10 cases per 1000 live births, with even higher rates in low-birth-weight neonates. Hospital acquired infections in neonatal intensive care units may also occur as frequently as 30 infections per 100 patients. Mortality rates resulting from sepsis in newborns are 30– 50% [Perez, EM. & Weisman, LE. (1997)]. Sepsis is characterized by alterations in body temperature, hypotension, hypoperfusion with cellular damage which culminates in multiple organ failure [Antonielli, M. (1999)]. The initiating event in sepsis is the result of release of endotoxins [i.e. bacterial cell wall lipopolysaccharides (LPS)] from gram-negative and gram-positive pathogenic bacteria [Lush, CW. & Kvietys, PR. (2000)]. LPS triggers activation of inflammatory cells, including polymorphonuclear leukocytes (neutrophils; PMN), monocytes/macrophages and lymphocytes. LPS also initiates cellular and humoral aspects of the inflammatory immune response. The inflammatory response that occurs as the result of infection is the predominant determinant of outcome in sepsis [Cohen, J. (2002), Abraham, E. & Singer, M. (2007)]. A major feature of sepsis is tissue infiltration by phagocytic cells [Basit, A. et al. (2006), Cepinskas, G. et al. (2003), Ley, K. & Reutershan, J. (2006), Rawlingson, A. (2003), Razavi, HM. et al. (2005)]. When this occurs, PMN and monocytes/macrophages respond to septic stimulation by producing ROS and RNS [Mochida, S. et al. (2007)]. In addition, PMN release enzymes (e.g. elastase, cathepsin, etc.) and the MPO-derived oxidant, HOCl. These reactants contribute to PMN/macrophage-mediated killing of bacteria. However, if produced in excess during sepsis, the ROS/RNS and proteolytic enzymes cause microvascular dysfunction followed by organ shutdown. An inflammatory response to septic stimuli is crucial for host defense, because it up-regulates anti-inflammatory mediators (e.g. IL-1 receptor antagonist, IL-4, IL-10) and antioxidant enzymes (e.g. CAT, GPx and SOD). However, the excessive production of pro-inflammatory mediators in sepsis overwhelms the anti-inflammatory signaling processes leading to a suppression of innate immune functions (especially those of PMN) and causing immunoparalysis and subsequently an increased susceptibility to infection [Riedemann, NC. et al. (2003)]. It is important to note that, besides immune cells, microvascular endothelial cells also become activated in sepsis which contributes to amplification of the inflammatory response [Lush, CW. & Kvietys, PR. (2000), Ley, K. & Reutershan, J. (2006), Liu, L. & Kubes, P. (2003)]. It is known that septic stimuli (e.g. LPS, TNF-a) initiate activation of transcription factors including NFjB and AP-1, resulting in transcriptional activation of multiple genes. This leads to the release of pro-inflammatory cytokines (e.g. TNF-a, IL-1b, etc), and elevates the expression of adhesion molecules (e.g. E-selectin, ICAM-1, VCAM-1) and chemokines by endothelial cells [Ley, K. & Reutershan, J. (2006), Liu, SF. & Malik, AB. (2006), Abraham, E. (2003), Rao, RM. et al. (2007)]. The central role of ROS/RNS in modulation of the endothelial cell proinflammatory phenotype is well documented [Janssen-Heininger, YM. et al. (2000)]. Despite a large amount of research, little progress has been made in improving the outcome of septic newborns [Riedemann, NC. et al. (2003)]. Efforts to block one or more aspects of the sepsis-associated inflammatory pathways have had little impact on patient survival. Of many drugs tested, few have demonstrated efficacy [Panacek, EA. et al. (2004), Bernard, GR. et al. (2001), Abraham, E. (2005), Ely, EW. et al. (2002)]. Clinical reports are consistent with the involvement of ROS/RNS in neonatal sepsis and its complications. Batra et al. [Batra, S. et al. (2000)] documented increased production of oxygenderived reactants in septic neonates. Also, Seema et al. [Seema, KR. et al. (1999)] found newborns with sepsis have significantly higher levels of TNF-a and increased activity of antioxidative enzymes, SOD and GPx. Finally, Kurt et al. [Nese Citak, KA. et al. (2007)] demonstrated that serum IL-1b, IL 6, IL-8, and TNF-a are mediators of inflammation and can be used at the diagnosis and at the evaluation of the therapeutic efficiency of drugs used to treat neonatal sepsis.

2.2 Oxidative stress and resuscitation with ambient air VS pure oxygen

The traditional method of resuscitation of newly born infants is with pure oxygen [Kattwinkel, J. et al. (1999), Niermeyer, S. et al. (2000)]. However, this therapy was introduced without any preceding randomised trials being conducted. It was assumed, without any supporting data, that 100% O2 would be the optimal oxygen concentration [Lefkowitz, W. (2002)]. There is, however, reason to believe that oxidative stress is elevated when resuscitation is performed with pure oxygen compared with ambient air. For this reason, SAUGSTAD and AASEN [Saugstad, OD. & Aansen, AO. (1980)] warned that the use of high concentrations of supplemental O2 might be detrimental for resuscitation. Several experimental as well as clinical studies seem to confirm this [Armstead, WM. et al. (1988), Bagenholm, R. et al. (1998), Kondo, M. et al. (2000), Kutzsche, S. et al. (2002), Vento, M. et al. (2001), Saugstad, OD. (2001)]. In addition to animal studies, clinical trials have importantly shown that ambient air is at least as efficient as pure O2 for resuscitation of the newly born [Ramji, A. et al. (1993), Saugstad, OD. et al. (1998), Vento, M. et al. (2001, 2003), Ramji, S. et al. (2003)].

In 1993, RAMJI et al. [Ramji, A. et al. (1993)] published a single-centre study from New Dehli with the aim of investigating the feasibility of using 21% O2 for resuscitation. A total of 42 infants resuscitated with 21% and 42 with 100% O2 were enrolled with the following inclusion criteria: cardiac frequency, 80 bpm and or apnoea/ poor response. Birth weight ,1,000 g and or lethal congenital anomalies were exclusion criteria. Restoration of cardiac frequency, Apgar score, acid base and blood gases were not different between the two groups. A second investigation in this area was the Resair 2 study [Saugstad, OD. et al. (1998)], a multicentre study comprising ,600 infants from Egypt, Estonia, India, Norway, Philippines and Spain recruited from 10 centres. The study was pseudo-randomised and not blinded. No significant differences in the primary outcome measure, which was early neonatal death and/or hypoxic ischaemic encephalopathy grade 2 or 3, were found. However, there was a statistically insignificant tendency to higher neonatal survival in the infants resuscitated with 21% versus 100% O2. Time to first breath and first cry was significantly delayed in those reoxygenated with pure oxygen. Since then, three more studies by Resair 2 collaborators have been published, two from Spain [Vento, M. et al. (2001, 2003)] and one from India [Ramji, S. et al. (2003)]. When the results of these five studies were combined, a significant reduction in neonatal mortality (from 13 to 8%) in those resuscitated with ambient air compared with 100% O2 was found. Most of the 1,737 children were enrolled from developing countries; SAUGSTAD et al. [Saugstad, OD. et al. (2005)], therefore, separately analysed the Spanish babies. In this material, a 3% reduced mortality was found in favour of room-air infants (from 3.5 to 0.5%), indicating that, also in industrialised countries, a significant reduction in neonatal mortality can be achieved by not using pure oxygen for resuscitation. One surprising finding of these studies is that time to first breath and first cry is significantly reduced by 24 s; moreover, the 5-min Apgar score, as well as cardiac frequency at 90 bpm is also significantly higher in room-air-resuscitated infants compared with those resuscitated with pure oxygen.

For babies born at term, the Guidelines of 2005 recommend use of 100% supplemental O2 when a baby is cyanotic or when positive pressure ventilation (PPV) is required during neonatal resuscitation. However, research suggests that resuscitation with ,100% may be just as successful. If resuscitation is started with ,100% oxygen, supplemental oxygen up to 100% should be administered if there is no appreciable improvement within 90 s following birth. If supplemental oxygen is unavailable, the use of room air to deliver PPV is suggested. To reduce excessive tissue oxygenation in a very pre-term baby (less than ,32 weeks), use of an oxygen blender and pulse oximeter during resuscitation is recommended; in this case, begin

PPV with an oxygen concentration between room air and 100%. No studies justify starting at any particular concentration. Adjust O2 concentration up or down to achieve an oxyhaemoglobin concentration that gradually increases toward 90%, and reduce the oxygen concentration as saturations rise over 95%. If the cardiac frequency does not respond by increasing rapidly to .100 bpm, correct any ventilation problem and use 100% oxygen. If the facility does not have use of an oxygen blender and pulse oximeter in the delivery room, and there is insufficient time to transfer the mother to another facility, the resources and oxygen management described for a term baby are appropriate. There is no convincing evidence that a brief period of 100% oxygen during resuscitation is detrimental to the pre-term infant. In 2007, a summary of the results of three systematic reviews [Saugstad, OD. et al. (2005), Tan, A. et al. (2005), Raby, Y. et al. (2007)] of five trials and seven individual studies, including up to 2,011 newborn infants, indicated that neonatal mortality was reduced by 30–40% if resuscitation is carried out with 21% instead of 100% O2 [Saugstad, OD. (2007)]. Room-air resuscitation also leads to faster early recovery and a shorter duration of resuscitation. To date, there are sufficient data available to recommend that newborn resuscitation should generally not be carried out using 100% O2. In extremely low-birth-weight (ELBW) infants, arterial oxygen saturation (Sa,O2) levels should be kept between 85 and 93% or possibly between 88 and 95%, but should definitely not exceed 95%. Fluctuations should be avoided [Saugstad, OD. (2007)]. A recent prospective, randomised, clinical trial included infants of *ƒ*28 weeks of gestation who required active resuscitation and were randomly assigned to a low-oxygen group (fraction of inspired oxygen: 30%) or a high-oxygen group (fraction of inspired oxygen: 90%) [Escrig, R. et al. (2008)]. The fraction of inspired oxygen in the low-oxygen group was increased stepwise to 45% and that in the high-oxygen group was reduced to 45% to reach a stable pulse oxygen saturation of approximately 85% at 5–7 mins in both groups. No differences in oxygen saturation in minute-to-minute registers were found, independent of the initial fraction of inspired oxygen used 4 mins after cord clamping. Likewise, no differences in mortality rates in the early neonatal period were detected. The authors concluded that resuscitation can be safely initiated for ELBW neonates with a low fraction of inspired oxygen (30%), which then should be adjusted to the infant's needs, reducing the oxygen load to the neonate [Saugstad, OD. (2003)].

New Guidelines for Neonatal Resuscitation give reason to Saugstad, who had long been considered a historical mistake and an anachronism to continue to resuscitate infants with 100% O_2. For term infants it's recommended to use oxygen blenders and pulse oximeters during resuscitation; it's recommended the use of O_2 100% only when a child is cyanotic or when is required positive pressure ventilation, but it can be successful resuscitation with concentrations of O_2 <100%; it's recommended to start with 21% oxygen; if there is not an adequate response regarding heart rate within 90 s, add oxygen according to pulse oximetry if possible [Vento, M. & Saugstad, OD. (2010)]. For preterm infants (<32 wk.) it's recommended to begin PPV with O_2 concentrations in a range between 21% and 30%. If Sa O_2 is < 70% at 5 min of age, give oxygen. If heart rate is not increasing satisfactorily, oxygen should be given at any time to both groups. Babies with abnormal lungs, for instance after meconium aspiration, may need supplemental oxygen from early on [Vento, M. & Saugstad, OD. (2010)].

2.3 Oxidative stress and lung injury

Chronic lung disease (CLD) of the newborn is one of the definitive factors influencing the mortality and morbidity of VLBW infants [Banks, BA. et al. (1998)]. The aetiology of CLD is unknown, but many investigators have suggested that free radicals may have a key role in its development. The exposure of immature lungs to prolonged periods of high levels of inspired oxygen is accepted as an important contributor to the development of CLD through both free radical effects on endothelial and epithelial cell barriers that induce pulmonary oedema and trigger mechanisms that lead to activation and accumulation of inflammatory cells [Saugstad, OD. (1998)]. Unfortunately, CLD still develops in extremely premature infants that do not have significant ventilatory or supplemental oxygen needs in the acute course of prematurity. A new form of CLD is less fibrotic than its earlier counterpart, and there is a significant component of delayed alveolar development and perhaps permanent alveolar underdevelopment [Coalson, JJ. et al. (1999), Margraf, LR. et al. (1991)]. Currently, the mechanisms for the development of the new form of CLD have not been fully elucidated and the contribution of oxygen toxicity is debatable. The fact that premature infants develop CLD without being exposed to high concentrations of supplemental oxygen raises the question as to whether oxidative stress in fact contributes to the development of CLD. It is plausible, however, that even low concentrations of supplemental oxygen in premature patients with developmentally poorly prepared antioxidant defense mechanisms may generate significant oxidant stresses and lung injury secondary to oxidation of specific macromolecules [Welty, SE. (2000)]. In addition, inflammatory cell accumulation and activation in the lung may generate oxidants and oxidant stresses that also oxidise macromolecules which leads to CLD [Welty, SE. (2000)]. The literature provides evidence that premature infants who develop CLD have both qualitative and quantitative differences in oxidation of lipids and proteins when compared with infants who do not develop CLD. Such differences in oxidation patterns are the most obvious in the first few days of life [Welty, SE. (2001)]. In a study by OGIHARA et al. [Ogihara, T. et al. (1999)], plasma levels of lipid aldehydes were measured in the first week of life in premature infants. Plasma concentrations of heptanal, 2-nonenal and 4 hydroxynonenal were higher in the first 24 h of life in infants who develop CLD than in those that did not. In another study, elevated exhaled pentane levels were strongly associated with several adverse outcomes in premature infants. In fact, infants who developed CLD had higher exhaled pentane on the first day of life than did patients who did not develop CLD [Nycyk, JA. et al. (1998)]. Protein oxidation was also previously assessed in premature infants and correlated with the development of CLD. There is also an association between higher protein carbonyl contents in tracheal aspirates in the first week of life and the development of CLD [Varsila, E. et al. (1995)]. Moreover, RAMSAY et al. [Ramsay, PL. et al. (2001)] demonstrated that there were no differences in oxygen requirements of tracheal aspirate contents of total 2,4-dinitrophenylhydrazine reactive proteins between premature infants who did or did not develop CLD; however, infants who developed CLD did have more frequent oxidation of specific proteins than did infants who did not develop CLD. These results suggest that identifying specific proteins that are more frequently oxidised in infants who develop CLD may be important in determining specific mechanisms for the development of CLD. Other pathways of ROS generation include metabolism of catecholamines, the arachidonic acid cascade, and mitochondrial metabolism [Bracci, R. (1997)]. However, the main source of free radicals in the lungs seems to be phagocyte activation [Delacourt, C. et al. (1996), Pittet, JF. et al. (1997)]. The increase in phagocyte number and interleukin concentrations in BAL fluid obtained from premature infants with CLD indicates that oxygen toxicity and inflammation are involved in the development of lung injury [Groneck, P. et al. (1993)]. Infants destined to develop CLD have increased pro-inflammatory cytokine levels in airway samples [Bancalari, E. & Gonzales, A. (2000), Speer, CP. & Groneck, P. (1998)]; however, there is little information on when the pro-inflammatory indicators appear or how they progress in the pre-term lung subjected to mechanical ventilation. Moreover, in those infants, a large number of activated neutrophils are found in the air spaces within hours after birth [Arnoon, S. et al. (1993)].The contribution of airway inflammation to the development of CLD of prematurity has been extensively studied [Jonsson, B. et al. (1997), An, H. et al. (2004), Bancalari, E. (2000), Groneck, P. & Speer, CP. (1995), McColm, JR. & McIntosh, N. (1994)]. There is a dynamic and complex balance between pro- and anti-inflammatory cytokines in the human immune system. Previous studies on premature infants have shown that an increase of tumour necrosis factor (TNF)-a in tracheal secretions, among other pro-inflammatory cytokines, was associated with the duration of mechanical ventilation [Schultz, C. et al. (2003)] and the development of CLD [Deng, H. et al. (2000), Kotecha, S. (1996), Kotecha, S. et al. (1995)]. The role of the anti-inflammatory cytokines is less clear. Recent studies have demonstrated that pre-term infants with respiratory distress do produce significant amounts of IL-10 in the lower airways and the presence of this anti-inflammatory cytokine prevents the development of CLD of prematurity [McColm, JR. et al. (2000)]. JONES et al. [Jones, CA. et al. (1996)] were unable to detect interleukin (IL)-10 in most of the airway samples from pre-term infants. This observation agrees with a study showing that the control of airway inflammation by this cytokine is limited in infants [Dudley, DJ. et al. (1997)]. Of interest is that SAUGSTAD [Saugstad, OD. (2003)] claims that these changes are seen very early and are present only a few hours or days after birth in those infants who go on to develop CLD. This may support the suggestion that pre-natal factors, such as inflammation, are important for its development and that the changes leading to CLD are triggered before birth. If this is the case, it holds important implications for future therapeutic approaches [Saugstad, OD. (2003)]. The most common reason for neonates requiring respiratory support is RDS. In this disease, the pathophysiology is one of progressive loss of lung volume, intrapulmonary shunt and deflation instability. Animal and human models of RDS have clearly shown that ventilator strategies alter the clinical and pathological evolution of RDS. In addition, it is claimed that neonates with RDS are susceptible to lung injury and the subsequent development of related conditions. It is being increasingly realised that modes of mechanical ventilation that result in end-inspiratory alveolar over-stretching and/or repeated alveolar collapse and re-expansion disturb the normal fluid balance across the alveolo-capillary membrane. The effects of this include disturbance in the integrity of the endothelium and epithelium and impairment of the surfactant system; these changes are similar to those seen in acute RDS. Mechanical ventilation can injure pre-term lungs and multiple ventilation strategies have been attempted to reduce injury and improve outcomes. In 1999, CLARK et al. [Clark, RH. et al. (1999)] proclaimed that, "the concept of ventilator-induced lung injury has come of age". There are many data which suggest that ventilation can cause biotrauma associated with a "mediator storm" (perhaps cytokines) and that it is responsible for distal organ dysfunction, subsequent multiorgan failure and death. Although it has been shown that pulmonary cytokine levels also appear to be elevated in some neonates on assisted ventilation, the exact relationship to neonatal lung injury has yet to be defined. Pro-inflammatory mediators may be elevated because of fetal exposure to maternal inflammatory mediators, post-natal infections or due to release of mediators from the pre-term lung attributable to ventilator-induced injury. The pre-term lung is susceptible to injury with the initiation of ventilation because potential lung volumes are small, surfactant may be deficient, the lung matrix is not fully developed and the air spaces contain residual fetal lung fluid. Tidal volume (VT) during the resuscitation of pre-term infants is not monitored, and easily visible chest movements will result in VT in excess of that routinely needed to ventilate infants [Ikegami, M. et al. (2000)]. Preterm infants are often hyperventilated and low carbon dioxide tension (PCO2) values after birth correlate with an increased incidence of CLD [Gannon, M. et al. (1998)]. The most effective strategy is the avoidance of mechanical ventilation with the use of nasopharyngeal continuous positive airway pressure whenever possible. Barotrauma, volutrauma and oxygen toxicity, during intermittent positive pressure ventilation, are assumed to be important factors in the pathogenesis of CLD as they cause pulmonary damage, resulting in a release of multiple proinflammatory cytokines and production of extracellular matrix components and growth factors [Ehrenkranz, RA. & Mercurio, MR. (1992)]. The current orientation in the clinical practice is to emphasise the potential importance of reducing mechanical insults on acutely diseased lungs by using special modes of ventilation, e.g. high frequency oscillatory ventilation (HFOV), that limit the pressure and volume of gas delivered to the lungs [Zoban, P. & C ˇ erny, M. (2003)]. HFOV may reduce volutrauma by using a small tidal volume (VT), maintaining almost constant alveolar pressure, and optimising lung volume through the regulation of mean airway pressure [Bohn, DJ. et al. (1980), Gerstmann, DR. et al. (1990)]. Reducing volutrauma is important since damaged tissue generates free radicals and may become inflamed, a process that further contributes to the production of toxic oxygen derivatives. The results of randomised trials to date, conducted on human neonates comparing HFOV with conventional mechanical ventilation (CMV), have been inconclusive and the results are conflicting. Therefore, it remains an open question whether HFOV is more beneficial in preventing CLD than a high-rate, minimal-pressure, low VT, CMV strategy [Bollen, CW. et al. (2003)]. Also, in the Cochrane Database of 2007, the authors conclude that there is no clear evidence that elective HFOV offers important advantages over CMV when used as the initial ventilation strategy to treat pre-term infants with acute pulmonary dysfunction. There may be a small reduction in the rate of CLD with HFOV use, but the evidence is weakened by the inconsistency of this effect across trials and the overall borderline significance [Cools, F. et al. (2007)]. To develop less traumatic mechanical ventilation, with the aim of limiting lung volutrauma, guaranteed volume (GV) integrates various modalities to trigger ventilation with pressure control including assisted/controlled (A/C), synchronised intermittent mandatory ventilation (SIMV) and pressure support ventilation (PSV). GV is an uncommon ventilation method which controls pressure but provides a fixed current volume according to compliance variations, to resistance and to spontaneous activity. The ventilator corrects inspiratory pressure giving a current volume that tends to be the same as the set volume. The gradual improvement in compliance of a pulmonary pathology ventilated with GV follows a reduction of peak inspiratory pressure [Donn, SM. & Sinha, SK. (2003), Herrera, CM. et al. (2003)]. LISTA et al. [Lista, G. et al. (2004)] evaluated the lung inflammatory response in pre-term infants with RDS mechanically ventilated with or without GV, by measuring pro-inflammatory cytokines (IL-6, IL-8, and TNF-a) in tracheobronchial aspirate (TA) fluid. Their data suggest that a volume-targeted ventilatory strategy may play a role in reducing the acute inflammatory response, and thereby also limiting oxidative stress in pre-term infants with RDS. The outcome of this clinical trial shows that there are lower pro inflammatory cytokine levels (IL-6, IL-8, and TNF-a) in BAL of infants with severe RDS supported with PSV with GV compared with PSV only. The study of DANI et al. [Dani, C. et al. (2006)] was the first clinical trial demonstrating that the early treatment of RDS with HFOV is associated with the reduction of pulmonary inflammatory reaction in pre-term infants in comparison with the early application of another potentially lung-protective ventilations strategy such as PSV plus GV. While there are obviously conflicting findings in this field, it is generally accepted that antecedent lung inflammation or injury makes the lungs more susceptible to volutrauma and oxidant induced injury by the reactive species shown in figure 1. The resulting damage promotes inflammation that is not limited to the lung but that may also affect distant organs, and oxygen, when used at high concentration, can be toxic. Although there are a variety of modalities of ventilation that are non invasive, each ventilatory strategy has a potentially negative consequence in terms of tissue damage resulting from the production of both ROS and RNS. Small VT ventilation is associated with progressive low volume and surfactant dysfunction. Limiting VT requires higher levels of end-expiratory pressure and/or FI,O2 to maintain adequate oxygenation. Higher levels of FI,O2 can contribute to oxidant-induced lung injury. Thus, the use of lung protective strategies in the neonate requires proactive decisions that must be specific for disease pathophysiology and lung maturity, and that involve compromises between gas exchange goals and potential toxicities of the treatments. Besides the ventilatory strategies in common use to treat brochopulmonary dysfunction in newborns and because optimal oxygen saturation for use in these cases is difficult to achieve, other treatments have also been attempted. For example, inhalation of nitric oxide, administration of caffeine or surfactant and intramuscular injection of high doses of vitamin A have been used in infants with the hope of improving pulmonary physiology. Additionally, the utility of two antioxidants, i.e. Nacetylcysteine and superoxide dismutase, have been tested. None of these extra-ventilatory procedures has generally provided substantial benefit [Thomas, W. & Speer, CP. (2008)].

3. Melatonin and oxidative stress

Melatonin, an endogenously produced indoleamine, is a highly effective antioxidant, free radical scavenger, and a primary circadian regulator. Melatonin has important antioxidant properties owing to direct and indirect effects. It directly scavenges reactive oxygen and reactive nitrogen species, prevents molecular oxidation, improves mitochondrial physiology, and restores glutathione homeostasis. Its indirect antioxidant effects stem from its ability to stimulate the activities of the enzymes involved in the glutathione cycling and production. Melatonin, by reducing free radical damage, may be an effective protective agent for the fetus as it is in adults. Several clinical studies on melatonin have shown that it reduces oxidative stress in human newborns with sepsis, hypoxic distress, or other conditions, where there is excessive free radical generation. Several clinical studies that used melatonin showed that it reduces oxidative stress in newborns with sepsis, distress, or other conditions, where there is excessive ROS/RNS production [Gitto, E. et al. (2009)]. In one of these studies, the level of lipid peroxidation products and the nitrite + nitrate levels were measured in the serum of asphyxiated newborns before and after treatment with melatonin given within the first 6 hr of life [Fulia, F. et al. (2001)]. Serum levels of these measures in newborns with asphyxia were found to be significantly higher than those in normal infants; these levels were significantly reduced by melatonin treatment [Fulia, F. et al. (2001)]. The protective actions of melatonin in these situations likely relate to the antioxidant properties of the indole and its metabolites as well as to the ability of melatonin to increase the efficiency of mitochondrial electron transport, thereby reducing electron leakage and free radical generation [Hardeland, R. (2005), Leon, J.; Acun˜a-Castroviejo, D. et al. (2004), Leo´n, J. et al. (2005), Reiter, RJ. et al. (2008)].

A seminal study examined the changes in the clinical status and serum levels of lipid peroxidation products [MDA and 4-hydroxylalkenals (4-HDA)] in septic newborns treated with melatonin given within the first 12 hr after diagnosis [Gitto, E. et al. (2001)]. Ten other septic newborns in a comparable state were used as _septic_ controls, while 10 healthy newborns served as normal controls. Serum MDA + 4-HDA concentrations in newborns with sepsis were significantly higher than those in healthy infants without sepsis; in contrast, in septic newborns treated with melatonin, there was a significant reduction of MDA + 4- HDA levels compared to the values measured in the normal controls at both 1 and 4 hr after the initiation of melatonin treatment. Melatonin also improved the clinical outcome of the septic newborns as judged by measurement of sepsis related serum parameters after 24 and 48 hr. We have also tested whether melatonin treatment would lower IL-6, IL-8, TNFa, and nitrite/nitrate levels in 24 newborns with respiratory distress syndrome (RDS) of III or IV grade (radiographically confirmed) diagnosed within the first 6 hr of life [Gitto, E. et al. (2004)]. Compared with the melatonin treated RDS newborns, in the untreated infants, the concentrations of IL-6, IL-8, and TNFa were significantly higher at 24, 72 hr, and at 7 days after onset of the study. In addition, nitrite/nitrate levels at all time points were higher in the untreated RDS newborns than in the melatonin treated babies. Following melatonin administration, nitrite/ nitrate levels decreased significantly, whereas they remained high and became further elevated in the RDS infants not given melatonin. In a clinical trial, the levels of proinflammatory cytokines (IL6, IL-8, and TNFa) and the clinical status of 110 preterm newborns with RDS ventilated with different modalities [conventional ventilation, pressure-support ventilation (PSV) and with guaranteed volumes (GV), and high-frequency oscillatory ventilation] were evaluated before and after treatment with the antioxidant melatonin [Gitto, E. et al. (2005)]. Compared with the melatonin-treated RDS newborns, the concentrations of inflammatory cytokines were significantly elevated in the newborns given only the diluent. When serum levels of IL-6, IL-8, and TNFa for the two groups were compared, melatonin treatment clearly had anti-inflammatory effects. In particular, it was noted that newborns mechanically ventilated in PSV mode with GV presented a greater reduction of serum levels of inflammatory cytokines than did newborns ventilated in conventional mode or with oscillatory ventilation. The measured inflammatory cytokines were most markedly elevated in infants mechanically ventilated but not given melatonin. Newborns not treated with melatonin, who developed chronic lung disease (CLD), have much higher concentrations of proinflammatory cytokines than infants without CLD [Gitto, E. et al. (2004)]. It was also found that melatonin lowered interleukin IL-6, IL-8, TNF-a, and nitrite/nitrate levels and modified serum inflammatory parameters in surgical neonates, thereby improving their clinical course [Gitto, E.; Romeo, C. et al. (2004)]. In animals, the anti-inflammatory actions are thoroughly described [Rodrı´guez, MI. et al. (2007)].

4. Conclusion

Toxic derivatives of oxygen are referred to as free radicals and are either oxygen (ROS) or nitrogen-based (RNS) reactants. ROS/RNS are destructive to all key molecules, i.e. lipids, proteins and DNA, within all cells. Since the lungs of newborn infants are highly susceptible to oxidative damage by ROS/ RNS, care should be taken in the use of pure oxygen during resuscitation of infants. Also, avoidance of mechanical ventilation with the use of nasopharyngeal continuous positive air pressure may reduce respiratory tissue damage resulting from ROS/RNS.

Oxygen, which is obviously vital to survival, can obviously be highly damaging to tissues such as the lungs of newborns which are known to be poorly equipped to neutralise its toxic derivatives. Thus, the exposure of the newly born infant respiratory tree to oxygen at a higher percentage than exists in normal ambient air, i.e. 20%, or at a positive pressure should be performed with caution especially since it may be minimally or no better than using ambient air. Also, the use of antioxidants to quell molecular damage by ROS/RNS could be considered in situations in which pure oxygen or positive pressure are used. One antioxidant that may be useful in these situations is melatonin; this indoleamine has been shown to be useful to combat oxygen toxic in newborns [Gitto, E. et al. (2009)].

5. References

Abraham, E. & Singer, M. (2007) *Mechanisms of sepsis-induced organ dysfunction.* Crit Care Med; 35:2408–2416.

Abraham, E. (2003) *Nuclear factor-kappa B and its role in sepsis associated organ failure.* J Infect Dis; 187(Suppl. 2):S364–S369.

Abraham, E. (2005) *Effects of recombinant human activated protein C in human models of endotoxin administration.* Proc Am Thorac Soc; 2:243–247.

An, H.; Nishimaki, S.; Ohyama, M. et al. (2004) *Interleukin-6, interleukin-8, and soluble tumor necrosis factor receptor-I in the cord blood as predictors of chronic lung disease in premature infants.* Am J Obstet Gynecol; 191: 1649–1654.

Antonielli, M. (1999) *Sepsis and septic shock: pro-inflammatory or anti-inflammatory state?* J Chemother; 6:536–540.

Archer, SL.; Peterson, D.; Nelson, DP. et al. (1989) *Oxygen radicals and antioxidant enzymes alter pulmonary vascular reactivity in the rat lung.* J Appl Physiol; 66: 102–111.

Armstead, WM.; Mirro, R.; Busija, DW. et al. (1988) *Postischemic generation of superoxide anion by newborn pig brain.* Am J Physiol; 255: H401–H403.

Arnoon, S.; Grigg, J. & Silverman, M. (1993) *Pulmonary inflammatory cells in ventilated preterm infants: effects of surfactant treatment.* Arch Dis Child; 69: 44–48.

Atamer, Y.; Kocyigit, Y.; Yokus, B. et al. (2005) *Lipid peroxidation, antioxidant defense, status of trace metals and leptin levels in preeclampsia.* Eur J Obstet Gynecol Reprod Biol; 119:60–66.

Auguelles, S.; Markado, MJ.; Ayala, A. et al. (2006) *Correlation between circulating biomarkers of oxidative stress of maternal and umbilical cord blood at birth.* Free Radic Res; 40:565–570.

Bagenholm, R.; Nilsson, UA., Gotborg, CW. et al. (1998) *Free radicals are formed in the brain of fetal sheep during reperfusion after cerebral ischemia.* Pediatr Res; 43: 271–275.

Bancalari, E. & Gonzales, A. (2000) *Clinical course and lung function abnormalities during development of neonatal chronic lung disease.* In: Bland RD, Coalson JJ, eds. Chronic Lung Disease in Early Infancy. New York, Marcel Dekker; pp. 41-64.

Bancalari, E. (2000) *Epidemiology and risk factors for the "new" bronchopulmonary dysplasia.* NeoReviews; 1: 2-5.

Banks, BA.; Ischiropoulos, H.; McClelland, M. et al. (1998) *Plasma 3- nitrotyrosine is elevated in premature infants who develop bronchopulmonary dysplasia.* Pediatrics; 101: 870-874.

Banks, BA.; Ischiropoulos, H.; McClelland, M.; Ballard, PL. & Ballard, RA. (1998) *Plasma 3-nitrotyrosine is elevated in premature infants who develop bronchopulmonary dysplasia.* Pediatrics; 101:870-874.

Basit, A.; Reutershan, J.; Morris, MA. et al. (2006) *ICAM-1 and LFA-1 play critical roles in LPS-induced neutrophil recruitment into the alveolar space.* Am J Physiol Lung Cell Mol Physiol; 291:L200-L207.

Batra, S.; Kumar, R.; Seema, KR. et al. (2000) *Alterations in antioxidant status during neonatal sepsis.* Ann Trop Pediatr; 20:27-33.

Beckman, JS. & Koppenol, WH. (1996) *Nitric oxide, superoxide, and peroxynitrite: the good, the bad, and ugly.* Am J Physiol; 271:C1424-C1437.

Berger, R. & Garnier, J. (2000) *Perinatal brain injury.* J Perinatol Med; 28:261-285.

Berger, R.; Gjedde, A.; Heck, J et al. (1994) *Extension of the 2- deoxyglucose method to the fetus in utero: theory and normal values for the cerebral glucose consumption in fetal guinea pigs.* J Neurochem; 63:271-279.

Bernard, GR.; Vincent, JL.; Laterre, PF. et al. (2001) *Efficacy and safety of recombinant human activated protein C for severe sepsis.* N Engl J Med; 344:699-709.

Bhandari, V.; Mauli, KN. & Kresch, M. (2000) *Hyperoxia causes an increase in antioxidant enzyme activity in adult and fetal rat type II pneumocytes.* Lung; 178:53-60.

Boda, D.; Nemeth, I. & Pinter, S. (1998) *Surface tension, glutathione content and redox ratio of the tracheal aspirate fluid of premature infants with IRDS.* Biol Neonate; 74:281-288.

Bohn, DJ.; Miyasaka, K.; Marchack, BE. et al. (1980) *Ventilation by highfrequency oscillation.* J Appl Physiol; 48: 710-716.

Bollen, CW.; Uiterwaal, CSPM. & van Vught, AJ. (2003) *Cumulative metaanalysis of high-frequency versus conventional ventilation in premature neonates.* Am J Respir Crit Care Med; 168: 1150- 1155.

Bracci, R. (1997) *Free oxygen radicals and surfactant.* Biol Neonate; 71: Suppl. 1, 23-27.

Buonocore, G., Gioia, D.; De Filippo, M.; Piccolini, E. & Bracci, R. (1994) *Superoxide anion release by polymorphonuclear leukocytes in whole blood of newborns and mothers during the peripartal period.* Pediatr Res; 36:619-622.

Buonocore, G.; Zani, S.; Sargentini, I.; Gioia, D.; Signorini, C. & Bracci, R. (1998) *Hypoxia-induced free iron released in the red cells of newborn infants.* Acta Pediatr; 87:77-81.

Cepinskas, G.; Savickiene, J.; Ionescu, CV. & Kvietys, PR. (2003) *PMN transendothelial migration decreases nuclear NFkappaB in IL-1beta-activated endothelial cells: role of PECAM-1.* J Cell Biol; 161:641-651.

Clark, RH.; Slutsky, AS.; Gerstmann, DR. (1999) *Lung protective strategies of ventilation in the neonate: what are they?* Pediatrics; 105: 112-114.

Clyman, RI.; Saugstad, OD. & Mauray, F. (1989) *Reactive oxygen metabolites relax the lamb ductus arteriosus by stimulating prostaglandin production.* Circ Res; 64: 1-8.

Coalson, JJ.; Winter, VT.; Siler-Khodr, T. et al. (1999) *Neonatal chronic lung disease in extremely immature baboons.* Am J Respir Crit Care Med; 160: 1333–1346.

Cohen, J. (2002) *The immunopathogenesis of sepsis.* Nature; 420:885–891.

Cools, F.; Henderson-Smart, DJ.; Offringa, M. et al. (2007) *Elective high frequency oscillatory ventilation versus conventional ventilation for acute pulmonary dysfunction in preterm infants.* Cochrane Database Syst Rev; 18: CD000104.

Crow, JP. & Beckman, JS. (1995) *The role of peroxynitrite in nitric oxide-mediated toxicity.* Curr Top Microbiol Immunol; 196:57–73.

Crow, JP. & Beckman, JS. (1996) *The importance of superoxide in nitric-oxide-dependent toxicity: evidence for peroxynitritemediated injury.* Adv Exp Med Biol; 387:147–161.

Dani, C.; Bertini, G.; Pezzati, M. et al. (2006) *Effects of pressure support ventilation plus volume guarantee vs. high frequency oscillatory ventilation on lung inflammation in preterm infants.* Pediatric Pulmonol; 41: 242 249.

Delacourt, C.; D'Ortho, M-P.; Maquin-Mavier, I. et al. (1996) *Oxidantantioxidant balance in alveolar macrophages from newborn rats.* Eur Respir J; 9: 2517–2524.

Dellinger, RP. (1999) *Inhaled nitric oxide in acute lung injury and acute respiratory distress syndrome. Inability to translate physiologic benefit to clinical outcome benefit in adult clinical trials.* Intensive Care Med; 25:881–883.

Deng, H.; Mason, SN.; Auten, RL Jr. (2000) *Lung inflammation in hyperoxia can be prevented by antichemokine treatment in newborn rats.* Am J Respir Crit Care Med; 162: 2316–2323.

Donn, SM. & Sinha, SK. (2003) *Can mechanical ventilation strategies reduce chronic lung disease?* Semin Neonatol; 8: 441–448.

Dudley, DJ.; Hunter, C.; Mitchell, MD. et al. (1997) *Amniotic fluid interleukin- 10 (IL-10) concentrations during pregnancy and with labor.* J Reprod Immunol; 33: 147–156.

Ehrenkranz, RA. & Mercurio, MR. (1992) *Bronchopulmonary dysplasia. In: Sinclair JR, Bracken MB, eds. Effective Care of the Newborn Infant.* Oxford, Oxford University; pp. 399–424.

Ely, EW.; Bernard, GR. & Vincent, JL. (2002) *Activated protein C for severe sepsis.* N Engl J Med; 347:1035–1036.

Escrig, R.; Arruza, L.; Izquierdo, I. et al. (2008) *Achievement of targeted saturation values in extremely low gestational age neonates resuscitated with low or high oxygen concentrations: a prospective randomized trial.* Pediatrics; 121: 875–881.

Esteban, J.; Morcillo, JE. & Cortjo, J. (1999) *Oxidative stress and pulmonary inflammation: pharmacological intervention with antioxidants.* Pharmacol Res; 40:393–404.

Ferrali, M.; Signorini, C.; Ciccoli, L. & Comporti, M. (1992) *Iron release and membrane damage in erythrocytes exposed to oxidizing agents, phenylhydrazine, divicine and isouramil.* Biochem J; 285:295–301.

Fogel, I.; Pinchuk, I.; Kupferminc, MJ.; Lichtenberg, D. & Fainarn, O. (2005) *Oxidative stress in the fetal circulation does not depend on mode of delivery.* Am J Obstet Gynecol; 193:241–246.

Fridovich, I. (1998) *Oxygen toxicity: a radical explanation.* J Exp Biol; 201: 1203–1209.

Fulia, F.; Gitto, E.; Cuzzocrea, S. et al. (2001) *Increased levels of malondialdehyde and nitrite/nitrate in the blood of asphyxiated newborns: reduction by melatonin.* J Pineal Res; 31:343–349.

Gannon, M.; Wiswell, TE. & Spitzer, AR. (1998) *Volutrauma, Pa,CO2 and neurodevelopmental sequelae following assisted ventilation.* Clin Perinatol; 25: 159–175.

Gerstmann, DR.; Fouke, JM.; Winter, DC. et al. (1990) *Proximal, tracheal, and alveolar pressures during high-frequency oscillatory ventilation in a normal rabbit model.* Pediatr Res; 28: 367-373.

Gitto, E.; Karbownik, M.; Reiter, RJ. et al. (2001) *Effects of melatonin treatment in septic newborns.* Pediatr Res; 6:756- 760.

Gitto, E.; Pellegrino, S.; Gitto, B. et al. (2009) *Oxidative stress in the newborn in the pre- and post-natal period and the clinical use of melatonin.* J Pineal Res; 46: 128-139.

Gitto, E.; Reiter, RJ.; Amodio, A. et al. (2004) *Early indicators of chronic lung disease in preterm infants with respiratory distress syndrome and their inhibition by melatonin.* J Pineal Res; 36:250-255.

Gitto, E.; Reiter, RJ.; Cordaro, SP. et al. (2004) *Oxidative and inflammatory parameters in respiratory distress syndrome of preterm newborns: beneficial effects of melatonin.* Am J Perinatol; 21:209-216.

Gitto, E.; Reiter, RJ.; Karbownik, M. et al. (2002) *Causes of oxidative stress in the pre-and perinatal period.* Biol Neonate; 81: 146-157.

Gitto, E.; Reiter, RJ.; Sabatino, G. et al. (2005) *Correlation among cytokines, bronchopulmonary dysplasia and modality of ventilation in preterm newborns: improvement with melatonin treatment.* J Pineal Res; 39:287-293.

Gitto, E.; Romeo, C.; Reiter, RJ. et al. (2004) *Melatonin reduces oxidative stress in surgical neonates.* J Pediatr Surg; 39:184-189.

Groneck, P. & Speer, CP. (1995) *Inflammatory mediators and bronchopulmonary dysplasia.* Arch Dis Child Fetal Neonatal; 73: F1-F3.

Groneck, P.; Reuss, D.; Gotze-Speer, B. et al. (1993) *Effects of dexamethasone on chemotactic activity and inflammatory mediators in tracheobronchial aspirates of preterm infants at risk for chronic lung disease.* J Pediatr; 22: 938-944.

Gupta, S.; Agarwal, A. & Sharma, RK. (2005) *The role of placental oxidative stress and lipid peroxidation in preeclampsia.* Obstet Gynecol Surv; 60:807-816.

Halliwell, B. & Gutteridge, JC. (1990) *Role of free radicals and catalytic ions in human disease: an overview.* Methods Enzymol; 186:1-85.

Halliwell, B. (1992) *Oxygen radicals as key mediators in neurological disease: Fact or fiction?* Ann Neurol; 32: S10-S15.

Halliwell, B. (1999) *Free radicals, antioxidants and human disease: Curiosity, cause, or consequence?* Lancet; 344: 721-724.

Hardeland, R. (2005) *Antioxidant protection by melatonin: multiplicity of mechanisms from radical detoxification to radical avoidance.* Endocrine; 27:119-130.

Harris, ED. (1992) *Regulation of antioxidant enzymes.* FASEB J; 6:2675-2683.

Haynes, RL.; Folkerth, RD.; Keefe, RJ. et al. (2003) *Nitrosative and oxidative injury to premyelinating oligodendrocytes in periventricular leukomalacia.* J Neuropathol Exp Neurol; 62: 441-450.

Herrera, CM.; Gerhardt, T.; Claure, N. et al. (2003) *Effect of volume guaranteed synchronized intermittent mandatory ventilation in preterm infants recovering from respiratory failure.* Pediatrics; 110: 529-533.

Hracsko, Z.; Safar, Z.; Orvos, H.; Novak, Z.; Pal, A. & Varga, IS. (2007) *Evaluation of oxidative stress markers after vaginal delivery or caesarean section.* In Vivo; 21:703-706.

Hubel, CA. (1999) *Oxidative stress in the pathogenesis of preeclampsia.* Proc Soc Exp Biol Med; 222:222-235.

Huertas, JR.; Palomino, N.; Ochoa, JJ. et al. (1998) *Lipid peroxidation and antioxidant erythrocyte membranes of full-term and preterm newborns.* Biofactors; 8:133–137.

Ikegami, M.; Kallapur, S.; Michna, J. & Jobe, AH. (2000) *Lung injury and surfactant metabolism after hyperventilation of premature lambs.* Pediatr Res; 47:398–404.

Ikegami, M.; Kallapur, S.; Michna, J. et al. (2000) *Lung injury and surfactant metabolism after hyperventilation of premature lambs.* Pediatr Res; 47: 398–404.

Inoue, S. & Kawanishi, S. (1995) *Oxidative DNA damage induced by simultaneous generation of nitric oxide and peroxide.* FEBS Lett; 371:86–88.

Janssen, YMW.; Soultanakis, R.; Steece, K. et al. (1998) *Depletion of nitric oxide causes cell cycle alterations, apoptosis and oxidative stress in pulmonary cells.* Am J Physiol; 275:L1100–L1109.

Janssen-Heininger, YM.; Poynter, ME. & Baeuerle, PA. (2000) *Recent advances towards understanding redox mechanisms in the activation of nuclear factor kappa B.* Free Radic Biol Med; 28:1317–1327.

Jones, CA.; Cayabyab, RG.; Kwong, KY. et al. (1996) *Undetectable interleukin (IL)-10 and persistent IL-8 expression early in hyaline membrane disease: a possible developmental basis for the predisposition to chronic lung inflammation in preterm newborns.* Pediatr Res; 39: 966–975.

Jonsson, B.; Tullus, K.; Brauner, A. et al. (1997) *Early increase of TNF alpha and IL-6 in tracheobronchial aspirate fluid indicator of subsequent chronic lung disease in preterm infants.* Arch Dis Child Fetal Neonatal; 77: F198–F201.

Kattwinkel, J.; Niermeyer, S., Nadkarni, V. et al. (1999) *ILCOR advisory statement: resuscitation of the newly born infant. An advisory statement from the pediatric working group of the International Liaison Committee on Resuscitation.* Circulation; 99: 1927– 1938.

Kim, K.; Whitin, JC.; Sukhova, NM. & Cohen, HJ. (1999) *Increases in extracellular glutathione peroxidase in plasma and lungs of mice exposed to hyperoxia.* Pediatr Res; 46:715–721.

Kondo, M.; Itoh, S.; Isobe, K. et al. (2000) *Chemiluminescence because of the production of reactive oxygen species in the lungs of newborn piglets during resuscitation periods after asphyxiation load.* Pediatr Res; 47: 524–527.

Kotecha, S. (1996) *Cytokines in chronic lung disease of prematurity.* Eur J Pediatr; 155: Suppl. 2, S14–S17.

Kotecha, S.; Chan, B.; Azam, N. et al. (1995) *Increase in interleukin-8 and soluble intercellular adhesion molecule-1 in bronchoalveolar lavage fluid from premature infants who develop chronic lung disease.* Arch Dis Child Fetal Neonatal Ed; 72: F90–F96.

Kothecha, S. (2000) *Lung growth: implication for the newborn infant.* Arch Dis Child Fetal Neonatal; 82:F69–F74.

Kutzsche, S.; Ilves, P.; Kirkeby, OJ. et al. (2002) *Hydrogen peroxide production in leukocytes during cerebral hypoxia and reoxygenation with 100% or 21% oxygen in newborn piglets.* Pediatr Res; 49: 834–842.

Lamb, NJ.; Gutteridge, JMC.; Baker, C et al. (1999) *Oxidative damage to proteins of bronchoalveolar lavage fluid in patients with acute respiratory distress syndrome: evidence for neutrophil- mediated hydroxylation, nitration and chlorination.* Intensive Care Med; 25:1738–1744.

Laurie, S.; Mataz, Z.; Boaz, M.; Fux, A.; Golan, A. & Sadan, O. (2007) *Different degrees of fetal oxidative stress in elective and emergent caesarean section.* Neonatology; 92:111–115.

Lefkowitz, W. (2002) *Oxygen and resuscitation: beyond the myth.* Pediatrics; 109: 517–519.

Leo´n, J.; Acun˜a-Castroviejo, D.; Escames, G. et al. (2005) *Melatonin mitigates mitochondrial malfunction.* J Pineal Res; 38:1-9.

Leon, J.; Acun˜a-Castroviejo, D.; Sainz, RM. et al. (2004) *Melatonin and mitochondrial function.* Life Sci; 75:765-790.

Ley, K. & Reutershan, J. (2006) *Leucocyte-endothelial interactions in health and disease.* Handb Exp Pharmacol; 176(Pt2):97- 133.

Lista, G.; Colnaghi, M.; Castoldi, F. et al. (2004) *Impact of targeted-volume ventilation on lung inflammatory response in preterm infants with respiratory distress syndrome (RDS).* Pediatr Pulmonol; 37: 510-514.

Liu, L. & Kubes, P. (2003) *Molecular mechanisms of leukocyte recruitment: organ-specific mechanisms of action.* Thromb Haemost; 89:213-220.

Liu, SF. & Malik, AB. (2006) *NF-kappa B activation as a pathological mechanism of septic shock and inflammation.* Am J Physiol Lung Cell Mol Physiol; 290:L622-L645.

Lush, CW. & Kvietys, PR. (2000) *Microvascular dysfunction in sepsis.* Microcirculation; 7:83-101.

Many, A.; Hubel, CA.; Fisher, SJ. et al. (2000) *Invasive cytotrophoblasts manifest evidence of oxidative stress in preeclampsia.* Am J Pathol; 156:321-331.

Margraf, LR.; Tomashefski, JF Jr.; Bruce, MC. et al. (1991) *Morphometric analysis of the lung in bronchopulmonary dysplasia.* Am Rev Respir Dis; 143: 391-400.

McColm, JR. & McIntosh, N. (1994) *Interleukin-8 in bronchoalveolar lavage samples as predictor of chronic lung disease in premature infants.* Lancet; 343: 729.

McColm, JR.; Stenson, BJ.; Biermasz, N. et al. (2000) *Measurement of interleukin 10 in bronchoalveolar lavage from preterm ventilated infants.* Arch Dis Child Fetal Neonatal; 82: F156-F159.

Metnitz, PGH.; Bartens, C.; Fisher, M. et al. (1999) *Antioxidant status in patient with acute respiratory distress syndrome.* Intensive Care Med; 25:180-185.

Mochida, S.; Matsura, T.; Yamashita, A. et al. (2007) *Geranylgeranylacetone ameliorates inflammatory response to lipopolysaccharide (LPS) in murine macrophages: inhibition of LPS binding to the cell surface.* J Clin Biochem Nutr; 41:115-123.

Nese Citak, KA.; Denizmen, AA.; Godekmerdan, A.; Kurt, A.; Dogan, Y. & Yilmaz, E. (2007) *Serum IL-1b, IL-6, IL-8, and TNF-a levels in early diagnosis and management of neonatal sepsis.* Mediators Inflamm; 2007:31397.

Niermeyer, S., Kattwinkel, J.; Van Reempts, P. et al. (2000) *International Guidelines for Neonatal Resuscitation: an excerpt from the Guidelines 2000 for Cardiopulmonary Resuscitation and Emergency Cardiovascular Care: International Consensus on Science. Contributors and Reviewers for the Neonatal Resuscitation Guidelines.* Pediatrics; 106: e29.

Nycyk, JA.; Drury, JA.; Cooke, RWI. (1998) *Breath pentane as a marker for lipid peroxidation and adverse outcome in preterm infants.* Arch Dis Child Fetal Neonatal Ed; 79: F67-F69.

Ogihara, T.; Hirano, K.; Morinobu, T. et al. (1999) *Raised concentrations of aldehyde lipid peroxidation products in premature infants with chronic lung disease.* Arch Dis Child Fetal Neonatal Ed; 80:F21-F25.

Ogihara, T.; Hirano, K.; Morinobu, T. et al. (1999) *Raised concentration of aldehyde lipid peroxidation products in premature infants with chronic lung disease.* Arch Dis Child Fetal Neonatal Ed; 80: F21-F25.

Ogihara, T.; Okamoto, R.; Kim, H. et al. (1996) *New evidence for the involvement of oxygen radicals in triggering neonatal chronic lung disease.* Pediatr Res; 39: 117-119.

Palmer, C.; Brucklalcher, RM.; Christensen, MA. et al. (1990) *Carbohydrate and energy metabolism during the evolution of hypoxic-ischemic brain damage in the immature rat.* J Cereb Blood Flow Metab; 10:227–235.

Panacek, EA.; Marshall, JC.; Albertson, TE. et al. (2004) *Efficacy and safety of the monoclonal anti-tumor necrosis factor antibody F(ab_)2 fragment afelimomab in patients with severe sepsis and elevated interleukin-6 levels.* Crit Care Med; 32:2173–2182.

Perez, EM. & Weisman, LE. (1997) *Novel approaches to the prevention and therapy of neonatal bacterial sepsis.* Clin Perinatol; 24:213–225.

Phelps, DT.; Ferro, TJ.; Higgins, PJ et al. (1995) *TNF-a induces peroxynitrite-mediated depletion of lung endothelial glutathione via protein kinase C.* Am J Physiol; 269:551–559.

Pittet, JF.; Mackersie, RC.; Martin, TR. et al. (1997) *Biological markers of acute lung injury: prognostic and pathogenetic significance.* Am J Respir Crit Care Med; 155: 1187–1205.

Poranen, AK.; Ekblad, U.; Uotila, P. & Ahotupa, M. (1996) *Lipid peroxidation and antioxidants in normal and pre-eclamptic pregnancies.* Placenta; 17:401–405.

Raby, Y.; Rabi, D. & Yee, W. (2007) *Room air resuscitation of the depressed newborn: a systematic review and meta analysis.* Resuscitation; 72: 353–363.

Ramji, A.; Ahuja, S.; Thirupuram, S. et al. (1993) *Resuscitation of asphyxic newborn infants with room air or 100% oxygen.* Pediatr Res; 34: 809–812.

Ramji, S.; Rasaily, R.; Mishra, PK. et al. (2003) *Resuscitation of asphyxiated newborns with room air or 100% oxygen at birth: a multicentric clinical trial.* Ind Pediatr; 40: 510–517.

Ramsay, PL.; DeMayo, FJ.; Hegemier, SE. et al. (2001) *Clara cell secretory protein oxidation and expression in premature infants who develop bronchopulmonary dysplasia.* Am J Respir Crit Care Med; 164: 155–161.

Rao, RM.; Yang, L.; Garcia-Cardena, G. & Luscinskas, FW. (2007) *Endothelial-dependent mechanisms of leukocyte recruitment to the vascular wall.* Circ Res; 101:234–247.

Rawlingson, A. (2003) *Nitric oxide, inflammation and acute burn injury.* Burns; 29:631–640.

Razavi, HM.; Wang, L.; Weicker, S. et al. (2005) *Pulmonary oxidant stress in murine sepsis is due to inflammatory cell nitric oxide.* Crit Care Med; 33:1333–1339.

Reiter, RJ.; Paredes, SD.; Korkmaz, A. et al. (2008) *Melatonin combats molecular terrorism at the mitochondrial level.* Interdisc Toxicol; 1:137–149.

Riedemann, NC.; Guo, RF. & Ward, PA. (2003) *Novel strategies for the treatment of sepsis.* Nat Med; 9:517–524.

Rodrı´guez, MI.; Escames, G.; Lo´pez, LC. et al. (2007) *Chronic melatonin treatment reduces the age-dependent inflammatory process in senescence-accelerated mice.* J Pineal Res; 42:272–279.

Salgo, MG.; Bermuzed, E.; Squadrito, G. & Pryor, W. (1995) *DNA damage and oxidation of thiol peroxynitrite causes in rat thymocytes.* Arch Biochem Biophys; 322:500–505.

Sanderud, J.; Bjoro, K. & Saugstad, OD. (1993) *Oxygen radicals stimulate thromboxane and prostacyclin synthesis and induce vasoconstriction in pig lungs.* Scand J Clin Lab Invest; 53: 447–455.

Sarker, AH.; Watanabe, S.; Seki, S. et al. (1995) *Oxygen radical-induced single-strand DNA breaks and repair of the damage in a cell-free system.* Mutat Res; 337: 85–95.

Saugstad, OD. & Aansen, AO. (1980) *Plasma hypoxanthine levels as a prognostic aid of tissue hypoxia.* Eur Surg Res; 12: 123–129.

Saugstad, OD. (1988) *Hypoxanthine as an indicator of hypoxia: its role in health and disease through free radical production.* Pediatr Res; 23: 143–150.

Saugstad, OD. (1996) *Mechanisms of tissue injury by oxygen radicals: implications for neonatal disease.* Acta Paediatr; 85: 1-4.

Saugstad, OD. (1998) *Chronic lung disease: the role of oxidative stress.* Biol Neonate; 74: Suppl. 1, 21-28.

Saugstad, OD. (2001) *Is oxygen more toxic than currently believed?* Pediatrics; 108: 1203-1205.

Saugstad, OD. (2001) *Resuscitation of newborn infants with room air or oxygen.* Semin Neonatol; 6: 233-239.

Saugstad, OD. (2003) *Bronchopulmonary dysplasia – oxidative stress and antioxidants.* Semin Neonatol; 8: 39-49.

Saugstad, OD. (2003) *Bronchopulmonary dysplasia-oxidative stress and antioxidants.* Semin Neonatol; 8: 39-49.

Saugstad, OD. (2003) *Oxygen toxicity at birth: the pieces are put together.* Pediatr Res; 789-783.

Saugstad, OD. (2005) *Oxidative stress in the newborn. A 30-year perspective.* Biol Neonate; 88: 228-236.

Saugstad, OD. *Optimal oxygenation at birth and in the neonatal period.* (2007) Neonatology; 91: 319-322.

Saugstad, OD.; Ramji, S. & Vento, M. (2005) *Resuscitation of depressed newborn infants with ambient air or pure oxygen: a metaanalysis.* Biol Neonate; 87: 22-34.

Saugstad, OD.; Rootwelt, T. & Aalen, O. *Resuscitation of asphyxiated newborn infants wiyh room air or oxygen: an international controlled trial the Resair 2 study.* (1998) Pediatr Res; 102: e1.

Scher, M. (2001) *Perinatal asphyxia: timing and mechanisms of injury in neonatal encephalopathy.* Curr Neurol Neurosci Rep; 1:175-184.

Schultz, C.; Tautz, J.; Reiss, I. et al. (2003) *Prolonged mechanical ventilation induces pulmonary inflammation in preterm infants.* Biol Neonate; 84: 64-66.

Seema, KR.; Mandal, RN.; Tandon, A. et al. (1999) *Serum TNF-a and free radical scavengers in neonatal septicaemia.* Ind J Pediatr; 66:511-516.

Shoji, H. & Koletzko, B. (2007) *Oxidative stress and antioxidant protection in the perinatal period.* Curr Opin Clin Nutr Metab Care; 10:324-328.

Speer, CP. & Groneck, P. (1998) *Oxygen radicals, cytokines, adhesion molecules and lung injury in neonates.* Semin Neonatal; 3: 219-228.

Szabo, C. & Oshima, H. (1997) *DNA damage induced by peroxynitrite: subsequent biological effects.* Nitric Oxide; 1:373-385.

Szabo, C., Cuzzocrea, S.; Zingarelli, B.; O_Connor, M. & Salzman, AL. (1997) *Endothelial dysfunction in endotoxic shock: importance of the activation of poly (ADP ribose) synthetase (PARS) by peroxynitrite.* J Clin Invest; 100:723-735.

Tan, A.; Schulze, A.; O'Donnell, CP. et al. (2005) *Air versus oxygen for resuscitation of infants at birth.* Cochrane Database Syst Rev; 18: CD002273.

Thomas, W. & Speer, CP. (2008) *Nonventilatory strategies for prevention and treatment of bronchopulmonary dysplasia – what is the evidence?* Neonatology; 94: 150-159.

Vanderlelie, J.; Venardos, K.; Clifton, VL. et al. (2005) *Increased biological oxidation and reduced antioxidant enzyme activity in preeclamptic placentae.* Placenta; 26:53-58.

Vannucci, RC.; Christensen, MA. & Yager, JY. (1993) *Nature, timecourse and extent of cerebral edema in the perinatal hypoxicischemic brain damage.* Pediatr Neurol; 9:29-34.

Varsila, E.; Pesonen, E. & Andersson, S. (1995) *Early protein oxidation in the neonatal lung is related to development of chronic lung disease.* Acta Paediatr; 84: 1296-1299.

Vento, G.; Mele, MC.; Mordente, A. et al. (2000) *High total antioxidant activity and uric acid in tracheobronchial aspirate fluid of preterm infants during oxidative stress: an adaptive response to hyperoxia?* Acta Paediatr; 89:336–342.

Vento, M.; Asensi, M.; Sastre, J. et al. (2001) *Resuscitation with room air instead of 100% oxygen prevents oxidative stress in moderately asphyxiated term neonates.* Pediatrics; 107: 642–647.

Vento, M.; Asensi, M.; Sastre, J. et al. (2001) *Six years of experience with the use of room air for the resuscitation of asphyxiated newly born term infants.* Biol Neonate; 79: 261–267.

Vento, M.; Sastre, J.; Asensi, M. et al. (2003) *Oxidative stress in asphyxiated term infants resusciteted with 100% oxygen.* J Pediatr; 142: 240–246.

Vento, M.; Saugstad, OD. (2010) *Resuscitation of the term and preterm infant.* Seminars in Fetal & Neonatal Medicine 15 216-222.

Walsh, SW. & Wang, Y. (1993) *Deficient glutathione peroxidise activity in preeclampsia is associated with increased placental production of thromboxane and lipid peroxides.* Am J Obstet Gynecol; 169:1456–1461.

Walsh, SW. & Wang, Y. (1993) *Secretion of lipid peroxides by the human placenta.* Am J Obstet Gynecol; 169:1462–1466.

Walsh, SW. & Wang, Y. (1995) *Trophoblast and placental villous coreproduction of lipid peroxides, thromboxane, and prostacyclin in preeclampsia.* J Clin Endocrinol Metab; 80:1888–1893.

Walsh, SW.; Vaughan, JE.; Wang, Y. & Roberts, LJ. (2000) *Placental isoprostane is significantly increased in preeclampsia.* FASEB J; 14:1289–1296.

Walsh, SW.; Wang, Y. & Jesse, R. (1993) *Peroxide induces vasoconstriction in the human placenta by stimulating thromboxane.* Am J Obstet Gynecol; 169:1007–1012.

Wang, Y. & Walsh, SW. (1996) *Antioxidant activities and mRNA expression of superoxide dismutase, catalase, and glutathione peroxidase in normal and preeclamptic placentas.* J Soc Gynecol Investig; 3:179–184.

Welty, SE. (2000) *Is Oxidant stress in the causal pathway to BPD?* NeoReviews; e6–e10.

Welty, SE. (2001) *Is the role for antioxidant therapy in bronchopulmonary dysplasia.* J Nutr; 131: 947S–950S.

Wisdom, SJ.; Wilson, R.; Mckillop, JH. & Walker, JJ. (1991) *Antioxidant systems in normal pregnancy and in pregnancy hypertension.* Am J Obstet Gynecol; 6:1701–1705.

Yager, JY.; Brucklalcher, RM. & Vannucci, RC. (1992) *Cerebral energy metabolism during hypoxia-ischemia and early recovery in immature rats.* Am J Physiol; 262:H672–H677.

Yitig, S., Yurdakok, M., Kilinc, K., Oran, O.; Erdem, G. & Tekinalp, G. (1998) *Serum malondialdehyde concentrations as a measure of oxygen free radical damage in preterm infants.* Turk J Pediatr; 40:177–183.

Zoban, P. & C ˇ erny, M. (2003) *Immature lung and acute lung injury.* Physiol Res; 52: 507–516.

6

Pain Management and Nursing Approaches in Pediatric Oncology

Nejla Canbulat[1] and Ayşe Sonay Kurt[2]
[1]Karamanoglu Mehmetbey University,
Karaman School of Health, Karaman,
[2]Selcuk University, Faculty of Health Science, Konya,
Turkey

1. Introduction

Pain is defined as "an unpleasant sensory and emotional experience associated with actual or potential tissue damage, or described in terms of such damage (Higginson&Murtagh 2010). Defining "pain" in a succinct manner is a great challenge. What is pain? It has been described as an emotional state, a physical experience, a spiritual sacrament, and a complex set of interconnected subcellular signals (Mirchandani et al., 2011). According to the International Association for the Study of Pain (IASP), pain is defined as "an unpleasant sensory and emotional experience which we primarily associate with tissue damage or describe in terms of such damage, or both (Portenoy&Kanner 1996). In different places and in different points over time, both Eastern and Western medical traditions have included a concept of imbalance as an important etiology of painful symptoms (Helms, 1998) ... the difference between the body of a living man and that of a dead man is just like the difference between (Bias&Cope, 2011). Cancer pain may be either acute or chronic. Acute pain; acute pain is initially treated with short-acting non-opioid pharmacologic agents or combination opioid drugs. Acute versus chronic pain is important to clearly differentiate. Acute pain is rapid in onset, self-limiting, a symptom of the disease, and the patient often presents in acute distress. Examples of acute pain include postoperative pain, obstetrical labor pain, and trauma or injury-related pain and characteristically is described as sudden, sharp, and localized pain. It is usually self-limited and may be associated with physiologic changes such as diaphoresis and increases in heart rate and blood pressure (Mirchandani et al 2011). Chronic pain; chronic pain is long-term pain classified as acute, moderate, and severe. It is often differentiated as malignant or non-malignant pain. Chronic pain is often described as gnawing, aching, and diffuse and is more gradual in onset and cessation than acute pain, which can also be simultaneously superimposed on top of the former. It can vary in intensity, may remit briefly, and has definite impact psychologically and socially. Pain characteristics: Acute and chronic was given Table 1. The treatment for such pain is often successful with traditional pharmacologic measures; however, often less traditional drugs and even non-pharmacologic therapies are necessary to achieve relief (Mirchandani et al., 2011).

Acute pain	Chronic pain
1. Usually obvious tissue damage 2. Distinct onset 3. Short, well-characterized duration 4. Resolves with healing 5. Serves a protective function 6. Effective therapy is available	1. Multiple causes (malignancy, benign) 2. Gradual or distinct onset 3. Persists after 3–6 months of healing 4. Can be a symptom or diagnosis 5. Serves no adaptive purpose 6. May be refractory to treatment

Table 1. Pain characteristics: acute and chronic (Mirchandani et al., 2011)

Over time and across cultures, the understanding and expression of pain reflects the contemporary spirit of the age. Universally, the human experience begins through the painful process of birth, and throughout our lifetimes (Dedeli&Karadeniz, 2009). Factors mediating children's pain was given Fig. 1.

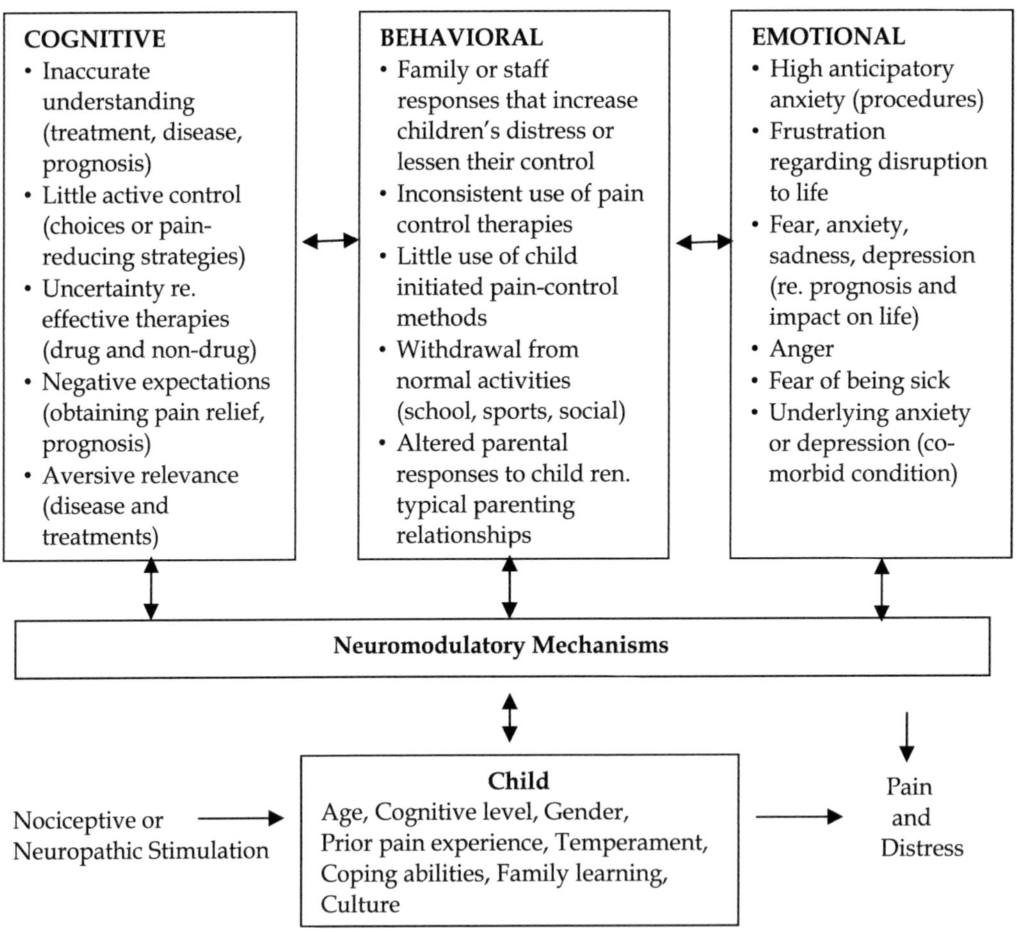

Fig. 1. Situational factors mediating children's pain (McGrath&Crawford, 2010)

Physiologic pain is defined as rapidly perceived non-traumatic discomfort of very short duration, alerting the individual of a dangerous stimulus. This is adaptive and initiates the withdrawal reflex that prevents and/or minimizes tissue injury. Physiologic pain can be divided into neuropathic pain and nociceptive pain (Mirchandani et al., 2011). Physiologic pain types of pain was given Table 2.

Two Major Types of Pain	
I. Nociceptive Pain	II. Neuropathic Pain
A. Somatic Pain B. Visceral Pain	A. Centrally Generated Pain B. Peripherally Generated Pain
I. Nociceptive Pain: Normal process of stimuli that damages normal tissues or has the potential to do so if prolonged; usually responsive to non-opioids and/or opioids. A. Somatic Pain: Arises from bone, joint, muscle, skin, or connective tissue. It is usually aching or throbbing in quality and is well localized. B. Visceral Pain: Arises from visceral organs, such as the GI tract and pancreas. This may be subdivided: 1. Tumor involvement of the organ capsule that causes aching and fairly well-localized pain. 2. Obstruction of hollow viscus, which causes intermittent cramping and poorly localized pain.	**II. Neuropathic** Pain: Abnormal processing of sensory input by the peripheral or central nervous system; treatment usually includes adjuvant analgesics. A. Centrally Generated Pain 1. Deafferentation pain: Injury to either the peripheral or central nervous system. Examples: Phantom pain may reflect injury to the peripheral nervous system; burning pain below the level of a spinal cord lesion reflects injury to the central nervous system. 2. Sympathetically maintained pain: Associated with dysregulation of the autonomic nervous system. Examples: May include some of the pain associated with reflect sympathetic dystrophy/causalgia (complex regional pain syndrome, type I, type II). B. Peripherally Generated Pain 1. Painful polyneuropathies: Pain is felt along the distribution of many peripheral nerves. Examples: diabetic neuropathy, alcohol-nutritional neuropathy, and those associated with Guillain-Barre syndrome. 2. Painful mononeuropathies: Usually associated with a known peripheral nerve injury, and pain is felt at least partly along the distribution of the damaged nerve. Examples: nerve root compression, nerve entrapment, trigeminal neuralgia.

Table 2. Physiologic pain types

The four predominant etiologies of cancer pain are: (1) that directly produced by the tumor; (2) that due to the various modalities of cancer therapy; (3) that related to chronic debility; and (4) that due to an unrelated, concurrent disease process (Eidelman&Carr, 2006). Tumor-Related Pain; Most cancer-related pain is directly produced by the malignancy itself. The neoplasm may extend into surrounding tissue and exert pressure on nociceptors in diverse organs, as well as nerves. Furthermore, recent studies have found evidence that pain-gene rating mediators are directly released from certain tumors or from surrounding tissue in response to tumor invasion or metastasis such as to bone (Eidelman&Carr, 2006; Unuvar, 1999). Treatment-Related Pain; The various modalities of cancer therapy may paradoxically cause pain. Cancer patients may experience acute discomfort following surgery or other invasive procedures. Also, there are numerous postsurgical chronic pain syndromes. The administration of chemotherapy itself may cause immediate acute pain (e.g., intravenous infusion pain, abdominal discomfort during intraperitoneal infusion) or painful sequelae such as mucositis, arthralgias, and headaches. Moreover, chemotherapeutic agents, including vinca alkaloids, cisplatin, and paclitaxel, are associated with peripheral neuropathies. Radiation therapy may injure soft tissue or neuronal structures, resulting in mucositis, proctitis, enteritis, osteonecrosis, peripheral neuro pathies, or plexo pathies. Furthermore, novel anti cancer agents such as hormonal or immunotherapy may produce pain (Eidelman&Carr, 2006; Unuvar, 1999). Debility-Related Pain; Many cancer patients may be inactive or suffer debilities that are associated with painful conditions. Many cancer patients may be inactive or suffer debilities that are associated with painful conditions. For instance, patients who have received immunosuppressive therapy or have hematologic malignancies are at increased risk for developing postherpetic neuralgia. Also, many malignancies are associated with an increased incidence of thrombosis, which may present as pain and swelling in the affected site (Eidelman&Carr, 2006). Non-Malignant Concurrent Disease; Patients with cancer may experience discomfort as a direct consequence of a concurrent, benign disease process (e.g., degenerative joint disease or diabetic neuropathy). Therefore, it is important to review patients' past medical histories and to consider any coexisting nonmalignant condition as a potential source of symptoms (Eidelman&Carr 2006).

2. Epidemiology

2.1 Frequency

World Health Organization (WHO) states that 25% of cancer patients suffer pain, 33% of such patients suffer pain during treatment of the diseases, the rate of pain is between 75-90% in advanced and terminal period of the disease, 70% of such pain is directly associated with cancer, 20% of such pain is also based on cancer treatment (Aslan, 2006).

When pain reasons of the patients consulted with a algology clinic in Turkey were analyzed, it was found that cancer pain ranked the first (Aslan, 2006). The prevalence of cancer pain in patients with advanced or terminal disease was given Table 3.

Even when WHO guidelines are followed, failure to achieve satisfactory pain relief occurs in 10%-20% of patients. For these instances, some authors have proposed descriptors such as "opioid-poorly responsive pain" or "opioid-irrelevant pain." Therefore, there is a need both in clinical practice and in the standardized comparison of research findings for a systematic approach to identify and categorize factors associated with a poor prognosis (O' leary et al., 2010).

2.2 Pain assessment methods

Pain assessment and pain measurement in children is challenging. These challenges depend on permanent changes in process of child's perception, interpretation and expression with regards to age, growth phase, previous pain experience and other environmental factors (Manworren&Hynan, 2003; Unuvar, 1999). Pain assessment in children is given in the fig. 2 (Ramamurthy, 2006)

Study type	Disease definition and tumor type	Sample size	Prevalence	Reference
Retrospective study	Caregivers of general cancer population	170	- 86% stated pain was a problem, 61% reported a great deal or quite a bit of pain, 25% had some or little pain	Bucher et al., 1999
			_ 82% reported data on pain relief intervention, 46% of which made pain stop/get better, 56% of which made pain a little better or had no effect or made it worse	
Prospective study	Advanced cancer patients admitted to hospice	232	- 81% had pain at the time of admission - Pain severity worsened in the 48 hours before death (prevalence not reported)	Chiu et al., 2000
Retrospective case note review	Patients referred to palliative care services - hospice, community, hospital, and outpatient (95% with cancer; of these, 71% had advanced disease)	400	- 64% had pain at first assessment - In the hospice, 62% of patients had pain - In the community setting, 56% had pain - In the hospital service, 63% had pain - In the outpatient service, 75% had pain	Potter et al., 2003
Cross-sectional survey	Patients with metastatic cancer or stage IV lymphoma in hospital for 72 hours for complications not treatment	66	- 78% of patients had pain (assessed using the Memorial Symptom Assessment Scale)	Tranmer et al., 2003
Prospective survey	In- and outpatients with metastatic or recurrent cancer	655	- 70.8% had some pain in the previous 24 hours - 63.3% rated their pain at 5 or higher on a visual analogue scale of 0–10	Yun et al., 2003

Table 3. The prevalence of cancer pain in patients with advanced or terminal disease, or who are at the end of life

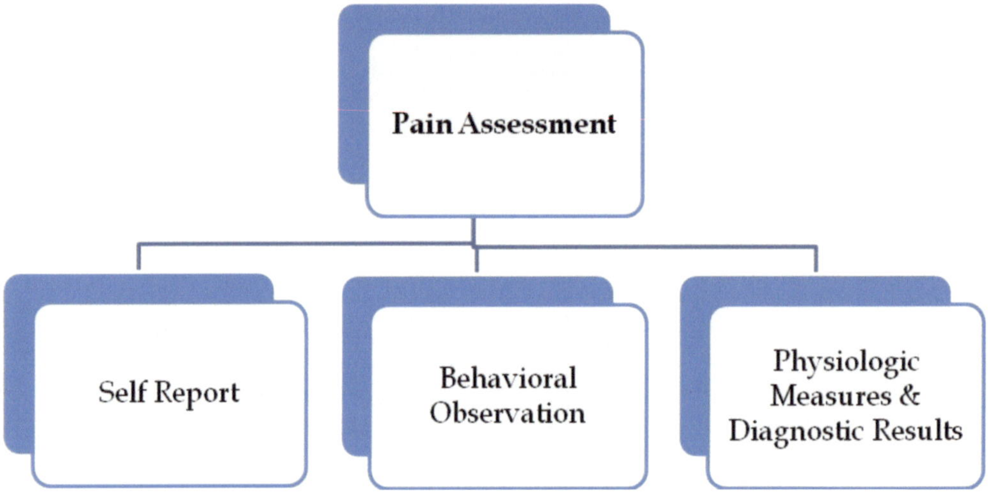

Fig. 2. Pain assesment stages (Hockenberry-Eaton et al., 1999)

The "ABCs" of pain assessment in children are:

- Assess: Always evaluate a child with cancer for potential pain. Children may experience pain, even though ther may be unable to expree the fact in words. Infans and toddlers can show their pain only by how they look and act: older children may deny their pain for fear of more painful treatment.
- Body: Be careful to consider pain as an integral part of the physical examination. Physical examination should include a comprehensive check of all body areas for potential pain sites. The child's reactions during the examination-grimacing, contracture, rigidity, etc.- may indicate pain.
- Context: Consider the impact of family, health-care, and environmental factors on the child's pain.
- Document: Record the severity of a child's pain on a regular basis. Use a pain scale that is simple and appropriate both for the developmental level of the child and fort he cultural context in which it is used.
- Evaluate: Assess the effectiveness of pain interventions regularly and modify the treatment plan as necessary, until the child's pain is alleviated or minimized.

Selection of method to be used for pain assessment in children should be made considering child's age, general status, pain recognition (Manworren&Hynan, 2003; Unuvar, 1999). Children show their pains in different ways according to age group. Newborn children move less than normal, cry more frequently and are highly restless, may look pale and sweaty when they have pain. They do not eat as much as they eat normally. They cry if they are touched or moved (Manworren&Hynan, 2003). Toddler; painful toddler may cry more than normal, is restless and moves less than normal like newborn children. Toddler may show location of the pain even though it may not state explicitly when she/he has pain. When toddlers are spoken about the pain, they may understand this. Do not think that you have known your child's pain location. In a study carried out, it is claimed that "FLACC" (Face ,Legs, Activity, Cry, Consolability) pain assessment scale which is conducted by assessing child's facial express, position of legs, movements, crying and being relieved is quite useful in paediatric nurse's assessing pain and pain approach in preverbal patients. In this study, patient's pains were graded with scores ranging between 0 to 10 by using "FLACC" score and the effects of oral and IV analgesics were evaluated. FLACC scores prior to use of analgesic drug were found significantly higher as compared to an assessment carried out subsequent to use of analgesic drug (Manworren&Hynan, 2003). Young children; young children think of their pains until they are able to speak. Child may be asked about the location of the pain. Child should be given help to find the location of the pain. Child might be asked to paint the location of the pain by showing him a picture as indicated below (Fig. 3).

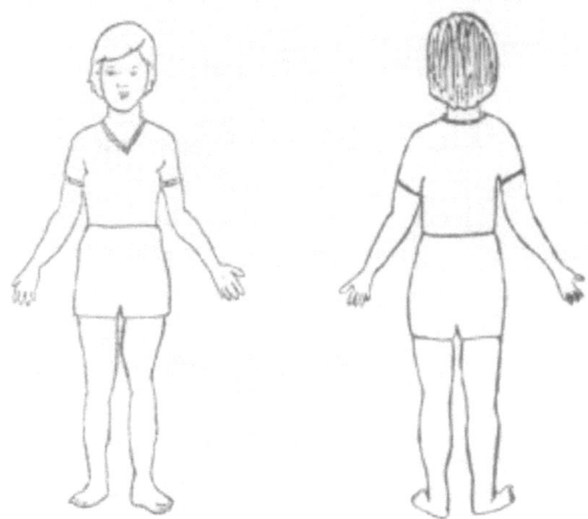

Fig. 3. Location of the pain in children

After determination of presence and location of the pain, it is required to determine the level of the pain. Pain might be measured with 3 different methods since it is subjective and individual (Fig. 2) (Unuvar, 1999). First of these methods is personal expressions. This method is the most important one in pain assessment which attempts to assess the cognitive component of the pain. It is necessary to know well the words which children use in describing the pain. The most frequently used method is face scale (Fig. 4) (Hockenberry-Eaton et al., 1999).

Pain Scale	**Descriptive**	**Recommended age**
FACES Pain Rating Scale	Consists of six cartoon faces ranging from a smiling face for "no pain" to tearful face for "worst pain"	Children as young as 3 years

0	**1**	**2**	**3**	**4**	**5**
No Hurt	**Hurts Little Bit**	**Hurts Little More**	**Hurts Even More**	**Hurts Whole Lot**	**Hurts Worst**

Fig. 4. Face scale (Hockenberry-Eaton et al., 1999)

The other methods depend on behaviour pattern (such as tone of voice, facial expression and gestures) and biological parameters (such as heart rate, falling of peripheral oxygen saturation). Personal expression is the best measurement method if can be obtained and is accepted as "golden rule" in pain measurement (Unuvar, 1999). Behavioral pain assessment scale for young children was given in the Table 4.

FLACC Scale Scoring			
Categories	0	1	2
Face	No particular expression or smile	Occasional grimace or frown, withdrawn, disinterested	Frequent to constant quivering chin, clenched jaw
Legs	Normal position or relaxed	Uneasy, restless, tense	Kicking, or legs drawn up
Activity	Lying quietly, normal position, moves easily	Squirming, shifting back and forth, tense	Arched, rigid or jerking
Cry	No cry (awake or asleep)	Moans or whinpers; occasional complaint	Crying steadily, screams or sobs, frequent complaints
Consolability	Content, relaxed	Reassured by occasional touching, hugging or being talked to, distractible	Difficult to console or comfort

Total is scored from 0-10.

Table 4. Behavioral pain assessment scales for young children (Hockenberry-Eaton et al., 1999)

Adolescents; adolescents give reactions similar to adults. They may look calm, have sleeping problems, loss of appetite, avoid from friends or family, be nervous or angry. They may not say when they have pain since they are afraid of getting addicted to narcotics. The best method determine the pain of adolescent patients is scales which have assessment criteria ranging 0 to 5 (0= presence of no pain, 5= presence of intense unbearable pain). Expression of pain according to age groups was given Table 5.

3. Pain control methods

The necessary nature of pain treatment has long been categorized among other basic human rights, and in 1999 the Joint Commission on Accreditation of Healthcare Organizations formalized pain standards to ensure to all patients their right to appropriate assessment and management of their pain, describing pain as the "fifth vital sign" (Lanser, 2001). Intrinsic to our capacity to treat pain is possession of perspective of themany cultural beliefs, philosophical ideologies, and scientific discoveries that have influenced and evolved into the modern Western conceptualization of pain. Cancer pain can not be treated sufficiently. In analysis of 11 reports including 2000 cancer patients in 1986, it was found that pains could not be healed in 50-80% of the patients in developed country. Pain may be healed with simple methods in 90% of cancer patients. However, it was also detected that pains could not be healed with acceptable methods in 10% of these patients. American National Cancer Institute attracted attention to be importance of issue with message that "being unable to treat cancer pain is a serious and unacceptable community health problem" (Aslan, 2006).

Developmental group	Expressions of pain
Infants	May: - Exhibit body rigidity or thrashing may include arching - Exhibit facial expression of pain (brows lowered and drawn together, eyes, tightly closed, mouth open ans squarish) - Cry intensely/loudly - Be inconsolable - Draw knees to chest - Exhibit hypersensitivity or irritability - Have poor oral intake - Be unable to sleep
Toddlers	May: - Be verbally aggressive, cry intensely - Exhibit regressive behavior or withdraw - Exhibit physical resistance by pushing painful stimulus away after it is applied - Guard painful area of body - Be unable to sleep
Preschoolers/ Young Children	May: - Verbalize intensity of pain - See pain as punishment - Exhibit thrashing of arms and legs - Attempt to push stimulus away before it is applied - Be uncooperative - Need physical restrain - Cling to parent, nurse, or significant other - Request emotional support (e.g. hugs, kisses) - Understand that there can be secondary gains associated with pain - Be unable to sleep
School-Age Children	May: - Verbalize pain - Use an objective measurement of pain - Be influenced by cultural belief - Experience nightmares related to pain - Exhibit stalling behaviors (e.g., "Wait a minute" or " I'm not ready") - Have muscular rigidity such as clenched first, white knuckles, gritted teeth, contracted limbs, body stiffness, closed eyes, or wrinkled forehead - Include all behaviors of preschoolers/young children - Be unable to sleep
Adolescents	May: - Localize and verbalize pain - Deny pain in presence of peers - Have changes in sleep patterns or appetite - Be influenced by cultural beliefs - Exhibit muscle tension and body control - Display regressive behavior in presence of family - Be unable to sleep

Table 5. Expression of pain in children

The WHO Analgesic Stepladder is a multi-step approach to treating pain, and is a guide for initiating analgesic drugs and dosages that correspond to the patient's reported level of pain (Fig. 5). The ladder starts with non-opioid oral drugs for mild pain and progresses to strong opioids, adjuvants and invasive therapies for severe and/or intractable pain (Hockenberry-Eaton et al., 1999).

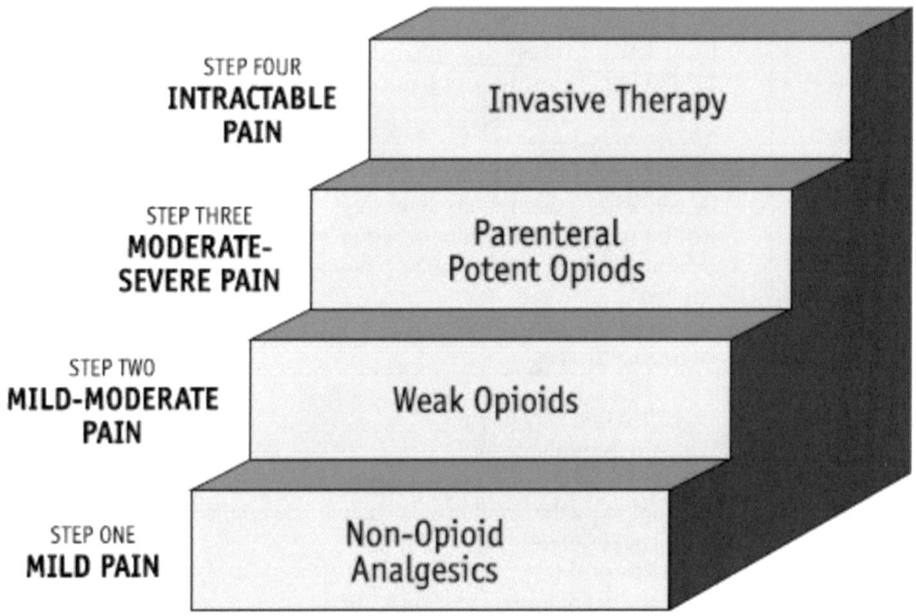

Fig. 5. Therpeutic ladder for pain management (Hockenberry-Eaton et al., 1999)

3.1 Pharmacological pain management

Western oncology group states that although cancer patients have taken analgesic, 67% of them have pain, 36% of them have so severe pains as to deteriorate their daily functions, 42% of them have not taken sufficient analgesic treatment. Tolerance and fear of addiction prevents cancer treatment (Aslan, 2006). While planning pain treatment, location, level, quality of pain, presence and features of the diseases causing pain, age of patient, present clinical facilities should be taken into consideration. In the light of all these features, treatment method is decided (Bedre& Sethna, 2002; Krauss& Gren, 2000). Drug treatment is the most frequently used method in treatment of acute and chronic pains in children. Analgesic drugs can be used singly or in a drug combination way (Golianu et al., 2000). For this purpose, non-opioid analgesics, opioid analgesics and adjuvant analgesics are used. In recent years, significant developments have been made in this field by adjustment of doses of these drugs and knowing their efficiency and pharmacologic differences in children. The most significant steps in this field have been taken by WHO. In consequence of studies concerning drug use especially in children with cancer pain, WHO published a guide book titled cancer pain treatment and palliative care (WHO, 1998). Medical management of cancer pain was given Fig. 6.

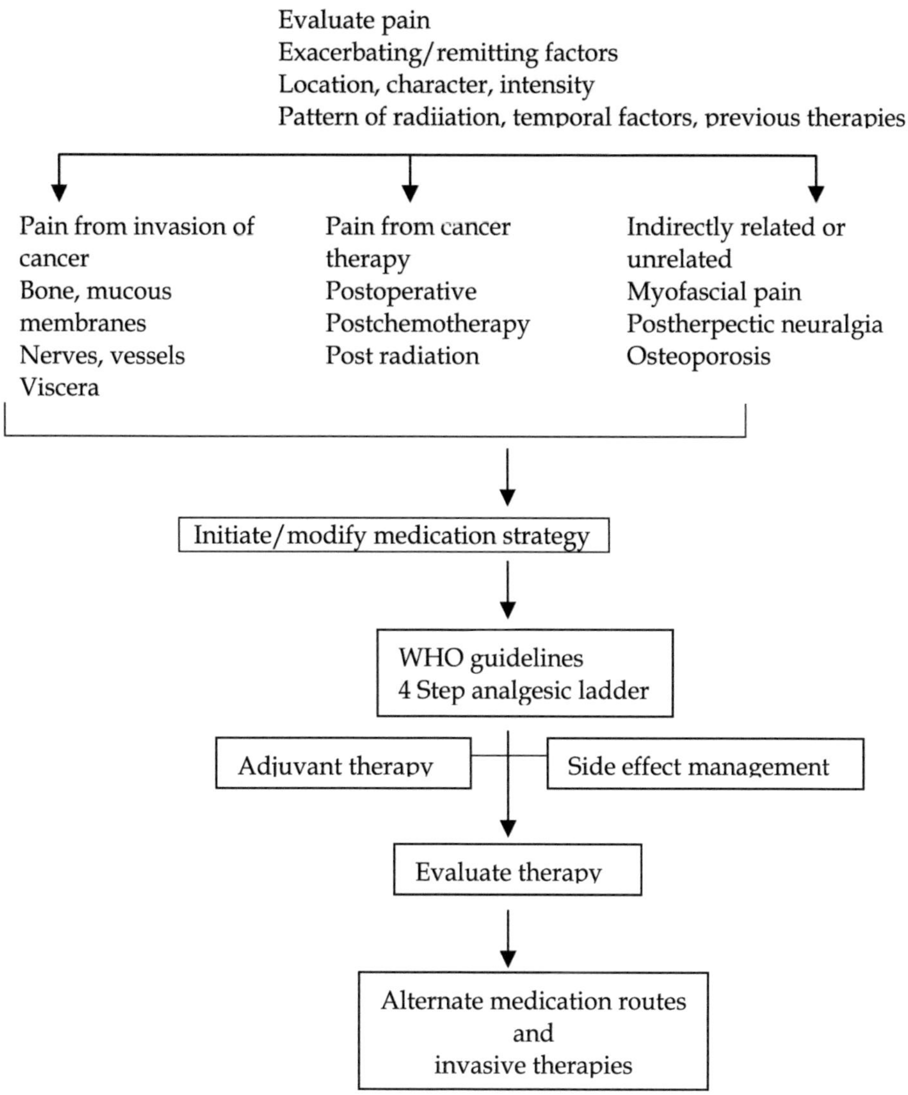

Fig. 6. Medical management of cancer pain (Gindrich, 2006)

3.1.1 Opioid (narcotic) analgesics

The word "opioid" contains all components associated with opium. Use of pure alkaloids has become widespread in whole world since second half of 19th century after Serturner isolated morphine from opium for the first time in 1806 (Cizmeci& Babacan, 2007). The first preference should be oral route in implementation of analgesic drugs, which is the first pain control method in algorithms used in treatment of chronic pains. Where oral intake is not possible, intravenous, intramuscular, subcutaneous, transdermal, intrathecal, or epidural route might be used (Golianu et al., 2000). Opioids are used for removal of severe pains. Opioids such as morphine, meperidine, methadone, fentanyl, codeine and hydromorphone are included in this group and are the most frequent used morphines. Gradually increasing doses might be needed in order to prevent pain due to tolerance occurring against opioids. Tolerance and development of addiction dependent on morphine use occur in children less than in adults. Morphine, intravenous, intramuscular are used with oral route, while nasal, intratecal are used with epidural route (Bedre& Sethna 2002).

The most commonly used 2 drugs;

- Morphine, given at 0,1 mg/kg IV 5-10 minutes before the procedure or 0,3 mg/kg orally 1 hour before the procedure.
- Fentanyl, 0.5-2 µg/kg given 5-10 minutes before the procedure.

The combined use of opioids and benzodiazepines should be evaluated for for efficacy and for any potential adverse effects at the peak of their action to guide subsequent titration (WHO, 1998). Schema related to using opiods was given Fig. 7.

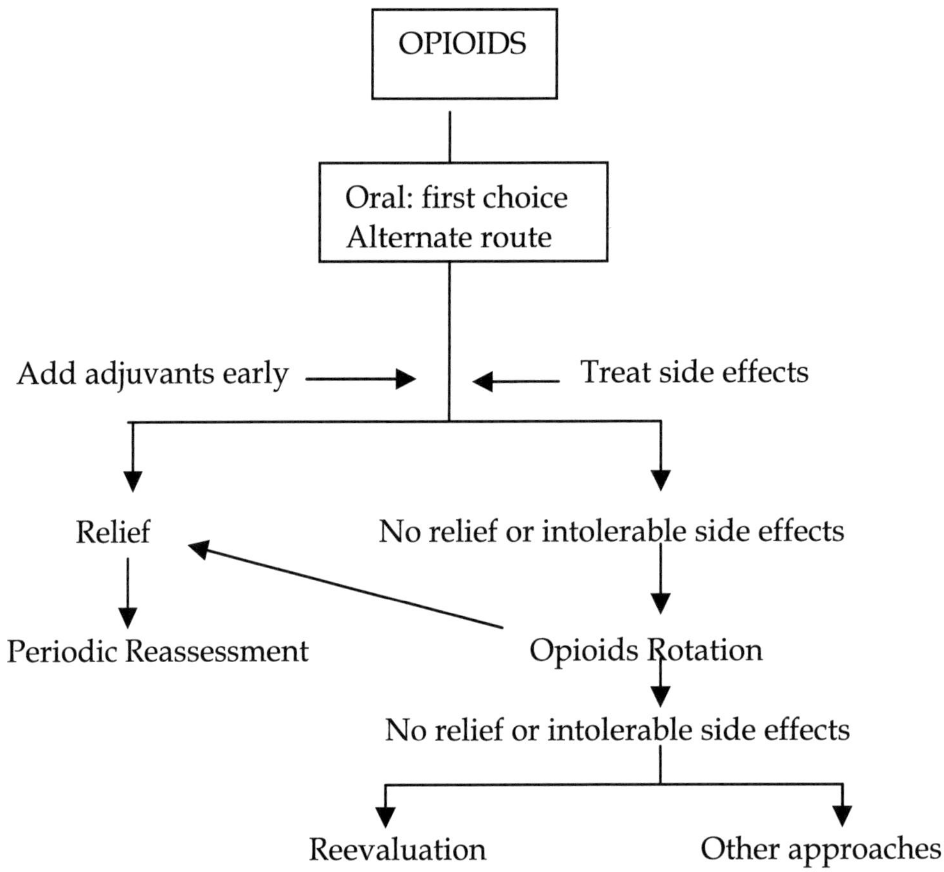

Fig. 7. Scheme of using opioid (Alanmanou, 2006a)

3.1.2 Non-opioid analgesics

Non-opioid analgesics are used singly in light pains or by combining with opioids in mild pains. The most frequent used non-opioids are paracetamol, aspirin and nonsteroid anti-inflammatory (Bedre&Sethna, 2002; Golianu et al., 2000). Pharmacodynamic and pharmacokinetic features of paracetamol, salicylates and nonsteroid anti-inflammatory drug (NSAID) in children are not different from adults except for neonatal period. Drug selection changes depending on various factors such as action time of drug, whether asked for anti-inflammatory effect or not, oral or IV route preference and adverse effects of drug. While majority of drugs in this group have both three of analgesic, antipyretic, anti-inflammatory effects, the others have just analgesic and antipyretic effects. Selections of analgesic are made in line with pain level according to step principle. According to WHO's three steps principle, nonsteroid anti-inflammatory drugs are given in light pains, weak opioids in addition to NSAIDs are given in mild pains, strong opioids are also given additionally in severe pains. Moreover, adjuvant drugs can be added in all steps (Eyigor et al., 2007). Schema related to using NSAIDs was given Fig. 8.

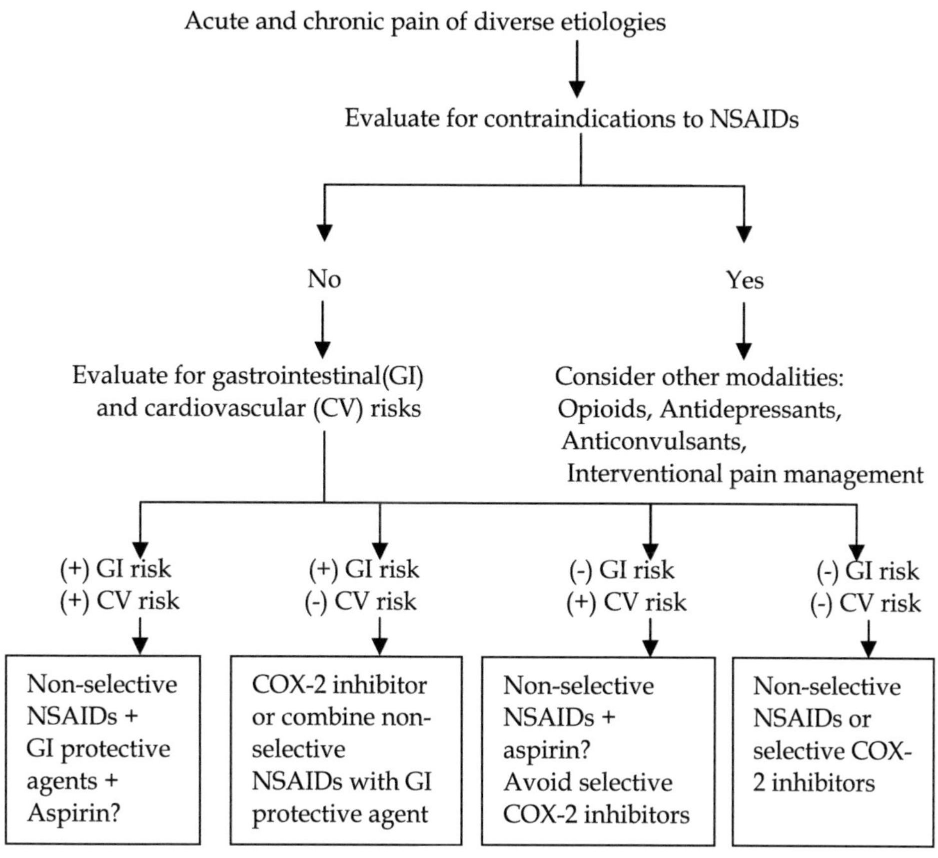

Fig. 8. Scheme of using nonsteroidal antiinflamatory drugs (Alanmanou, 2006b)

3.1.3 Adjuvant agents

Adjuvant analgesics are used for potantializing analgesic effects and improving symptoms accompanying pain. In this group, drugs such as anticonvulsants, antidepressants, oral local anesthetics, neuroleptics, myorelaxants, ntihistaminics, psychostimulants, corticosteroids and calcium channel blockers are used (Bedre&Sethna, 2002, Eyigör et al., 2007). Unless drugs are useful in removing pain in children, invasive attempts might be applied. The fundamental reason for childhood regional anaesthesia and analgesia implementations' not attracting attention might be listed as lack of experience in this field, adverse effect fear and not establishing dialog with the patient during attempt. Anatomical differences such as being different heights and anatomical structures of children during adolescence, extension of dura and spinal cord to lower segments in newborn children, being tight of epidural field, not yet completing of myelination following the birth, being thin of ligaments and fascias might lead to technical difficulties in regional implementations (Yaster&Hardart 2002; Desparment-Sheridan, 2000). Schema related to using steroids was given Fig. 9.

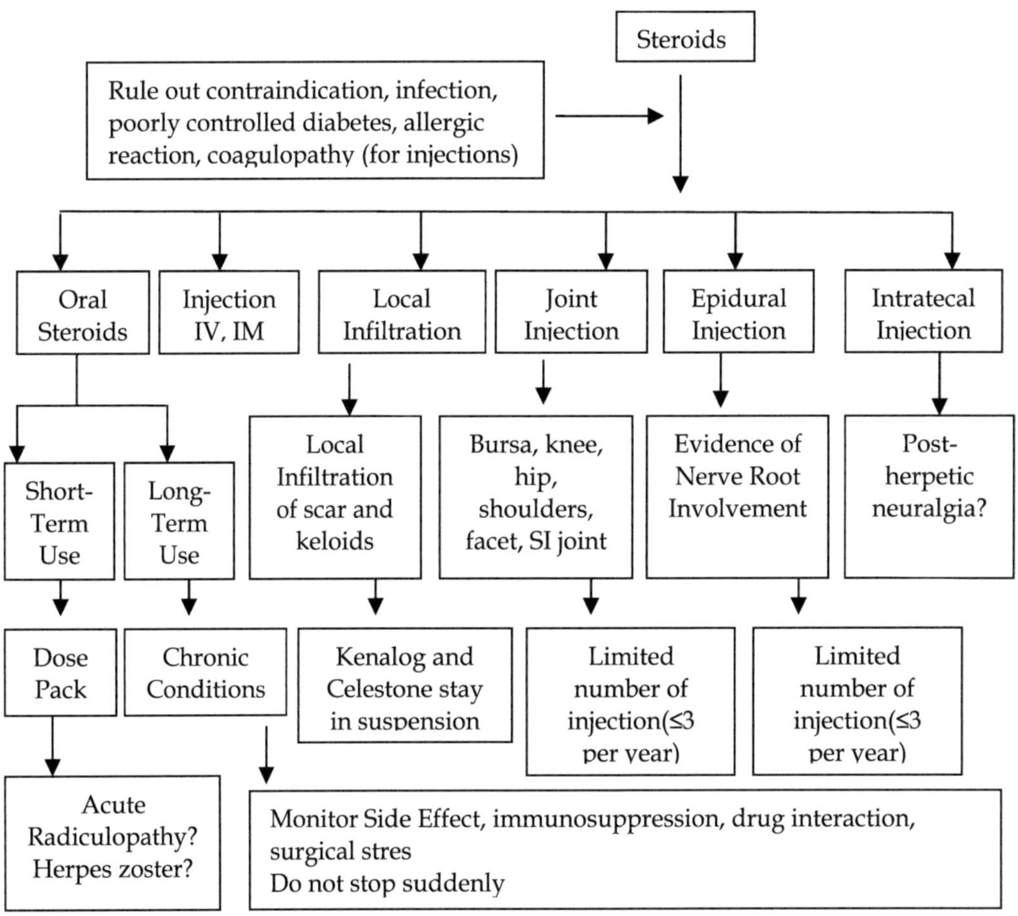

Fig. 9. Scheme of using steroids (Ramamurthy&Alanmanou, 2006)

In general, pain assessment and treatment steps were given in fig. 10.

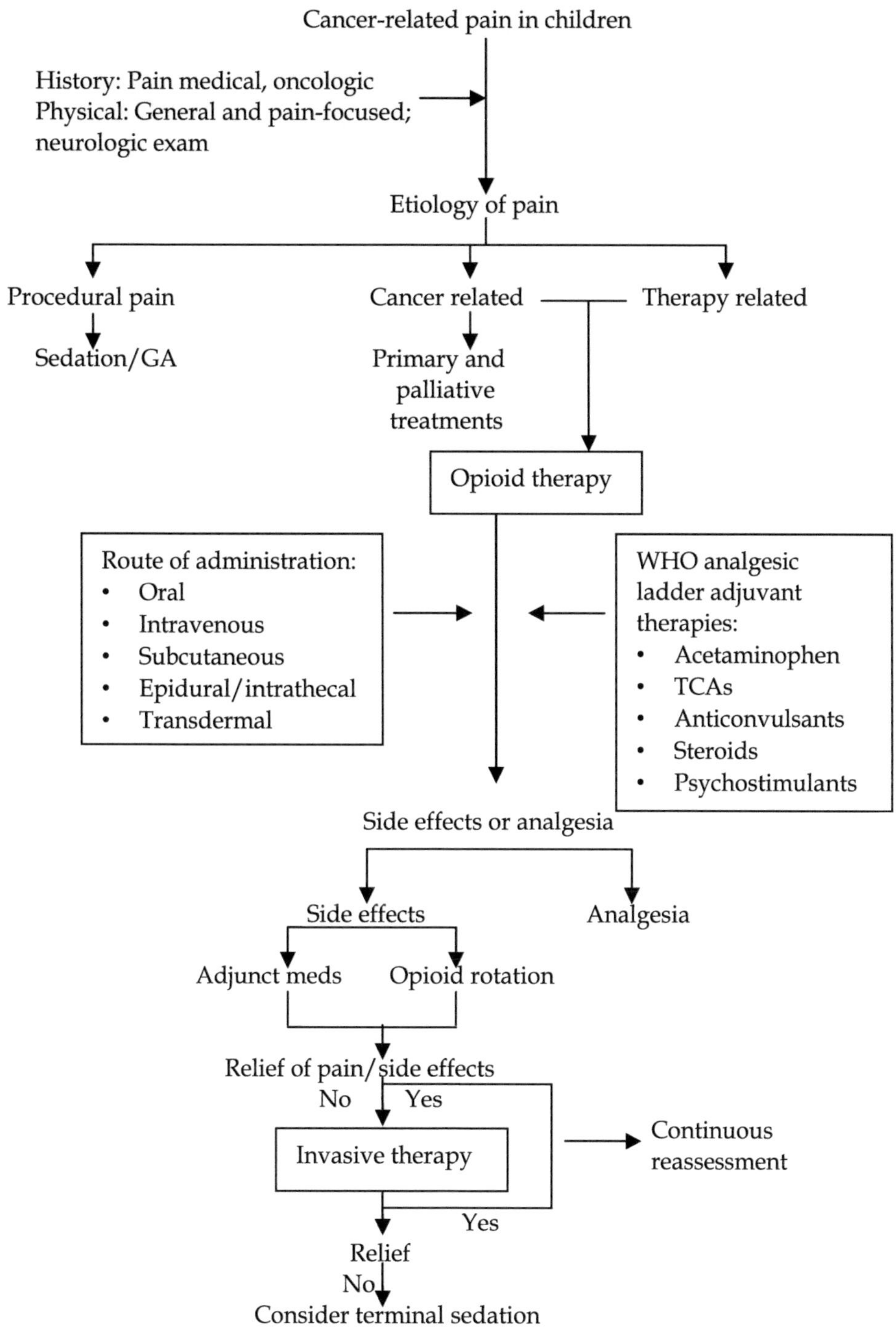

Fig. 10. Pain assessment and treatment practices (Weidner et al,. 2006)

3.2 Nonpharmacologic pain management

Nonpharmacologic methods must be integral part of the management of children's cancer pain, beginning at the time of diagnosis and continuing throughout treatment (WHO, 1998). Nonpharmacologic methods in the management of pain have been found to be highly effective for some children and for some procedures. These techniques are easy to learn and should be used when possible to give the child some control in the management of pain. The examples given for distraction, muscle relaxation, and guided imagery are easy techniques to learn and can be used with young children (Hockenberry-Eaton, M et al; 1999). Non-drug approaches should supplement, but not replace, appropriate drug treatment (Hockenberry-Eaton et al., 1999; WHO, 1998). In selection of nonpharmacologic method use, child's age, behavioral factors, coping ability, fear/anxiety and type of pain experience play role. Nonpharmacologic pain management implementations are divided into 4 groups as supportive, cognitive, behavioral and physical methods. In Table 6, non-pharmacologic methods used in relieving pain are summarized (WHO, 1998).

Supportive	**Cognitive**	**Behavioral**	**Physical**
Family-centre care	Distraction	Deep breathing	Touch
Information	Music	Relaxation	Heat and cold*
Empathy	Imagery		Transcutaneous electrical nerve stimulation (TENS)
Choices	Hypnosis		
Play			

*Heat and cold should not be used with infants because of the risk of injury

Table 6. Nonpharmacologic methods of pain relief (WHO 1998)

3.2.1 Supportive methods

Supportive methods are intended to promote the good psychosocial care of children. The first principle is that care is family-centered, that is, it is based on the needs of both family and child. Parental involvement in decision-making, and in providing comfort to children, is particularly important. Parents need a perceptive environment and they may require instruction in how best to help their child. The family includes everyone who is intimately associated with the child. In most cases it is the parents who know their children best and can therefore become allies in treatment, but they may need to be taught how they can help manage their children's pain and anxiety. Family centered care encourages them to choose how to participate in treatment, giving them culturally appropriate information and teaching them coping techniques. It also helps family members to understand the cultural, spiritual, financial, social, interpersonal, and emotional impact of the diagnosis of cancer in a child.Making the clinic or hospital environment friendly to families is another important aspect of family-centre care, and liberal visiting arrangements and a physical atmosphere conducive to family participation in treatment should be encouraged. It is essential that a child's family and friends are made to feel welcome. Both children and families need information to prepare them for what will happen during the course of the disease end its treatment. If families are not accurately informed about the diagnosis and the treatment plan, they cannot participate. Information is accepted best if it is tailored to the needs of the child and family. Some children and families seek out information; others may find that too much information increases their anxiety. Health care provides should therefore try to individualize their dealings with families. An empathic approach is essential, and information should be given a little at a time, repeated as frequently as needed. Booklets, videos, drawings, and dolls can be useful tools in this process. Children should never be lied to about painful procedures; they will distrust and fear what will be done to them in the future. Health-care workers must be genuinely fond of children and know how to deal with them. Ideally, children should be given choices about which techniques to use to control pain. They should be given choices about which techniques to use to control pain. They should also be allowed to make decisions that do not interfere with treatment, such as which finger to prick for blood samples. Play is an essential part of every child's daily life and even the sickest child can be helped to play. Playing enables children to understand their world and to relax and forget their worries. All children must therefore have the time and place to play, and painful procedures must not be carried out in play areas. Normal activities such as school, hobbies, and visits by friends should be encouraged. Psychosocial treatment is an integral part of cancer pain treatment. It should be used in all painful or potentially painful situations, often combined with analgesic drug therapy (WHO, 1998).

3.2.2 Cognitive methods

Cognitive treatment methods are intended to influence a child's thoughts and images. Parents are often very skilled at using these methods because they know their children's preferences (WHO, 1998). Distraction is used to focus the child's attention away from the pain (Hockenberry-Eaton, 1999). Active distraction of children's attention is important: the more involved a child becomes in an activity, the greater the distraction from pain (WHO, 1998). For children, simple distraction techniques can be very effective in decreasing pain (Hockenberry-Eaton, M 1999). Infants and young children require concrete events or objects to attract their attention; interesting toys that provide something to see, hear, and do are best. Older children benefit from concentrating on a game, conversation, or special story (WHO 1998). In studies conducted, it was reported virtual reality was useful in distracting attention in painful medical interventions and decreasing pain and distress and child's selection should be attached importance in implementation (Gershon et al., 2004, Nilsson et al., 2009). Music, even as simple as a mother's lullaby, is a universal soother and distractor (WHO, 1998). Listening to music is an important tool which decreases heart rate, body temperature, blood pressure and breathing rate, distracts patient's attention, lowers the nausea depending on chemotherapy and especially increases the life quality of the patients in terminal period (Chase, 2003; Deng et al., 2004; Halstead&Roscoe, 2002; Hiilliard, 2003; Kaminski&Hall, 1996; Mccaffery, 2000). In a study performed by Burns et al. (2001) on cancer patients, it was reported that well-being and relaxion increased in the patients in music listening process, and tension decreased. In the study carried out by Chan et al. (2003) on the patients to whom colposcopy was applied, pain and anxiety level of the group listening to music was found lower. Nguyen et al. (2010) found that pain score, heart and breathing rate were lower in the group listening to music during and after lumbar puncture implementation in children with cancer. Listening to music was found to increase endorphin secretion by inducing alpha wands and to play a role in not only decreasing the pain by creating a state of relaxion but also in decreasing blood pressure, heart rate and other physiological responses (Henry, 1995). It is also quite important that child selects his/her own music (Nilsson S et al. 2009). Moreover, there are studies concerning influence of the music belonging to children's own culture (Balan et al., 2009; Ngyen et al. 2010). Imagery is the process in which a child concentrates on the image of a pleasant and interesting experience instead of on the pain. A child can be helped by an adult to become absorbed in a previous positive experience or an imaginary situation or adventure. Colors, sounds, tastes, smells and atmosphere can all be experienced in imagination (WHO, 1998; Hockenberry-Eaton, 1999). Storytelling is a powerful way to engage the imagination and provide distraction; children may enjoy old favorites or new stories told from books or from memory (WHO, 1998). What should be taken into account in assisted imagining is not to use images causing fear and anxiety in patient (such as water, forest) (Black&Matassarin Jacobs, 1997). Children should be encouraged to use their imagination by their parents. In their studies in which Kuttner et al. (1988) compared medical treatment, occupation and imagination techniques under hypnosis during bone marrow aspiration, they found imagination method was more useful in children between 3-6, both occupation and imagination method was more effective in 7-10 group. Besides, it was determined that one or more sessions were required in order to learn coping abilities of the group to which occupation method was applied. Occupation methods which children may like according to their age groups are given in Table 7.

Age	Methods
0-2 years	Touching, stroking, patting, rocking, playing music, using mobiles over the crib
2-4 years	Puppet play, storytelling, reading books, breathing, blowing bubbles
4-6 years	Breathing, storytelling, puppet play, talking about favorite places, TV shows, activities
6-11 years	Music, breathing, counting, eye fixation, thumb squeezing, talking about favorite places, activities on TV shows, humor

Table 7. Distraction techniques in children (Hockenberry-Eaton, M 1999)

True hypnosis requires specialized training, but pain can be modified by words of comfort and relief spoken in a particular way. Firstly, a child should be encouraged to relax and focus attention on a favorite activity, on deep breathing, or on a pain-free part of the body. Children can also imagine they are closing pain "switches" or "gates" or that they have the "magical" powers of their popular heroes to make their pain become less (WHO, 1998). Hypnotic ability is limited in children younger than 3, they begin at 5-6 and climb up to the highest level at 7-14. In the study conducted by Liossi et al (2006) on pediatric cancer patients, it was found that hypnosis decreased pain and anxiety level of the patients (Liossi et al., 2006). However, there are many clinic researches and systemic reviews concerning efficiency of hypnosis in decreasing distress related to chemotherapy and interventions (lumbar puncture, bone marrow aspiration, venepuncture etc.) which cause pain in especially pediatric cancer patients (Accardi&Milling, 2009; Liossi et al., 2006, Liossi et al. 2009; Richardson et al., 2006; Rogovik&Goldman, 2007; Tsao&Zeltzer 2005; Zelter et al. 2001). Also, it was found that distress management implementations had useful and positive effect in coping with pain in the future (Rocha et al., 2009). Imagination scenes which children like are given in Table 8.

Visual Imagery	Auditory Imagery	Movement Imagery
Favorite places	Conversations with significant others	Flying
Animals	Favorite song	Swimming
Flower gardens	Playing a musical instrument	Skating
TV or movies	Listening to music	Amusement rides
Favorite room	Environmental sounds (waves, etc.)	Any activity
Favorite sport		

Table 8. Favorite imagery scenes for children (Hockenberry-Eaton, M 1999)

3.2.3 Behavioral methods

Deep breathing is a simple way to help a child to reduce pain and gain self-control. It focuses the attention, reduces muscular tension, relaxes the diaphragm, and oxygenates the body. It is best to start teaching this technique by asking the child to breathe out, and tol et go of the tension, or "scary" feelings, with each breath. Deep breathing is the easiest technique to use with young children. Younger children can be taught to breathe deeply by blowing bubbles from soap solution or by using party blowers (WHO, 1998). For school age children, asking them to hold their breath during a painful procedure transfers their focus to their breathing and not on the procedure (Hockenberry-Eaton, 1999). Older children can use more sophisticated breathing techniques such as breathing in and out, each fort he count of three (WHO, 1998). Muscle relaxation Muscle relaxation is used to decrease mental and physical tension. It is used most effectively in older children and adolescents because it involves the relaxation of voluntary skeletal muscles. Slowly each muscle is tensed and then relaxed in a systematic way. Attention is placed on breathing which causes the individual to be aware of the feelings of tension and relaxation (Hockenberry-Eaton, 1999). Relaxation is often combined with suggestion and deep breathing, and these methods can reduce anticipatory anxiety and help to reduce nausea and vomiting (Hockenberry-Eaton, 1999; WHO, 1998). In the study Anderson et al. (2006) carried out on cancer patients, it was found that less pain was suffered in the group to which relaxion technique was applied. Walco et al (2005) reported significant decrease in heart rate using cognitive-behavioral method in preventing procedural distress in children with cancer. In systemic reviews of Ellis&Spanos (1994), it was reported that cognitive-behavioral methods had critical importance in decreasing pain during painful procedures such as bone marrow aspiration and lumbar puncture. Cognitive-behavioral methods are the most frequently used methods to increase coping ability of the child and decrease children's distress in medical procedures (Collins et al., 2008).

3.2.4 Physical methods

Touch is important for all children, particularly the pre-verbal child, who understands the world to a large extent through touching and feeling. Touch must be appropriate for the child's needs, that is, not too invasive either physically or psychologically. Touching includes stroking, holding and rocking, caressing, massaging hands, back, feet, head, and stomach as well as swaddling. Vibration and tapping can also be comforting. When talking is too much effort for the child, touch can be the best form of communication. When a child must be touched for medical purposes, e.g. palpation of the abdomen, care must be taken to use warm hands, to proceed gently, and to talk quietly with the child about what is being done. Sources of heat and cold are often easily available. Ice wrapped in a cloth can be used to soothe disease pain or inflammation, or to reduce the pain of a procedure such as intramuscular injection. Heat is useful for muscle pain. However, neither cold nor heat should be used on infants because there is a risk of injury. The physical methods applied in removal of pain and their definitions are given in Table 9. Transcutaneous electrical nerve stimulation (TENS) is achieved with a battery-operated device that delivers electrical stimulation through electrodes placed on the skin. It possibly acts by cutaneous stimulation of large-diameter nerve fibres, reducing pain transmission at the spinal level. Children often experience TENS as tingling or tickling; it must not become painful. The technique is simple to use, is effective, and requires little preparation (WHO, 1998). Acupuncture has been used therapeutically in China for thousands of year, its importance in Europe and USA increases gradually. It was reported to be especially efficient in decreasing chemotherapy-related nausea/vomiting and cancer-related pain in the patients. However, number of studies carried out on pediatric patients is low (Hockenberry-Eaton, 1999; Jindal et al., 2008). In their study, Reindl et al. (2006) reported that acupuncture decreased the need of antiemetic treatment in preventing chemotherapy-related nausea in pediatric patients.. It is recommended to apply acupuncture with methods such as hypnosis and massage (Jindal et al 2008). Zelter et al (2002) applied hypnotherapy with acupuncture to children with chronic pain their study and reported no adverse effect, on the contrary parents and children reported significant improvements concerning pain and treatment. However, since there was no control group available in the study, efficiency of acupuncture / hypnotherapy was not specified.

Comfort Measure	Description
Massage	Includes stroking, rubbing or deep manipulation of muscles.
Music	Can help to provide the child with a familiar environment; children often come to the hospital or hospice with their own music.
Heat	Warm compress or use of a heating pad, to the painful site (moist or dry heat).
Cold/Ice	Cold compress or ice pack. Precaution: assure ice pack is wrapped allowing comfortable sensation of cold without damaging the skin by freezing tissue. Limit ice application to10 minutes, then rotate site. If skin becomes blanched, discontinue cold treatment.

Table 9. Comfort measures (Hockenberry-Eaton, M 1999)

4. Nursing approach

As in all the other fields of pediatrics, supportive methods have indisputable importance in pediatric oncology. Family-centered care which is the fundamental element of supportive methods forms the integrative role of pediatric nursing. Parents should be encouraged to participate in care of their children at hospital in accordance with their readiness so that family-centered care implementations can be carried out and the care given should be controlled. Nurse training and consultancy roles should be used effectively. Parents should be allowed to ask question so that they could understand the diagnosis and treatment methods applied to their children and parents' opinion should be asked in decisions related to child's treatment. In this regard, nurse should encourage the parents to ask question and be open in communication with them. Pediatric nurse is responsible for training the parents about the care of the child. It is important that such training continues until child is discharged from the hospital. Nurse should make sure that family has gained the knowledge and skills required in respect of child's care and do these correctly. Nurse should prepare the parents about care of child at home by ensuring parents' participation in care and controlling the care they give at hospital (Boztepe, 2009). Nurses should conduct proper assessment and treatment of the pain which is a necessary part of children's care for optimal treatment of the child with pain. The pain which is not treated or taken under control might lead to long-term chronic pain. Having limited knowledge about effective assessment and treatment options might be a reason for being unable to take the pain under control. However, attitude, belief and previous experiences may affect their decisions. Nurses should spare time for themselves in order to equip themselves with up-to-date knowledge concerning assessment and treatment of the pain (Clark, 2011). Nurses play a critical role in efficient pain management of the patient. Nurse should permanently inform the patient and patient's family about pain management methods. They should be encouraged to participate in efficient pain management and trained about how pain management and methods to increase their life qualities will be (Williams, 2011). Also, nurses should ensure inclusion of effective behavioral methods in routine care of the children with cancer (McCarthy et al., 1996). Pain is a subjective experience and each and every child should be treated as an individual. Multimodal approach (together with pharmacologic and nonpharmacologic pain management) is the best way to optimize pain control with least negative effects. Even the smallest children deserve ensuring the best pain control in a safe manner (Clark, 2011).

5. References

Accardi, M.&Milling L.S. (2009) The effectiveness of hypnosis for reducing procedure-related pain in children and adolescents: a comprehensive methodological review. *Journal of Behavioral Medicine*, Aug;32(4), pp. 328-39. ISSN (printed): 0160-7715.

Alanmanou, E. (2006a). Opioids. In: *Decision making in pain management.* Somayaji Ramamurthy, Euleche Alanmanou, James Rogers, (Ed.). pp. 255, 2nd Edition, Elsevier Mosby, ISBN 13: 978-0-323-01974-3

Alanmanou, E. (2006b). Nonsteroidal antiinflamatory drugs. In: *Decision making in pain management.* Somayaji Ramamurthy, Euleche Alanmanou, James Rogers, (Ed.). pp. 247, 2nd Edition, Elsevier Mosby, ISBN 13: 978-0-323-01974-3

Anderson, K.O., Cohen, M.Z., Mendoza, T.R., Guo, H., Harle, M.T. et al. (2006). Brief cognitive-behavioral audiotape interventions for cancer-related pain: Immediate but not long-term effectiveness. *Cancer*, 107(1), pp.207-214, ISSN 1097-0142

Aslan, F.E. (2006). Tarihsel Süreçte Ağrı. In: *Ağrı, doğası ve kontrolü*. Fatma Eti Aslan (Ed.). Avrupa Tıp Kitapcılık Ltd. Şti, pp. 3-9, ISBN 975-6257-17-2, İstanbul

Balan, R., Bavdekar, S. B., & Jadhav, S. (2009). Can Indian classical instrumental music reduce pain felt during venepuncture? *Indian Journal of Pediatrics, 76*, pp. 469-473. ISSN 0019-5456

Bedre, C.B. & Sethna, N.F.(2000). Analgesics for the treatment of pain in children. *The New England Journal of Medicine* Vol. 347, pp. 1094- 1103 ISSN 0028-4793

Bial, E. & Cope, D.K. (2011). Introduction to pain management, historical perspectives, and careers in pain management. In: . In: . *Essentials of pain management.* Naili Vadivelu, Richard D. Urman & Roberta L. Hines (Ed.). Springer Science+Business Media. pp. 3-7, ISBN 978-0-387-87578-1 New York.

Black, J.M.&Matassarin Jacobs, E. (1997). Pain, In: *Medical Surgical Nursing: clinical management for continuity of care,* Thomas Eoyang (Ed) 5. edition, W.B. Saunders Company, pp: 342-365, ISBN 9780721663999, Philadelphia

Boztepe, H. (2009), Family Centered Care in Pediatric Nursing: Review, *Turkiye Klinikleri Journal of Nursing,* 1(2). pp. 88-93, ISSN: 1308-092X

Bucher, J.A., Trostle, G.B. & Moore, M. (1999). Family reports of cancer pain, pain relief, and prescription access. *Cancer Practice,* Vol. 7, No.2, pp.71–77, ISSN 1065-4704

Burns, S.J.I., Harbuz, M.S., Hucklebridge, F. & Bunt, L. (2001). A pilot study into the therapeutic effects of music therapy at a cancer help center, *Alternative Therapies in Health and Medicine,* 7(1), pp. 48-56. ISSN 1078- 6791

Chan, Y.M., Lee, P.W., Ng TY Ngan, H.Y.&Wong, L.C. (2003). The use of music to reduce anxiety for patients undergoing colposcopy: a randomized trial, *Gynecologic Oncology,* 9(1), pp. 213-217. ISSN 0090-8258

Chase, K.M. (2003). Multicultural music therapy: a review of literature, *Music Therapy Perspectives,* 21(2), pp. 84-88. ISSN: 0734-6875.

Chiu, T.Y.; Hu, W.Y. & Chen, C.Y. (2000). Prevalence and severity of symptoms in terminal cancer patients: a study in Taiwan. *Support Care in Cancer,* Vol. 8, No.4, pp. 311–313, ISSN 0941-4355

Cizmeci, P. & Babacan, A.(2007). Analjezikler ve Analjezik Kullanım İlkeleri. *Clinic Medicine.* (Pain Special Issue -2), pp. 9-14

Clark, L, (2011) Pain management in the pediatric population, *Critical Care Nursing Clinics of North America*is 23, pp. 291–301

Collins, J.J., Stevens, M.M., Berde, C.B. (2008) Pediatric cancer pain, In: *Clinical Pain Management, Cancer Pain,* Andrew Rice (Ed) 2nd edition, Hodder & Stoughton Limited, pp: 345-355, London

Dedeli, Ö. & Karadeniz, G. (2009). Kanser ağrısının kontrolü ile psikososyal-spiritüel modelin birleştirilmesi, *Ağrı,* Vol. 21, No. 2, pp. 45-53, ISSN 1300-0012

Deng, G., Cassileth, B.R. & Yeung, K.S. (2004). Complementary therapies for cancer-related symptoms, *Journal of Support Oncology,* 2(5), pp. 427-429.

Desparmet- Sheridan, J.F. (2000). Pain in Children, In: *Practical Management of Pain,* PP Raj (Ed.), Mosby, ABD, pp. 295-315

Eidelman, A. & Carr, D.B. (2006). Taxonomy of Cancer Pain. In: *Cancer Pain: Pharmacologic, intervention, and palliative approaches.* De Leon-Casasola, O.A. (Ed.). Elsevier Inc. pp. 3-6

Ellis, J.A. & Spanos, N.P. (1994). Cognitive-behavioral interventions for children's distress during bone marrow aspirations and lumbar punctures: a critical review. *Journal of Pain and Symptom Management,* Feb;9(2), pp. 96-108. ISSN: 0885-3924

Eyigör, C.; Pirim, A. & Uyar, M. (2007). Çocuklarda Ağrı Tedavisi. *Clinic Medicine.* (Pain Special Issue -2), pp. 15-22.

Gershon, J., Zimand, E., Pickering, M., Rothbaum, B.O., & Hodges, L. (2004). A pilot and feasibility study of virtual reality as a distraction for children with cancer. *Journal of the American Academy of Child and Adolescent Psychiatry,* Oct;43(10), pp. 1243-9 ISSN:0890-8567

Gingrich, T. (2006). Medical management of cancer pain. In: *Decision making in pain management.* Somayaji Ramamurthy, Euleche Alanmanou, James Rogers, (Ed.). pp. 127, 2nd Edition, Elsevier Mosby, ISBN 13: 978-0-323-01974-3

Golianu, B., Krane, E.J., Galloway, K.S. & Yaster, M. (2000). Pediatric acute pain management. *Pediatric Clinics of North America,* Vol.47, No.3, pp. 559-587, ISSN 0031-3955

Halstead, M.T. ve Roscoe, S.T. (2002). Restoring the spirit at the and of life: music as an intervention for oncology nurses, *Clinical Journal of Oncol Nursing,* 6(6), pp. 332- 336. ISSN: 1462-3889

Helms, J.M. (1998). An overview of medical acupuncture. *Altern Ther.* (May). Vol. 4, No.3 , pp. 32-45

Henry, L.L. (1995). Music therapy: a nursing intervention for the control of pain and anxiety in the ICU: a review of the research literature, *Dimension Critical Care Nursing,* 14(6), pp. 295-304, ISSN: 1538-8646

Higginson, I.J. & Murtagh, F. (2010). Cancer pain epidemiology. In: *Cancer Pain Assessment and Management.* Eduardo D. Bruera, Russell K. Portenoy (Ed.). Second edition. Cambridge University Press. pp. 37-52, ISBN 0 521 77332 6, USA

Hiilliard, R.E. (2003). The effect of music therapy on the quality and length of life people diagnosed with terminal cancer, *Journal of Music Therapy,* 40(2), pp. 113-117. ISSN: 0022-2917

Hockenberry-Eaton, M.; Barrera, P.; Brown, M.; Bottomley, S.J. & O'Neill, J.B. (1999). *Pain management in children with cancer.* Texas Cancer Council. pp. 9-25, 50-54, Texas

Jindal, V., Ge, A.,&Mansky, P.J. (2008). Safety and Efficacy of Acupuncture in Children A Review of the Evidence. *Journal of Pediatric Hematology/ Oncology.* June; 30(6), pp. 431–442. ISSN: 1077-4114

Kaminski, J. & Hall, W. (1996). The effect of soothing music on neonatal behavioral states in the hospital newborn nursery, *Neonatal Network,* 25(1), pp. 45-54. ISSN 0730-0832

Krauss, B. & Gren, S.M. (2000). Sedation and analgesia for procedures in children. The *New England Journal of Medicine.* Vol. 342:, pp. 938-945, ISSN 0028-4793

Kuttner, L., Bowman, M. & Teasdale, M. (1988). Psychological treatment of distress, pain, and anxiety for young children with cancer. *Journal of Developmental and Behavioral Pediatrics.* 9, pp. 374–81.

Liossi, C., White, P. & Hatira, P. (2006). Randomized clinical trial of local anesthetic versus a combination of local anesthetic with self-hypnosis in the management of pediatric procedure-related pain. *Health Psychology,* 25(3), pp. 307-315.

Liossi, C., White, P. & Hatira, P. (2009). A randomized clinical trial of a brief hypnosis intervention to control venepuncture-related pain of paediatric cancer patients. *Pain*. Apr;142(3), pp. 255-63

Manworren , R.C.B. & Hynan, L.S. (2003). Clinical Validation of FLACC: Preverbal patient pain scale. *Pediatric Nursing*, Vol.29, pp. 140-146. ISSN 1744-6155

Mccaffery, R.G. (2000). The lived experience of listening to music while recovering from surgery. *Journal of Holistic Nursing*, 18(4), pp. 378-390. ISSN 0898-0101

McCarthy, A.M., Cool, V.A., Petersen, M., & Bruene, D.A. (1996). Cognitive behavioral pain and anxiety interventions in pediatric oncology centers and bone marrow transplant units. *Journal of Pediatric Oncology Nursing*. Jan;13(1), pp. 3-12; discussion 13-4. ISSN 1043-4542

McGrath, P.A. & Crawford, E.J. (2010). Evaluating pain for children with cancer. . In: *Cancer Pain Assessment and Management*. Eduardo D. Bruera, Russell K. Portenoy (Ed.). Second edition. Cambridge University Press. pp. 131, ISBN 0 521 77332 6, USA

Mirchandani, A., Saleeb, M. & Sinatra, R. (2011). Acute and Chronic Mechanisms of Pain. In: *Essentials of pain management*. Nalini Vadivelu, Richard D. Urman, & Roberta L. Hines, (Ed.). Springer Science+Business Media. pp. 45-48, ISBN 9780387875781, New York

Nguyen, T.N., Nilsson, S., Hellström, A.L., & Bengtson, A. (2010). Music therapy to reduce painand anxiety in children with cancer undergoing lumbar puncture: A randomized clinical trial, *Journal of Pediatric Oncology Nursing*, 27, pp. 146-155, ISSN 1043-4542

Nilsson, S., Finnstrom, B., Kokinsky, E., & Enskar, K. (2009). The use of virtual reality for needle-related procedural pain and distress in children and adolescents in a paediatric oncology unit. *European Journal of Oncology Nursing, 13*, pp. 102-109, ISSN 1462-3889

Nilsson, S., Kokinsky, E., Nilsson, U., Sidenvall, B., & Enskar, K. (2009). School-aged children's experiences of postoperative music medicine on pain, distress, and anxiety. *Paediatric Anaesthesia*, 19, pp. 1184-1190. ISSN 1155-5645

O'leary, N.; Stone, C. & Lawlor, P.G. (2010). Multidimensional assessment: pain and palliative care. . In: *Cancer Pain Assessment and Management*. Eduardo D. Bruera, Russell K. Portenoy (Ed.). Second edition. Cambridge University Press. pp. 110, ISBN 0 521 77332 6, USA

Plotnick, A.B., & O'Grady G.J. (1991). Hypnotic responsiveness in children. In: *Clinical hypnosis with children*, William C. Wester, Donald J. O'Grady (Ed), Brunner/Mazel, pp. 19-33. New York

Portenoy, R.K. & Kanner, R.M. (1996). Definition and assessment of pain. In: *Pain management: Theory and Practice*. F.A. Davis (Ed.). Company, Philadelphia, pp. 3-17

Potter, J., Hami, F., Bryan, T. & Quigley, C. (2003). Symptoms in 400 patients referred to palliative care services: prevalence and patterns. *Journal of Palliative Medicine*, Vol.17, pp. 310–314, ISSN 1096-6218

Ramamurthy, S. & Alanmanou, E. (2006). Steroids. In: *Decision making in pain management*. Somayaji Ramamurthy, Euleche Alanmanou, James Rogers, (Ed.). pp. 249, 2nd Edition, Elsevier Mosby, ISBN 13: 978-0-323-01974-3

Reindl, T., Geilen, W., Hartmann, R., Wiebelitz, K.R., Kan, G., Wilhelm, I., Lugauer, S., Behrens, C., Wieberlenn, T., Hasan, C., Gottschling, S., Wild-Bergner, T., Henze, G., & Driever, P.H. (2006). Acupuncture against chemotherapy-induced nausea and vomiting in pediatric oncology. Interim results of a multicenter crossover study. *Support Care in Cancer,* 14, pp. 172–176. ISSN 1433-7339

Richardson, J., Smith, J.E., McCall, G., & Pilkington, K. (2006). Hypnosis for procedure-related pain and distress in pediatric cancer patients: a systematic review of effectiveness and methodology related to hypnosis interventions. *Journal of Pain and Symptom Management.* 31, pp. 70–84. ISSN 0885-3924

Rocha, E. M., Marche, T. A., & von Baeyer, C.L. (2009). Anxiety influences children's memory for procedural pain. *Pain Research & Management, 14*(3), pp. 233–237. ISSN 1203-6765

Rogovik, A.L. & Goldman, R.D. (2007). Hypnosis for treatment of pain in children, *Canadian Family Physician,* 53, pp. 823-25, ISSN: 0008-350X

Steggles, S., Damore-Petingola, S., Maxwell, J. & Lightfoot, N. (1997). Hypnosis for children and adolescents with cancer: an annotated bibliography, 1985–1995. *American Journal of Clinical Hypnosis.* 39, pp. 187–200, ISSN 0002-9157

Tranmer, J.E., Heyland, D., Dudgeon, D., Groll, D., Squires-Graham, M. & Coulson, K. (2003) Measuring the symptom experience of seriously ill cancer and noncancer hospitalized patients near the end of life with the Memorial Symptom Assessment Scale. *Journal of Pain and Symptom Management,* Vol. 25, No.5, pp. 420–429, ISSN 0885-3924

Tsao, J.C.I. & Zeltzer, L.K (2005). Complementary and Alternative Medicine Approaches for Pediatric Pain: A Review of the State-of-the-science, *Evidence-Based Complementary and Alternative Medicine (eCAM),* 2(2), pp. 149–159

Unuvar, A. (2009). Ağrı. In: *Pediatrik Onkoloji.* Alp Özkan (Ed.). Nobel Medical Kitabevleri. pp. 1267-1271, ISBN 9789754206630, İstanbul

Walko, G.A., Conte, P.M., Labay, L.E., Engel, R., & Zeltzer LK, (2005) Procedural distress in children with cancer: self-report, behavioral observations, and physiological parameters. *The Clinical Journal of Pain.* 21(6), pp. 484-90, ISSN 1536-5409

Weidner, N.J.; Goldschneider, K.R. & Varughese ,A.M. (2006). Cancer-Related Pain in Children. In: *Decision making in pain management.* Somayaji Ramamurthy, Euleche Alanmanou, James Rogers, (Ed.). pp. 235, 2nd Edition, Elsevier Mosby, ISBN 13: 978-0-323-01974-3

Williams, E. (2011). Nursing perspective on pain management, In: *Essentials of pain management.* Nalini Vadivelu, Richard D. Urman, & Roberta L. Hines, (Ed.). Springer Science+Business Media. pp. 374, ISBN 9780387875781, New York

World Health Organization (1998), Cancer Pain Relief and Palliative Care in Children, Geneva, pp:18-22

Yaster, M. & Hardart, R.A. (2002). Pediatric pain management. In: *Text book of Regional Anesthesia.* P. Prithvi Raj (Ed.). Churchill Livingstone, pp. 1009-1032. ABD

Yun, Y.H., Heo, D.S., Lee, I.G., Jeong, H.S., Kim, H.J., Kim, S., Kim, Y.H., Ro, Y.J., Yoon, S.S., Lee, K.H. & Huh, B.Y. (2003). Multicenter study of pain and its management in patients with advanced cancer in Korea. *Journal of Pain and Symptom Management,* Vol.25, No.5, pp. 430–437, ISSN 0885-3924

Zeltzer, L.K., Dolgin, M.J., LeBaron, S., & LeBaron, C. (1991). A randomized, controlled study of behavioral intervention for chemotherapy distress in children with cancer. *Pediatrics.* 88, pp. 34–42. ISSN 0031-4005

Zeltzer, L.K., Tsao, J.C.I., Stelling, C., Powers, M., Levy, S., & Waterhouse, M. (2002). A phase I study on the feasibility of an acupuncture/hypnotherapy intervention for chronic pediatric pain. *Journal of Pain and Symptom Management,* 24, pp. 437–46. , ISSN 0885-3924

7

Snake Bites in Pediatric Patients, a Current View

M.E. De la O. Cavazos, C. Treviño Garza, G. Guajardo-Rodríguez, B.A. Hernández-Montelongo and F.F. Montes-Tapia
Hospital Universitario "Dr. José Eleuterio González"
Facultad de Medicina UANL,
México

1. Introduction

It has been estimated that worldwide about 5 million people (adults and children) are bitten by snakes every year (Kalantri et al., 2006), and 50,000 die according to data from the World Health Organization (Schaper, de Haro, Desel, Ebbecke, & Langer, 2004). However, it is well known that events related to snake bites are under-reported, especially in the author's country possibly because snakebites are not a very relevant cause of mortality. Nevertheless, they are a serious cause of morbidity, especially in children. Under-reporting of this important health issue can be blamed on the fact that the population is not well informed about snake classification causing them to not provide accurate information to healthcare personnel when a patient is taken for medical care after a snake attack. Children do not react to snake bites in the same way as adults. In children, this event is always more severe since they are exposed to a larger amount of venom per m^2 of body surface (De la O Cavazos 2006). A small child is more vulnerable to a given volume of venom than a larger individual (Hodge III & Tecklenburg, 2006) Also, there will be different presentations including neurotoxicity, myotoxicity, renal failure, edema, bleeding due to activation of clotting proteins, and intravascular hemolysis, because different kinds of snakes have different types of venom that cause different symptomatology. (Jeng & Glader, 2004).

On the other hand, there is very little information for primary care physicians and pediatricians and most of the time it is outdated. Hence, the need for a reliable source of information in the event of a snake bite in pediatric patients that is updated, easy to find and well-structured in a way physicians find it easy to read and to easily and rapidly translate it into clinical practice to assure a fact-based, accurate treatment and prompt recovery with the least possible amount of sequels.

2. Epidemiology

Snakebites are seriously under-reported all over the world. We currently do not have trustworthy studies or statistics to asses this problem. What we do have is information that can guide us and inform us about the most affected areas and the most common presentation. For example, studies such as the one by Ruiz Molina and cols. show not only a higher incidence in men (2.5:1) but also a reasonably high incidence in pediatric population between the ages of 11 and 16 (39.3%), followed closely by even younger children ages of 6-10 (32.1%). This may be related to the fact that in several under-developed tropical countries where snakebites represent a major health issue children take part in agricultural activities or are attacked due to their innate curiosity, which in turn, makes them victims more easily than adults. Snake bites remain a public health problem in most countries. This is especially true in countries where agricultural activities are predominant, since this is one of the occupations more often affected by snakebites (Chippaux, 1998). Once we get hold of he few statistics we have, we face a new problem: the disparity in the epidemiological data. This reflects different grades of reporting. The more industrialized the country, the more reliable the statistics are. Sadly, snake bites are a problem related to low-income countries that have frail health systems and a lower rate of reporting. Also, morbidity and mortality have low rates and are well documented in first-world countries, probably because of the health facilities and availability of newer and better treatments. This is yet another argument to sustain that snake envenoming is a disease of the underdeveloped countries. In the few studies we can relate to, a negative association between snakebite deaths and government expenditure on health services has been found. Because of this, mortality is highest in these countries, since the population has no access to proper and adequate treatment and the government is not able to provide it because they are just not capable of dealing with the financial burden of snakebites (Harrison, Hargreaves, Wagstaff, Faragher, & Lalloo, 2009).

In México, an average of 20 deaths per year are reported. However, very few accidents are reported in communities most at risk. These communities also have little access to health services. In fact, about 27 000 cases of snake envenomation and more than 100 deaths per year occur in México. Between 1994 and 1996, the Mexican Social Security Institute (IMSS) reported 1 961 venomous snake bites; thirty percent of patients were children. In the IMSS report, the age group most affected was 15 to 44 years, with 51.4% of cases. The immense majority of poisonings occurred between June and October and 70-90% of these bites were located in the legs.

Area of the Body Involved	Frequency (%)
Foot and Ankle	72
Thigh	14
Hand	13
Head	10

Table 1. Areas most commonly involved in snakebites.

For years, it has been accepted that snake attacks occur in the field and men are the most affected, but in the study by Sotelo-Cruz it was found that there is no predominance in gender and while it is true that most of the children attacked were from rural areas, these attacks occured nearby their living places in some cases even within their home. The seasons of the year when more attacks were reported were summer and autumn. This is because the summer season in these countries lasts nearly six months. The time of day when most of the attacks happened ranges from 2:00 and 7:00 p.m., although 12.7% of the attacks happened during the night, the injury site was located in the legs in 78.1% of cases (Sotelo 2004).

3. Snake identification

In the world there are over 2,500 snake species described, of these, only about 350 are considered poisonous and dangerous for humans. These 2,500 snake species are divided into 15 families and the following have enough species to be relevant or dangerous (Government of Canada, n.d.): Colubridae, Boidae, Viperidae, and Elapidae or Hydrophiidae. Just as we have countries where venemous snakes are a major health issue because of the large number of species they harbor, we also have countries where venemous snakes are virtually non-existent (except for imported snakes), such as New Zealand, Cuba, Haiti, Jamaica, Puerto Rico, Ireland, Polynesia, Hawaii and the polar regions.

In this chapter, we are going to be focusing on the snakes most commonly found in the Americas, more specifically in North America (the United States and Northern México), These snakes are from the Elapidae and the Viperidae families such as the pit viper, the rattlesnake, the water moccasin, and the copperhead, since they are responsible for about 99% of the cases reported. The coral snake, which can also be found in North America, is responsible for only 1% of the cases, along with the exotic imported species.

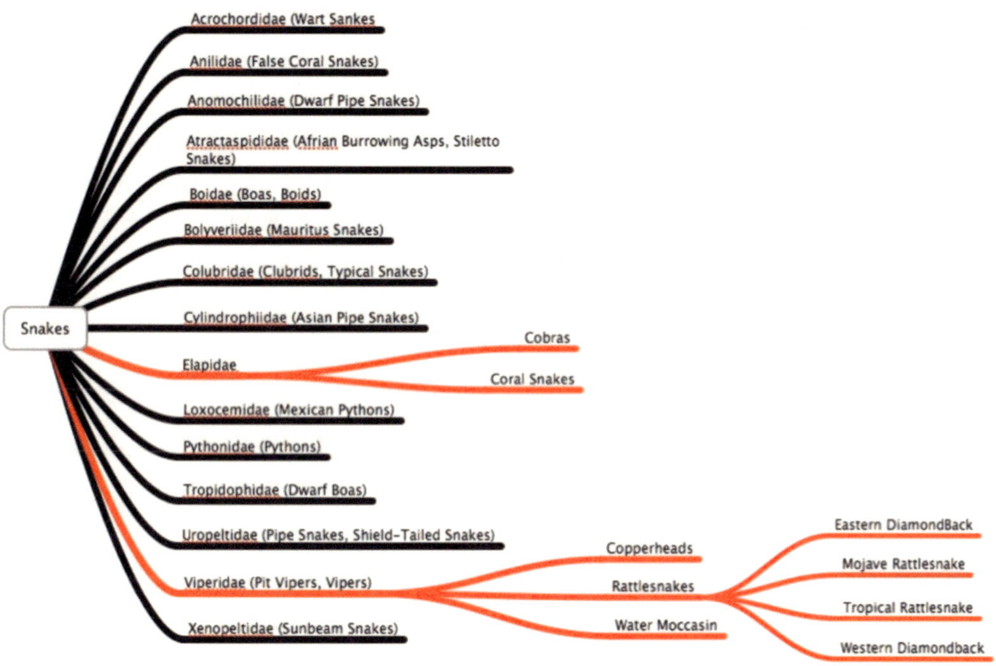

Fig. 1. Diagram that shows the fifteen families of snakes in the world. The families marked in red contain the most important and dangerous snakes in America.

A very important part of the process of providing the best medical care available resides in the identification of the snake. Important as this is, it is recommended not to go after the snake to try to identify it or kill it. We need to remember that most snakes only attack when they feel menaced in the first place, thus, going after a snake after it has already attacked would put us in more danger, risking a second bite or a first bite in a different person. If we are in an advantageous situation (adequate lighting, such as broad sunlight, regular, flat surface with minimal plant growth, etc.) there are several bits of information we should recall if we clearly see the snake:

3.1 Pit viper

These snakes have pits, one in each side of the face, located between the eye and the nostril. These pits, not found in the non-venomous species, contain heat-sensing organs, very important for these venomous snakes, since they have a very poor vision. If we have a good view of the snake, we can observe its pupils, which are different from non-poisonous snakes. Pupils in the pit viper are elliptical and vertically oriented. The fangs in venomous snakes are only superior, two in number and hollow. These are usually 5 to 20 mm long. These fangs are folded posteriorly in the palate and are shown only when the snake attacks. Regarding the head, in most poisonous snakes it is more triangular than in non-poisonous snakes. Last, if the snake is captured or killed, we can examine the anal plate. In poisonous snakes the scales are in a single row after the anal plate. In non-harmful snakes the anal plate ends in a cleft or a double row of scales. These snakes produce an hemotoxic venom.

3.1.1 Rattlesnakes

There are four kinds of rattlesnakes (Crotalus) in North America, this is the reason why this species is very heterogeneous regarding its colors and length. We have: the Eastern Diamondback, the Western Diamondback, the Mojave Rattlesnake and the Tropical Rattlesnake. The Eastern Diamondback is the most common. We can find it in the Southeast Coastal area of the United States (North Carolina, South Carolina, Louisiana and Florida). This snake can be up to two meters long and has a characteristic pattern of bright lines that form a symmetric diamond pattern. The Western Diamondback lives in the Southeast of the United States, mainly southeast California, Oklahoma, Arizona, New Mexico and Texas. It is a little shorter than the Eastern Diamondback measuring only up to 1.5 meters. The Mojave Rattlesnake can be found in the Southwestern United States, principally in the Mojave Desert in California, Nevada, Southeast Arizona, Texas and the north portion of Mexico. It prefers rocky desert areas and this species is only about 75 cm. Last, we have the Tropical Rattlesnake, which lives in crops and sandy areas in the Southern of Mexico, Central America and South America (except Chile). These can measure up to two meters long, even though it usually is 1.5 meters long. These snakes are responsible for approximately 60% of all pit viper attacks and for this reason emergency staff need to be familiar with the general characteristics of these snakes and always take into consideration the possibility of a rattlesnake attack when treating a patient that has been bitten by an unidentified snake in the United States and Northern Mexico (Hodge III & Tecklenburg, 2006). Rattlesnakes attract children because of the sound the rattle makes when the snake is ready to attack.

3.1.2 Copperheads

The copperhead (Agkistrodon contortrix) is a common poisonous snake that lives in the Southeast United States (from Florida to Massachusetts) and much of the Northeast (Oklahoma, Illinois, Kansas, Ohio) but it can reach westward to states such as Texas and Nebraska. This reptile accounts for approximately 30% of venomous snake bites but, luckily, it is seldom a serious threat to life or limb. Copperheads are usually 60 cm to 1 m in length and have a light pink to red-brown body with darker brown crossbands shaped like hourglasses. The head has a coppery tinge (Hodge III & Tecklenburg, 2006).

3.1.3 Water moccasin

The water moccasin, also known as the cottonmouth (Agkistrodon piscivorus), is a semiaquatic pit viper found in the Southeastern of the United States, including Southeast Virginia, West and Central Alabama, South Georgia, Illinois, East and central Kentucky, South and Central Oklahoma, Texas, North Carolina, South Carolina and Florida. These are larger and more belligerent snakes, often traveling with their heads in an aggressive 45-degree angle from the horizontal. Their body is olive brown to black, with darker markings on the sides that often fade over the dorsum. The ventral surface is lighter in color. The oral mucosa is distinctively white, hence the name cottonmouth. Like the copperhead, bites from this species are, in general, less serious than Crotalus species (Hodge III & Tecklenburg, 2006). The cottonmouth may alert the future victim of the imminent attack by mouth gaping and tail vibrations (Glaudas & Winne, 2007).

3.2 Coral snake

Coral snakes belong to the Elapidae family. This is a relatively shy and passive snake. It can be found in Southeast United States as far as west Texas, as well as in countries from Central and South America. Unlike the pit viper, coral snakes have round pupils, not so triangular heads and do not have pits with heat sensing organs between the eye and the nostril. They can measure approximately 60 cm. and are described as a brightly colored snake. They can attract young children, who end up being victims of this venomous snake. It can be easily confused with non-poisonous snakes because of their bright colors. If the snake is presented in a safe way we can observe red and black bands that alternate with narrow yellow rings. Whenever we see yellow rings next to red bands we should think of a coral snake. Non-poisonous similar snakes have yellow rings directly in touch with black (and not red) bands.

3.3 Snakes outside america

In Europe, Africa and Oceania, we have an enormous number of species as dangerous as the ones living in America. In Europe, the Common adder is distributed widely across the continent, even reaching the northern part of Morocco. Has a variable color, ranging from completely black specimens to different dark zigzag patterns, measuring around 45 centimeters. Inoculates hemotoxic venom, its victims usually are campers, hikers and field workers. Another hemotoxic venom inoculating snake in Europe, although not as common (found only in Italy, Yugoslavia, northern Albania, and Romania) is the Long-nosed adder, which is gray, brown, or reddish with a dark brown or black zigzag pattern running the length of its back. A dark stripe is usually found behind each eye. In the southeast Europe area we can find the Pallas' viper with hemotoxic venom that is rarely fatal.

Regarding Africa, the Boomslang a 60-centimeter green or brown snake with hemotoxic venom inhabits the sub-Saharan Africa. Through most of the African territory particularly Angola, Cameroon, Uganda, Kenya, and the Congo we can find the Bush viper, often called leaf viper because of its color and because it uses its prehensile tail to secure itself to branches. Its venom is hemotoxic and healthy adults rarely die from its bite. The feared Asiatic cobra is distributed from southeast to southwest Asia, including Indonesia. Its venom is highly neurotoxic, causing respiratory paralysis with some tissue damage. With even stronger neurotoxic venom and wider distribution (From southeast to southwest Asia, including Indonesia) we have the Egyptian cobra

4. Pathophysiology

In the pathophysiology of envenomation we can consider different factors that can be divided into human factors, which include the size of the victim, general health and wound characteristics, such as depth of fang penetration and location of the wound and snake factors which include the size of the snake, the amount of venom injected, and the strength of the particular species venom. Healthy, angered and hungry snakes unload more venom than a recently satiated and surprised snake (Hodge III and Tecklenburg 2006). Snake venom is a complex mixture of proteolytic enzymes, peptidases, proteinases, phospholipases and neurotoxins that are able to cause serious damage to the musculoskeletal, blood clotting, cardiopulmonary, renal and central nervous systems. Due to the venom, there is cell function degeneration and the final outcome depends on the type of venom injected. Generally, envenomation increases capillary permeability that results in blood and plasma loss from the intravascular to the extracellular space, creating edema, which, in case of being sufficiently important, may cause circulatory compromise and hypovolemic shock. Also, snake venom has citolytic properties, which cause local necrosis and secondary infection, which could result in sepsis and death (De la O Cavazos 2006). Venoms with neurotoxic activity produce paralysis and respiratory distress by binding the nicotinic acetylcholine receptors, and preventing the depolarizing action of acetylcholine. Hemotoxic effects induce hemolysis, fibrinogen proteolysis, and thrombocytopenia, which, along with activation of plasminogen, can lead to a bleeding diathesis in severe envenomation (Hodge III & Tecklenburg, 2006). Cardiotoxic effects lead to heart failure as well as myotoxicity and nephrotoxicity. Some are known poisons and it is important to know their mechanism of action for diagnosing anding accidents caused by these reptiles. It is also helped to unveil a number of physiological distrurbances caused by these venoms regarding neurotransmission, coagulation processes and mechanisms of inflammation. The most important effect of neurotoxins is to prevent the transmission of nerve impulses in cholinergic synapses. ALFA neurotoxins interfere with neurotransmitter release and cause muscle paralysis, respiratory failure and death by asphyxiation. Phospholipase A2 catalyzes the hydrolysis of phosphoglycerides creating phospholipids, which have detergent properties with a highly polar hydrophilic head and a hydrophobic tail and therefore they are capable of damaging cell membranes by breaking the continuity of its bilayer lipid . They have an important action in the phenomena of hemolysis, myonecrosis, neurotoxicity and anticoagulantion. The myotoxin-type crotalin protein acts through activation of sarcolemmal channels, inhibiting the activity of sarcoplasmic reticulum ATPase with significant depolarization and changes in the osmolarity of muscle fibers with vacuolization and lysis of myocytes and, local necrosis of skeletal muscle. The coagulants and anticoagulants such as the crotaline venoms cause a syndrome similar to disseminated intravascular coagulation (DIC) through an enzyme protein similar to thrombin, which prompts the formation of fibrin monomers, generating an abnormal mesh of fibrin, upon which the factor XIII can not act being lysed by the mechanisms of fibrinolysis as degradation products of fibrin D-dimer. It also contains inhibitors of factor X activation of prothrombin and thrombin and fibrinogenases.

5. Clinical manifestations

We can have diverse clinical manifestations when it comes to snakebites. The inapparent bites occur mainly when dealing with non-venomous snakes or when we have a bite by a venemous snake which did not cause symptoms. Due to the low frequency of poisoning by snake bites, it has been suggested that snakes who bite as a defensive move against humans do not inject enough venom to cause systemic symptoms, these are called dry bites.

Generally, local events occur in the time span of the first 10 to 30 minutes. Local pain is perceived along with the presence of edema, exudate and presence of bullae, accompanied by numbness of the tongue, jaw and scalp. There may be numbness around the bite with bleeding or a purpuric rash and/or necrosis or gangrene. As for the systemic manifestations, they start with the onset of fear and impending death feeling, which accelerates absorption of the venom. Other symptoms depend on the pathophysiological changes of the venom of certain species; neurotoxic venoms manifest as neuromuscular blockade resulting in flaccid paralysis, ptosis, and difficulty breathing; cardiotoxic venoms manifest as tachycardia, hypotension and ECG abnormalities, there may be fluctuations in heart rate, blood pressure and even heart failure in severe cases. There may be muscle necrosis resulting in myoglobinuria.

Different poisons trigger different clinical manifestations and it is important for healthcare staff to learn to recognize the general characteristics of every single of them or at least the more common, depending on their geographical localization.

5.1 Pit vipers

Pit viper snakes (rattlesnakes, copperheads, and water moccasins) produce hemotoxic venom. Local pain is typically intense, and a sensation of burning occurs within five to ten minutes. The pain is greater with ensuing edema and presumably increases with a larger inoculation of venom. Only in rare occasions the venom will sediment in the muscule compartment, in which cases the amount of edema will be minimal. In Diamondback rattlesnake bites, the limb may swell completely in just one hour. There can be local echymmosis and vesicles in the first hours. Lymphadenitis and some adenomegalies may become apparent. Victims of a significant rattlesnake bite often complain within minutes of perioral numbness, extending to the scalp and periphery. This parenthesis may be accompanied by a metallic taste in the mouth.

These patients also may have nausea, vomiting, weakness, chills, sweating, syncope, and other more ominous symptoms of systemic venom absorption. A copperhead envenomation produces less local symptoms, and systemic consequences are often minimal or nonexistent unless a small child, multiple bites, or a larger than average snake is involved. The water moccasin's effects are more variable.

5.2 Coral snakes

In Coral Snake bites, the inoculation of venom is neurotoxic. Clinical manifestations from a coral snake envenomation are mild pain (against intense pain from a pit viper snakebite), swelling, erythema and paresthesis in the area of the wound. The wound is represented by puncture marks, abrasions or scratches (D. L. Morgan, Borys, Stanford, Kjar, & Tobleman, 2007). Most snake bites do not leave important local signs other than one or two punctures and sometimes small teeth marks. Systemic effects appearing after several hours include nausea, vomiting, dizziness, malaise, slurred speech, muscle weakness, respiratory depression, or seizures (Hodge III & Tecklenburg, 2006).

6. Laboratory

The laboratory tests are of little importance to diagnose a snakebite, with the exception of the ELISA test, which is available to identify the species involved, based on venom antigens. These studies are expensive and are not fully available and are of no value except for epidemiological studies. In a hospital setting , laboratory studies are important to monitor poisoning victims, as well as when determining stages of treatment.

Changes in the blood include anemia, leukocytosis and thrombocytopenia, the blood smear may show evidence of hemolysis. Also, prolonged clotting times and decreased fibrinogen may be present. Among the metabolic changes we can find hypokalemia and respiratory acidosis if neuroparalysis occurs.

Urinalysis may reveal hematuria, proteinuria and hemoglobinuria. Electrocardiographic changes are usually nonspecific and may include rhythm disturbances, mainly bradycardia, AV block with ST segment elevation or depression. Cholesterol lowering has been documented and can be explained by transcapillary lipoprotein loss. There have been reports of changes in the electroencephalogram in up to 96% of patients with snake bites, but none showed clinical changes or encephalopathy. In 62% of the patients, the electroencephalogram showed grade I changes, 31% showed grade II changes. (Avila-Aguero: ML199).

7. Management and treatment

Science has made enormous advances regarding the pharmacologic treatment of children and adults who have been victims of snake bites. Successful treatment will always depend on the rapidness with which management begins, even at the scene of the attack, and, of course, once the patient arrives for appropriate management to a hospital.

7.1 Prehospital care

As we mentioned before, efforts should not be made to catch the snake, since this might result in wasted time and further bites. The basis in prehospital care is to limit the spread of venom throughout the body. Compressive bandages might be of help. These can be done with elastic bandages, if available, or torn clothing after removing clothes and jewelry. The extremity should be kept below the level of the heart. The bandage should be tight enough to help delay systemic absorption of the venom. Please be aware that incisions and suction are not indicated and could actually promote the development of further infections (D. L. Morgan et al., 2007). Remember that all bite wound are already considered contaminated wounds and that these invasive measures might actually worsen the problem unless performed in the first 30 minutes after the attack has taken place and in a sterile environment (Robert L Norris & Adler, 2011). Tourniquets that completely occlude vascular irrigation have created more problems than those solved, therefore, they are not recommended for their prehospitalary care.

7.2 Emergency room care

As soon as the patient reaches the hospital it is important to asses the CAB (circulation, airway and breathing) before starting any kind of treatment, this includes appropriate management of any active bleeding and of the airway to avoid respiratory failure or aspiration. Monitoring of vital signs can be useful to forecast complications and most of the times this can be done in the emergency room without sending the patient to the ICU. After these measures have been taken care of, hydration is next, since one of the effects of snake venoms is to mobilize intravascular fluid to the interstitial space, leaving the patient dehydrated. For this, normal saline or Ringer´s lactate is used. Laboratory tests that are useful in these settings are CBC, PT/PTT, serum electrolytes, CPK, urinalysis, BUN and creatinine and a cross-match for blood.

The wound should be inspected, if fang marks are found, the distance between them needs to be measured in order to get an idea of the size of the snake. The distance between fang punctures smaller than 8 mm suggests a small snake, between 8 and 12 mm a medium snake and a distance greater than 12 mm suggests a large snake. In the case of the patient being bitten by a rattlesnake, the fang punctures could be hidden by hemorrhagic blebs and edema. If no puncture wounds can be found, we need to consider the fact that scratches and abrasions could be envenomed wounds until we demonstrate otherwise. When a snake attacks and bites 10 % to 20% of the time it does not inject any venom (dry bite) and if we are dealing with a non-venomous snake we could observe a row of tiny teeth without fang punctures. As a precaution, the circumference of the limb should be measured every thirty minutes for 6 hours and every 4 hours until 24 hours have passed with the aim of preventing the development of complications related to important edema. If no systemic symptoms are evident, the wound should be cleansed, dressed and slightly elevated.

In the setting of not only the subject being bitten, but also suffering from envenomation, the use of antivenins is required. In the case of pit viper attacks, there are two antivenins, the Polyvalent Crotalic Antivenin (PCAV), which is the oldest, derived from horse's serum and highly antigenic, which is the reason for it to be discontinued from the United States market. In 2000, the FDA approved the Crotalic Polyvalent Fab Immune (FabAV) to manage patients with mild to moderate envenomations by American crotalus and since the Polyvalent Crotalic Antivenin is no longer marketed, the Fab Immune represents the only treatment option available in the United States, regardless of the severity of the envenomation. This alternative is derived from sheep's serum, a property that makes it less antigenic that its predecessor. FabAV appears to be effective in the management of severe crotaline snake envenomation (Lavonas, Schaeffer, Kokko, Mlynarchek, & Bogdan, 2009). It is available as a powder that needs to be reconstituted with normal saline. Regarding the use of PCAV, the dosing should be greater in children than in adults; for FabAV, since it can be eliminated before the venom emerges from tissues, therefore, a fixed dosing schedule is used. When using PCAV, a crash cart (including instruments to ensure airway patency, IV adrenaline, antihistaminics, steroids, etc) should be readily available because of the antivenin's elevated immunogenicity and risk of anaphylactic reactions. Skin testing should be performed and is done by injecting 0.02 ml of 1:10 diluted antivenin. Skin testing is not necessary for use of FabAV. Even though the use of antivenin is the only treatment for envenomations, its use is not free from adverse reactions, some of which could be life-threatening such as anaphylaxis. Some authors recommend the use of 0.25 ml of 1:1000 subcutaneous adrenaline to reduce the risk of acute adverse reactions to the serum (Premawardhena, C. E. de Silva, Fonseka, Gunatilake, & H. J. de Silva, 1999). If no adverse reactions appear, the full dosage should be administered (one vial with 10 ml saline solution) diluted in normal saline 1:4 as a slow infusion (1 or 2 ml per hour). Even after negative skin tests, one should be aware of the signs or symptoms of anaphylaxis within the first 10-20 minutes. If data suggestive of an anaphylactic reaction are not observed, the remaining volume should be passed on within two hours. The initial dose should be repeated until the swelling has stopped. There are reports in children of up to 75 bottles being used. In case of anaphylactic reaction, the infusion must be stopped and diphenhydramine administered (1 or 2 mg / kg IV). The infusion can be restarted at a slower rate, but a close watch should be kept and if symptoms of anaphylactic reaction reoccur treatment with antivenom should be discontinued.

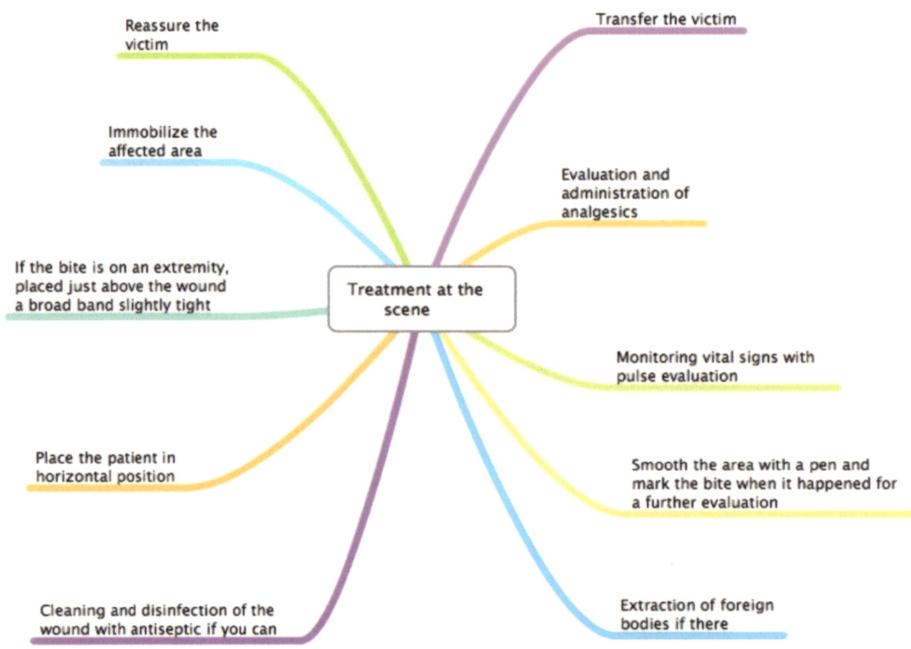

Fig. 2. Diagram that shows actions that should be taken care of when helping a snakebite victim.

In patients who receive FabAV, the starting dose consists of four to six bottles in a period of one hour. Each vial is reconstituted with 10 ml of sterile water mixed in a total dose in 250 ml of saline. The infusion is started slowly to see if there is a reaction to medication, if not, the rest of the load is administered in one hour. The initial dose is fixed, regardless of the degree of poisoning. Subsequent doses are administered depending on the progression of the clinical evolution.

Modified scale that correlates of clinical signs, edema and dose of antivenom in children					
(Christopher-Rodning)		Loading dose			Subsequent doses
Grade	Signs and symptoms	Direct (intra-venous) 1ml/min Normal saline	First hour 100 ml dilute solution (glucose-normal saline 2:1)	Following three hours in 250 ml mixed solution	Maintenance (value)
0	Evidence of bite without poisoning (probably dry bite)	0	0	0	
1	Mild poisoning, pain and edema less than 10 cm from the lesion.	2-3	4	Rate 4 bottles	Assess clinical status
2	Moderate poisoning: pain, edema greater than 15 cm from the lesion site, changes in skin, lymph regional.	5	10	6-8 bottles	Assess clinical status
3	Severe poisoning, swelling around the affected limb, vomiting, dizziness, fever, most notable changes in skin (ecchymosis, bullae, petechiae, numbness, oliguria)	5	20	6-8 bottles	4-5 bottles every 4 hours
4	Severe poisoning, bleeding bite marks, bruising and petechiae extensive data of disseminated intravascular coagulation, acute renal failure, respiratory distress, multiple organ failure.	25	25	10 bottles	4-5 bottles every 4 hours

Table 2. Modified scale correlation of clinical signs, edema and dose of antivenom in children.

When facing bites by Coral Snakes, the FDA extended the expiration date on the only product available in the United States to treat these envenomations. Wyeth's *Micrurus fulvius* Antivenin is no longer in production and there has been a need to obtain antivenoms produced in other countries (eg, Brazil, Costa Rica) for non-North American coral snakes. Mexico shares snake distribution with the United States. This country produces antivenom that is likely effective for coral snake bites in the United States. In the absence of such antivenom care must be entirely supportive. (R. L Norris, n.d.). Wound care should include irrigation, cleansing and dressings. Is convenient to consider tetanus prophylaxis and analgesia in case of need.

8. Complications

Compartmental syndrome is a limb threatening complication and it is considered a medical emergency that should be managed with fasciotomies. Fasciotomies are indicated in patients with signs and symptoms related to the syndrome, such as, pain to passive mobilization, hipostesia, weakness and elevated compartmental pressure, measured every hour with more than 30 mmHg regardless of elevation of the extremity and the administration of the antivenin. (Walter, Bilden, & Gibly, 1999)

9. Prevention

Snake bites are considered occupational accidents involving farmers, workers in plantations, sheepherders and fishermen (Alirol, Sharma, Bawaskar, Kuch, & François Chappuis, 2010). The Statistical Yearbook of the Méxican Ministry of Health (SSA) in the chapter on accidents and poisoning in the section of hospital morbidity does not appear to report cases of snakebites in the years 1995 to 2000. Clearly there is an underreporting of such injuries. This assertion is based on the IMSS 1994-1998 reported 2 620 cases with 23 deaths (0.8%). (Madrazo-Navarro M, Zarate-Aguilar A, 1998). Although in normal conditions victims are adults, we must take into account that children perform these activities in many third world countries. In performing these activities, people should wear appropriate clothing (heavy pants, rubber boots) and it could be helpful to limit activities that involve staying in areas with tall grass to hours with sunlight. Most of the times this is impossible, and in these cases is important to educate the population about the appropriate pre-hospital management in case of a snake bite. They should know the fastest routes to reach the nearest hospital and take into account that children engaged in these activities are at greater risk of bites by snakes and that the severity of these lesions is greater, even if they are exposed to the same amount of venom as an adult.

Open rooms with no windows or doors and some habits, such as sleeping on the ground exposes people to night snake attack (Alirol et al., 2010) and these practices must be eradicated whenever it is possible. Since the snake bites are more common in the legs, feet, to be more precise, the mere fact of having children wear shoes dramatically reduces the incidence of such bites, as well as keeping children away from sites where snakes may hide, especially in the evenings and early hours of the morning in summer and autumn seasons. (Hon, Kwok, & Leung, 2004)

There is very vague knowledge about the procedures to be followed when someone is attacked by a snake, below we present some guidelines that contrary to popular belief and misinformation should not be performed:

- No incisions in places where the bite is located, as excesive bleeding and the risk of infection are favored.
- Do not use tourniquets since they hinder blood flow and therefore cause more tissue damage.
- Do not apply ice, it worsens local lesions caused by poison.
- Do not administer electric shocks of any kind.
- Do not use any chemicals or extracts of plants or animals of any kind, so far none have been proven scientifically effective as treatment.
- Do not give alcoholic beverages.
- Do not suction with the mouth, this favors infections on the bite site and can be dangerous if you have a cavity or open lesion in your mouth. In addition there is no guarantee of how much venom you can withdraw with this method.

10. Conclusion

Snakebites are not an infectious disease, they do not have an epidemic potential and snakes themselves are not vectors that carry important diseases throughout the world. Nonetheless, the mortality caused by these attacks is greater than the mortality attributed to other diseases such as dengue hemorrhagic fever, cholera and Chaga's disease. At least 100 000 people die as a result of snake bites each year, and around three times as many amputations and other permanent disabilities are caused by snakebites annually and agricultural workers and children are the most affected (World Health Organization, n.d.). It is important to be familiar with first aid procedures as well as proper treatment in a hospital environment in order to decrease deaths and prevent complications and sequels derived from this very important health issue.

Science has made tremendous progress with regard to drug treatment for children and adults who have been bitten by snakes. Successful treatment will always depend on the speed with which you begin handling the victim from the outpatient level, as well as the availability of the drugs for proper treatment once the patient enters the hospital. Keep in mind that treatment recommendations published in 1999 could represent insufficient dosages and it is necessary an accurate clinical assessment to provide an effective therapy.

11. References

Alirol, E., Sharma, S. K., Bawaskar, H. S., Kuch, U., & François Chappuis. (2010). Snake Bite in South Asia: A Review. *PLoS Neglected Tropical Diseases*, 4(1), 1-9. doi:10.1371/journal.pntd.0000603

Avila-Agüero M. L.; Nuevos conceptos en el manejo de pacientes pediátricos mordidos por serpientes venenosas. *Acta Pediàtrica costarricense* V13 N13 San José 1999

Chippaux, J. P. (1998). Snake-bites: appraisal of the global situation. *Bulletin of the World Health Organization*, *76*(5), 515-524.

Consejo de Salubridad General. Cuadro Básico de Medicamentos, 2nd ed. México, D.F. : 1999. p. 23-29

Glaudas, X. G. X., & Winne, C. T. W. C. T. (2007). Do warning displays predict striking behavior in a viperid snake, the cottonmouth (Agkistrodon piscivorus)? *Canadian journal of zoology*, *85*(4), 574–578.

Government of Canada, A. & A.-F. C. (n.d.). Integrated Taxonomic Information System (ITIS);Biological Observations, Specimens and Collections (BiOSC) Gateway. Retrieved July 29, 2011, from http://www.cbif.gc.ca/pls/itisca/next?v_tsn=563895&taxa=&p_format=&p_ifx=cbif&p_lang=

Harrison, R. A., Hargreaves, A., Wagstaff, S. C., Faragher, B., & Lalloo, D. G. (2009). Snake envenoming: a disease of poverty. *PLoS Neglected Tropical Diseases*, *3*(12), e569. doi:10.1371/journal.pntd.0000569

Henderson B; Dujon E; (1973) Snake in bites. *Journal of Pediatric Surgery*, Vol. 8 No.5 (Octubre)

Hodge III, D., & Tecklenburg, F. W. (2006). Bites and Stings. *Textbook of Pediatric Emergency Medicine* (5th ed., pp. 1054-1061). 530 Walnut Street, Philadelphia, PA 19106, USA: Lippincott Williams & Wilkins.

Hon, K. L., Kwok, L. W., & Leung, T. F. (2004). Snakebites in children in the densely populated city of Hong Kong: a 10-year survey. *Acta Paediatrica (Oslo, Norway: 1992)*, *93*(2), 270-272.

Jeng, M. R., & Glader, B. (2004). Hemolysis Due to Venoms. *Wintrobe's Clinical Hematology* (11th ed., p. 1231). 530 Walnut Street, Philadelphia, PA 19106, USA: Lippincott Williams & Wilkins.

Kalantri, S., Singh, A., Joshi, R., Malamba, S., Ho, C., Ezoua, J., & Morgan, M. (2006). Clinical predictors of in-hospital mortality in patients with snake bite: a retrospective study from a rural hospital in central India. *Tropical Medicine & International Health: TM & IH*, *11*(1), 22-30. doi:10.1111/j.1365-3156.2005.01535.x

Lavonas, E., Schaeffer, T., Kokko, J., Mlynarchek, S., & Bogdan, G. (2009). Crotaline Fab antivenom appears to be effective in cases of severe North American pit viper envenomation: An integrative review. *BMC emergency medicine*, *9*(1), 13.

Morgan, D. L., Borys, D. J., Stanford, R., Kjar, D., & Tobleman, W. (2007). Texas coral snake (Micrurus tener) bites. *Southern Medical Journal*, *100*(2), 152-156.

Norris, R. L. (n.d.). *Snake envenomation, coral*. E-Medicine from WebMD. http://emedicine. medscape. com/article/771701-overview.

Norris, Robert L, & Adler, J. (2011, May 3). Coral Snake Envenomation. Medscape Reference. Retrieved from http://emedicine.medscape.com/article/771701-overview

Schaper, A., de Haro, L., Desel, H., Ebbecke, M., & Langer, C. (2004). Rattlesnake bites in Europe--experiences from southeastern France and northern Germany. *Journal of Toxicology. Clinical Toxicology*, *42*(5), 635-641.

Schaper, A., de Haro, L., Desel, H., Ebbecke, M., & Langer, C. (2004). Rattlesnake bites in Europe--experiences from southeastern France and northern Germany. *Journal of Toxicology. Clinical Toxicology*, 42(5), 635-641.

Sotelo N. (2003). Envenenamiento por mordedura de serpiente de cascabel, daños a la salud y su tratamiento en edad pediatrica, *Gaceta Medica de Mexico*, Vol 139, No. 4 (Julio-Agosto 2003) (317-324)

Vazques J., Hernandez J., Ayometzi M., (2002) Envenenamiento por Mordedura de Serpientes, *Urgencias en Pediatria* (5ta Edicion), Rodriguez R., Valencia P., (173-183) McGraw-Hill Interamericana, 970-10-3837-1, Mexico,D.F.

Walter, F. G., Bilden, E. F., & Gibly, R. L. (1999). Envenomations. *Critical Care Clinics*, *15*(2), 353-386, ix.

World Health Organization. (n.d.). WHO | Snake antivenoms. Retrieved August 17, 2011, from http://www.who.int/mediacentre/factsheets/fs337/en/index.html

8

What is the Role of Pediatricians on Oral Health?

Cigdem Elbek Cubukcu
Uludag University, School of Medicine,
Consultation Unit of Oral Diseases,
Turkey

1. Introduction

Good oral health and dentition is important for efficient mastication, speaking and cosmetically for smiling. If left untreated, dental pathologies can lead to pain and infection, reduced growth and development, speech disorders, and high treatment costs. Chronic infection around one or more teeth can result in damage to localized structures, such as the developing permanent teeth. Children who are medically compromised (such as being immunocompromised from a disease and/or therapy) are at increased risk of developing systemic complications from dental infections which can be fatal. Therefore, the author focuses on the role of the general pediatrician in promoting the importance of good oral health for all children and in particular those children receiving cancer therapy. Etiology, assessment, and prevention of dental caries and oral mucositis are presented, evidence based where available.

2. Dental caries development

Dental caries has historically been considered one of the most important global oral health burdens. It is still a major health problem in both developing and developed countries. 60-90 % of school-aged children are affected by the disease (Petersen, 2003). At present, the distribution and severity of dental caries vary in different parts of the world and within the same region or country. In permanent dentition, when dental caries experience is expressed as Significant Caries Index (SiC), the determined values are relatively high both for America region (SiC = 4.8) and the European region (SiC = 5.3) whereas the experience is lower in most African countries (SiC = 3.4) (World Health Organization [WHO], 2011). In developing countries, the prevalence rates of dental caries and its experience are now tending to increase probably due to the increasing consumption of sugars and inadequate exposure to fluorides. Conversely, a decline in caries has been observed in most developed countries as a result of a number of public health measures, including effective use of fluorides, together with changing living conditions, lifestyles and improved self-care practices. However, it must be emphasized that *dental caries as a disease of children has not been eradicated, but only controlled to a certain degree.*

2.1 Etiology of dental caries

Dental caries is a process that may take place on any tooth surface in the oral cavity where dental plaque (biofilm) is allowed to develop over a period of time. Plaque formation is a natural, physiological process. It is an example of a biofilm which means a community of microorganisms attached to a surface. The bacteria in the plaque are always metabolically active. Some of them are capable of fermenting a suitable dietary carbohydrate substrate (such as the sugars sucrose and glucose), to produce acid. The acid produced causes the plaque pH to fall to below 5 within 1-3 minutes. Repeated falls in pH may result in demineralization of the tooth surface in time. However, the acid is neutralized by saliva, so the pH increases and mineral may be regained. This is called remineralization. The cumulative results of de- and remineralization processes may be a loss of mineral and a carious lesion can be seen. Alternatively, the changes may be so slight that a carious lesion never becomes apparent (Kidd, 2005). *The formation of the biofilm and its metabolic activity cannot be prevented, but dental caries formation can be controlled, its progression in enamel tissue can be arrested and even advanced carious lesions (in dentin) may become inactive.*

2.2 Factors known to influence increased dental caries risk

Socio-economic factors or circumstances may influence increased caries risk. Factors such as social deprivation, unemployment, lower socio-economic status, low knowledge, low education of parents, and no regular dental check-ups are directly related to dental caries resulting in more cariogenic food consumption, less good oral hygiene, saliva problems (medications), and reduced fluoride support (WHO, 1994).

General health may also indicate increased caries risk. Some general diseases such as Sjögren's Syndrome or their treatments (medicines) affect saliva secretion. Also, the conditions can result in more cariogenic food and in less good oral hygiene (WHO, 2003).

Medicines can interfere with dental caries in two ways by leading to voluminous plaque-formation (containing fermentable carbohydrates) and by leading to a change in saliva production and composition. Medicines classified as follows have been proposed to cause xerostomia (oral dryness): antispasmodic, antidepressant, antipsychotic, skeletal muscle relaxant, parkinsonism therapy, antiarrythmic, antihistamine, appetite depressant, anticonvulsant, anxiolytic, antihypertensive, and diuretic. *Oral dryness is the third most common side-effect from using medicines* (Moore, 2008).

Diet is one of the key factors for dental caries and will be discussed in detail on section 4.1.

3. Assessment of dental development and referral for dental problems

Accurate chronologies of primary (deciduous) teeth calcifications as well as permanent dentition in particular first permanent molars are of clinical significance to the pediatricians (Table 1 and 2). It is often necessary to explain to parents the time sequence of calcification in utero and during infancy. The common observation of tetracycline pigmentation, developmental enamel defects, and generalized hereditary anomalies can be explained if the calcification schedule is known.

3.1 Chronologic development and eruption of the teeth

Evidence of development of the human tooth can be observed as early as the sixth week of embryonic life. Its life starts with initiation (bud stage) and follows with proliferation (cap stage), histodifferentiation and morphodifferentiation (bell stage), apposition, and

Upper Primary Teeth Development Chart		
Upper Teeth	When tooth emerges	When tooth falls out
Central incisor	8 to 12 months	6 to 7 years
Lateral incisor	9 to 13 months	7 to 8 years
Canine (cuspid)	16 to 22 months	10 to 12 years
First molar	13 to 19 months	9 to 11 years
Second molar	25 to 33 months	10 to 12 years
Lower Primary Teeth Development Chart		
Lower Teeth	When tooth emerges	When tooth falls out
Second molar	23 to 31 months	10 to 12 years
First molar	14 to 18 months	9 to 11 years
Canine (cuspid)	17 to 23 months	9 to 12 years
Lateral incisor	10 to 16 months	7 to 8 years
Central incisor	6 to 10 months	6 to 7 years

Table 1. Eruption and exfoliation timetable of primary human dentition. The first teeth begin to break through the gums at about 6 months of age. Usually, the first two teeth to erupt are the two bottom central incisors (the two bottom front teeth). Next, the top four front teeth emerge. After that, other teeth slowly begin to fill in, usually in pairs -- one each side of the upper or lower jaw -- until all 20 teeth (10 in the upper jaw and 10 in the lower jaw) have come in by the time the child is 2 ½ to 3 years old.

Upper Permanent Teeth Development Chart	
Upper Teeth	When tooth emerges
Central incisor	7 to 8 years
Lateral incisor	8 to 9 years
Canine (cuspid)	11 to 12 years
First premolar (first bicuspid)	10 to 11 years
Second premolar (second bicuspid)	10 to 12 years
First molar	6 to 7 years
Second molar	12 to 13 years
Third molar (wisdom teeth)	17 to 21 years
Lower Permanent Teeth Development Chart	
Lower Teeth	When tooth emerges
Third molar (wisdom tooth)	17 to 21 years
Second molar	11 to 13 years
First molar	6 to 7 years
Second premolar (second bicuspid)	11 to 12 years
First premolar (first bicuspid)	10 to 12 years
Canine (cuspid)	9 to 10 years
Lateral incisor	7 to 8 years
Central incisor	6 to 7 years

Table 2. Eruption and exfoliation timetable of permanent human dentition. Permanent teeth begin to come in around the age of 6. In some children, the first permanent molars are the first to emerge; in others, the incisors are the first to emerge.

calcification (AlQahtani et al., 2010). Ameloblasts will form enamel whereas odontoblasts will form dentin tissue. Following completion of all these stages the tooth will erupt. Primary teeth will shed (exfoliate) to their permanent successors. Although many theories have been advanced (Marks Jr., 1996; Philbrick et al., 1998; Wise et al., 2002), the factors responsible for the eruption of the teeth are not fully understood. The factors that have been related to the eruption of teeth include elongation of the root, forces exerted by the vascular tissues around and beneath the root, growth of the alveolar bone, growth of dentin, growth and pull of the periodontal membrane, hormonal influences (pituitary growth hormone, thyroid hormone, and parathyroid hormone-related protein), presence of a viable dental follicle, pressure from the muscular action, and resorption of the alveolar crest. A review article by Wise et al (Wise et al., 2002) focused on the molecular signals that initiate tooth eruption. They stated that tooth eruption is a complex and tightly regulated process involving cells of the tooth organ and surrounding alveolus. Mononuclear cells (osteoclast precursors) must be engaged into the dental follicle prior to the onset of eruption. These cells will turn into osteoclasts which resorb alveolar bone, and create an eruption pathway for the tooth to exist its bony container. Interaction of osteoblasts, osteoclasts and dental follicle involve a complex interplay of regulatory genes. It should be remembered that the time of eruption of both primary and permanent teeth varies greatly and variations of 6 months on either side of the usual eruption date may be considered normal for a given child. Demirjian and Levesque (1980) investigated a large sample of 5437 radiographs from a homogenous French-Canadian population, their analysis showed the similarity in timing between sexes for the early stages of tooth development (crown formation). However, their data indicated the importance of sexual dimorphism during the period of root development which girls were more advanced than boys by an average of 0.35 year for four teeth. For the stages of root development the mean difference between the sexes for all teeth was 0.54 year. The largest difference was for the canine (0.90 year). A study by Proffit and Fraizer-Bowers (2009) reviews the mechanism and control of tooth eruption. Finally an extensive review by Almonaitiene et al. (2010) analyzed the factors influencing permanent teeth eruption. Readers who wish to obtain more information about the details of the tooth eruption process are referred to these review articles.

3.2 Teething and difficult eruption

In general, the eruption of primary teeth comes before by increased salivation, and the child would want to put the hands and fingers into the mouth. Some young children become daytime restlessness, an increase in the amount of finger sucking or rubbing of the gum, an increase in drooling and some loss of appetite during the time of eruption of the primary teeth. *These observations may be the only indication that the teeth will soon erupt* (Macknin et al., 2000; Feldens et al., 2010). However, in some children a pronounced change in the mucosa often with small hemorrhages could be expected (Tasanen, 1968). Many conditions including croup, diarrhea, fever, convulsions, and primary herpetic gingivostomatitis have been *incorrectly* attributed to eruption (Dally, 1996). Leung (1989) reported that serious mistakes could be made in the care of infants and toddlers if their symptoms were ascribed to teething without completion of a thorough diagnostic evaluation and resulted in the overlooking of significant systemic disturbances. *Because of the tooth eruption is a normal physiologic process, the association with fever and systemic disturbances are not justified.* Inflammation of the gingival tissues before complete eruption of the tooth crown may cause a temporary painful condition which relieves within a few days. The eruption process may be hastened if the child is allowed to chew on a clean teething object. Using finger press technique upon where the tooth has been emerging will subside the probably fretful condition. The application of a nonirritating topical anesthetic may bring in temporary relief in the child has been experiencing extreme difficulty during the teeth eruption (Sood & Sood, 2010).

Primary teeth eruption facts for the pediatricians:

- A general rule of thumb is that for every 6 months of life, approximately 4 teeth will erupt
- Girls generally precede boys in tooth eruption
- Lower teeth usually erupt before upper teeth
- Teeth in both jaws usually erupt in pairs -- one on the right and one on the left Primary teeth are smaller in size and whiter in color than the permanent teeth that will follow
- By the time a child is 2 to 3 years of age, all primary teeth should have erupted Shortly after age 4, the jaw and facial bones of the child begin to grow, creating spaces between the primary teeth. This is a perfectly natural growth process that provides the necessary space for the larger permanent teeth to emerge.
- Between the ages of 6 and 12, a mixture of both primary teeth and permanent teeth reside in the mouth

If baby teeth fall out after a couple of years, why is it important to care for them?

- They reserve space for their permanent counterparts
- They give the face its normal appearance
- They aid in the development of clear speech
- They help attain good nutrition (missing or carious teeth make it difficult to chew causing children to reject foods)
- They help give a healthy start to the permanent teeth (caries and infection in baby teeth can cause dark spots on the permanent teeth developing beneath it).

3.2.1 Eruption hematoma (eruption cyst)

A bluish purple, elevated area of tissue called an *eruption hematoma* rarely develops a few weeks before the eruption of a primary or permanent tooth. It is actually a blood-filled cyst. It occurs most frequently in the primary second molar or the first permanent molar regions. The condition usually develops as a result of trauma to the soft tissue during mastication. The condition is self-limited and usually subsides in a few days following the break-through of the crown. Therefore, the treatment of the hematoma is rarely necessary. In order to expose the crown, surgical incision of the gingival tissue may rarely be needed (Tsiklakis & Patsakas, 1989).

3.2.2 Eruption sequestrum

The eruption sequestrum is seen occasionally at the time of eruption of the first permanent molar. It may develop from either osteogenic (Starkey & Shafer, 1963) or odontogenic tissue (Watkins, 1975; Pridds & Price, 1984). Regardless of its origin, the condition is usually of little or no clinical significance. As the tooth erupts, the fragment will sequestrate. However, it can be removed if it causes local irritation.

3.2.3 Ectopic eruption

A variety of local factors such as arch length inadequacy may influence a tooth to erupt or try to erupt in an abnormal position (Gupta et al, 2011).

3.3 Natal and neonatal teeth (prematurely erupted primary teeth)

The normal eruption of the primary teeth typically begins at six months of age. Natal teeth (teeth present at birth) and neonatal teeth (teeth that erupt during the first 30 days) are usually benign conditions (Cunha et al., 2001). Whatever the conditions they are, both of them considered as early eruption of primary teeth. Spouge and Feasby believe that the terms *natal teeth* and *neonatal teeth* constitute a relatively artificial distinction. Therefore, they have suggested that the terms *mature* and *immature* are more in keeping with the varying prognoses associated with such teeth in clinical point of view (Spouge & Feasby, 1966). The incidence of natal teeth ranges from 1:2000 to 1:3500 live births (Seminario & Ivancakova, 2004). The exact etiology is unknown. Infection, febrile states, trauma, malnutrition, superficial position of the tooth germ, hormonal stimulation and maternal exposure to environmental toxins has been implicated as causative factors (Cunha et al., 2001). It has been previously reported that heavily exposures to polychlorinated biphenyls and dibenzofurans caused to born infants with natal teeth in Taiwan (Gladen et al., 1990). However, Alaluusa et al. (2002) did not find any association between milk levels of polychlorinated biphenyls and dibenzofurans, and the occurrence of natal teeth. Early eruption of primary teeth might occur as a hereditary transmission of an autosomal dominant gene. A positive familial history has been reported in 8-62 % of natal teeth cases (Zhu & King, 1995). Natal teeth are present in 2 % of infants with unilateral cleft lip and palate and 10 % of infants with bilateral cleft lip and palate (de Almeida & Gomide, 1996). Natal teeth have been reported in association with syndromes such as Ellis-van Creveld, Jadassohn-Lewandowsky, Hallerman-Streiff, craniofacial dysostosis, steacystoma multiplex, Sotos, Wiedemann-Rautenstrauch, Meckel-Gruber and Pierre Robin (Seminario & Ivancakova, 1992; Uzamis et al., 1999; Marakoglu et al., 2004).

The most commonly affected teeth are the lower primary central incisors (85 %), followed by the maxillary incisors (11%), mandibular canines and molars (3 %), and maxillary canines and molars (1 %). Natal teeth usually occur in pairs (Zhu & King, 1995). However, an unusual case of an infant with fourteen natal teeth was reported by Masatomi et al. (1991). Natal teeth might resemble normal primary teeth in size and shape; however, the teeth are often smaller, conical and yellowish, and have hypoplastic enamel and dentin with poor or absent root development. Most prematurely erupted primary teeth are mobile because of limited root development. Some teeth may be supernumerary or mobile to the extent that there is danger of displacement of the tooth and possible aspiration. In such cases the removal (extraction) of the tooth is indicated. However, Zhu and King (1995) did not find any reported cases of aspirated natal or neonatal teeth in the literature. In some cases sharp incisal edge of the teeth may cause sublingual ulceration of the infant (Riga-Fede disease) or laceration of the mothers' breasts. If the teeth with rough edges are not hypermobile or not supernumerary; smoothing the sharp incisal edges of teeth or the placement of round smooth composite resin over the incisal edges is indicated. *However, if the tooth does not interfere with breastfeeding or not hypermobile, no intervention is necessary. Consultation with a pediatric dentist is strongly recommended in order to evaluate the preferred treatment and for differential diagnosis.* Eruption of teeth during the neonatal period causes fewer problems. These teeth can usually be maintained even tough root development is limited (Figure 1).

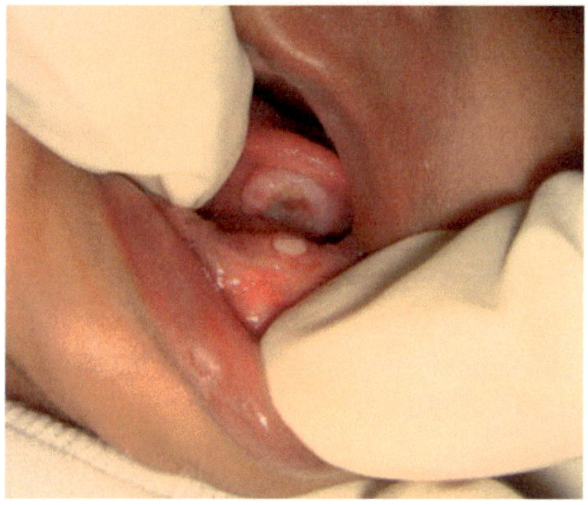

Fig. 1. Intraoral view showing a natal teeth and Riga-Fede disease (quoted from Padmanabhan et al. (2010) Neonatal sublingual traumatic ulceration - case report & review of the literature. *Dent Traumatol* 26, 6, Dec, 490-5.)

3.4 Epstein pearls, bohn nodules, and dental lamina cysts

Small, white or grayish white lesions on the alveolar mucosa of the newborn are identified as inclusion cysts. They are classified as the following three types according to their location in oral cavity: Epstein pearls are formed along the midpalatine raphe. Bohn nodules are formed along the buccal and lingual aspects of the dental ridges and on the palate away from the raphe. Dental lamina cysts are found on the crest of the maxillary and mandibular ridges. These lesions are usually multiple but do not increase in size. No treatment is indicated since the lesions will spontaneously be shed a few weeks after birth. These lesions may be incorrectly diagnosed as the natal teeth (Fromm, 1967; Cetinkaya et al., 2011).

3.5 Local and systemic factors that influence tooth eruption

Local factors which influence tooth eruption are ankylosed primary and permanent teeth, and ankylosis of primary molars with absence of permanent successors. Local factors generally cause delayed teeth eruption (Ertugrul et al., 2002). Referral to a pediatric dentist is recommended for appropriate treatment.

General factors associated with altered tooth eruption are Down syndrome (Trisomy 21 syndrome), cleidocranial dysplasia, congenital hypothyroidism (Cretinism), juvenile hypothyrodism, hypopituitarism, and achondroplastic dwarfism. Sporadic delayed eruption of teeth frequently occurs in children with Down syndrome. The first primary teeth may not appear until 2 years of age, and the dentition may not be complete until 5 years of age. The eruption generally follows an abnormal sequence and some of the primary teeth may be retained until 15 years of age (Jara et al., 1993; Ondarza et al., 1997). The prevalence and severity of early onset periodontal disease in children with Down syndrome are much higher compared to normal healthy and other mentally disabled children. A high prevalence of necrotizing ulcerative gingivitis is also reported (Carlstedt et al., 1996; Cichon et al., 1998). These higher prevalence relating periodontal diseases cannot only be explained by poor oral hygiene alone and may be the result of impaired immune responses and deficient phagocytic systems (Morinushi et al., 1997). Dental caries susceptibility is usually low in those with Down syndrome (Davidovich et al., 2010). Cleidocranial dysplasia (osteodentin dysplasia) has dental significance. The patients exhibit mandibular prognathism. The maxilla tends to be short vertically but not in sagittal way. The development of the dentition is delayed. One of the distinguishing characteristics is the presence of supernumerary teeth (Richardson & Deussen, 1994). The pediatric dentist serves as the coordinator of overall oral health care and disease prevention during an extended treatment regimen that usually includes two surgical interventions and three stages of orthodontic surgery. Hypothyroidism whether it occurs at birth or juvenile stage, causes delayed primary and permanent teeth eruption, and delayed primary teeth exfoliation (Mganga & Chindia, 1990). Hypopituitarism also causes delayed teeth eruption. Primary teeth may not undergo resorption but instead retained throughout the life of the patient. The underlying permanent teeth will develop but do not erupt (Conley et al., 1990). Delayed teeth eruption has been linked to other disorders, such as fibromatosis gingivae, chondroectodermal dysplasia, Gardner syndrome.

4. Provision of a caries control measurements

4.1 Cariogenic diet (reduction in the intake of freely fermentable carbohydrates)

Diet refers to the habitual allowance of food and drink taken by any person from day to day. Thus, the diet may exert an effect on caries locally in the mouth by reacting with the enamel surface and by serving as a substrate for cariogenic microorganisms. The food per se does not cause dental caries. Diet operates via the bacteria and the result may be a low pH at which the tooth starts to dissolve. The role of diet for proper tooth formation is a separate issue.

The consumption of sugar in substantial amounts is a recent trend in many areas of the world. Evidence linking caries and sugar has been evaluated from communities with low sugar consumption, and the results from severe dietary restrictions in many countries since 1940s. Another piece of evidence linking diet and caries concerns the rare hereditary disease fructose intolerance, which is caused by an inborn error of metabolism. Ingestion of foods containing fructose or sucrose causes severe nausea because of lack a certain liver enzyme. Consequently children with this disease avoid to eat these foods. The caries experience of them is considerably low, indicating that a group of children who are not able to tolerate many sugary foods are unlikely to develop much caries. There have been a number of non-interventional studies and animal experiments to relate dietary habits to the high prevalence of dental caries. According to a WHO study group, very little caries occurs in children when the national consumption level of sugar is below 10 kg per caput per annum (i.e., about 30 g/day), but a steep increase may occur from 15 kg upwards (WHO, 2003). Interventional human studies also designed in Sweden and Finland. Dentists now base much of dietary advice on the results of these two interventional studies, indicating that *the frequency of sugar intake should be reduced to confine sugar to meal times as much as possible.* The goal is not to exclude sugar from the diet but rather to make the patient eat sugar in a sensible way sugar discipline (reasonable amounts and mainly at meal times). This also introduces the concept that it may be possible to substitute sucrose by substances which will impart sweetness but are not cariogenic, which is covered in more detail in section 4.3. However, a comparable study on human subjects will probably never be repeated as it would now be regarded as unethical to alter diets experimentally in directions likely to increase caries. Sugars integrated into the cellular structure of food (e.g. in fruit) are called *intrinsic sugars*. Sugars present in a free form (e.g. table sugar) or added to food (sweets, biscuits, etc.) are called *extrinsic sugars*. These are more readily available for metabolism by the oral bacteria. Therefore, they are potentially more cariogenic. Milk contains lactose. It is not generally regarded as cariogenic. Cheese and yoghurts, without added sugars, may also considered safe for teeth (Ahola et al., 2002). Bread, peanuts (not for children under 5 years), and sugar-free drinks are some examples of foods and drinks with low potential for dental caries. Thus the most damaging sugars for dental health are *non-milk extrinsic sugars (NMES)* (Moynihan, 2002). Both frequency and amount of sugars are associated with dental caries. However, at the level of the individual patient, it is more practical to advise limiting frequency of intake. Since frequency and amount of sugar consumed are closely associated and repeated sugar intakes mean several acid attacks on the teeth giving demineralization, efforts to reduce frequency should be made. Additionally, selecting food products that only lead a slight and/or short pH drop (above critical pH at which the enamel starts to dissolve around pH 5.5) is another measurement to reduce the unwanted local effects of diet with respect to caries. Many common food products containing fermentable carbohydrates can lead to a pH of about 4 after their consumption.

Raw starch (e.g. raw vegetables) is of low cariogenity. Cooked and highly refined (e.g crisps) can cause caries, and combinations of cooked starch and sucrose (e.g. cakes, biscuits, sugared breakfast cereals) can be highly cariogenic. Fruits contain sugar (fructose, sucrose, and glucose) but fresh fruits appear to have low cariogenity. However, the same cannot be said for fruit juice. The juicing process releases the sugars from the whole fruit, and these drinks are potentially cariogenic. Dried fruits are also cariogenic since they are sticky, tending to adhere to teeth, and the drying process releases some of the intrinsic sugars (Moynihan, 2002). Some children have particular risk to caries because of dietary factors. These children should at least sound warning bells in the pediatrician's mind as well as dentist's (Fejerskov & Kidd, 2003; Vadiakas, 2008):

- Infant and toddlers with prolonged breast-feeding on demand
- Infants and toddlers provided with a feeding bottle at bedtime, or bottle hung up in the cot for use during the night with a sugar-containing liquid
- Children with an increased frequency of eating because of a medical problem, e.g. gastrointestinal disease, eating disorders, uncontrolled diabetes
- Children with an increased carbohydrate intake due to a medical problem, e.g. Chron's disease, chronic renal failure, other chronic illnesses, malnutrition, or failure to welfare
- Children who are on medications causing reduced salivary flow, irradiation to the region of salivary glands
- Children on long term and/or multiple medications: Are these sugar-based and/or do they cause dry mouth?.

Measures to reduce caries risk and/or to stop ongoing caries activity in children are:

- Number of meals and snacks should be kept on a low level.
- Low sugar consumption is desirable from a cariological point of view
- Sugars should be eliminated as fast as possible from the oral cavity. Foods needing active
- Chewing lead to an increased salivation, which is desirable.

It is neither necessary nor practical to stop children eating sweets completely. On the contrary, children should be encouraged to eat a balanced meal before any sweets are given. Friend and relatives should be encouraged to bring gifts rather than sweets. The consumption of bed-time snack or drink (other than water) should be strongly discouraged, since salivary flow is virtually absent at night and plaque pH may remain low for many hours.

All dental professionals are encouraged to share current best practice oral health prevention strategies with their local community medical providers especially with pediatricians (Huston & Wood, 2009).

4.2 Clinical use of fluorides

There is substantial evidence that fluoride, through different applications and formulas, works to control caries development. The first observations of fluoride's effects on dental caries were linked to fluoride naturally present in the drinking water, and then from controlled water fluoridation programs. Other systemic methods to deliver fluoride were later suggested, including dietary fluoride supplements such as salt and milk. These systemic methods are now being questioned due to the fact that many studies have indicated that fluoride'*s action relies mainly on its post-eruptive effect from topical contact with the tooth structure. It is known that even the methods of delivering* fluoride *known as 'systemic' act mainly through a topical effect when they are in contact with the teeth.* The effectiveness of water fluoridation in many geographic areas is lower than in previous eras due to the widespread use of other fluoride modalities. Nevertheless, this evidence should not be interpreted as an indication that systemic methods are no longer relevant ways to deliver fluoride on an individual basis or for collective health programs. *Caution must be taken to avoid excess ingestion of* fluoride *when prescribing* dietary fluoride *supplements for children in order to minimize the risk of* dental *fluorosis, particularly if there are other relevant sources of* fluoride *intake - such as drinking water, salt or milk and/or dentifrice* (Sampaio et al., 2011; Jimenez-Farfan et al., 2011). Safe and effective doses of fluoride can be achieved when combining topical and systemic methods. Before considering supplementing fluoride, recommendations on how to avoid excessive fluoride intake should be followed (Buzalaf & Levy, 2011).

4.2.1 Communal water fluoridation

Studies evaluating the effect of water fluoridation on dental caries show a reduction in both the primary and permanent dentitions of about 50%. Community water fluoridation is safe and cost-effective and therefore, should be introduced and maintained wherever socially acceptable and feasible. The optimum fluoride concentration will normally be within the range 0.5-1.0 mg/l (ppm). At this currently accepted optimal level, water fluoridation will result in some mild enamel fluorosis (McDonagh et al., 2000). The technical operation of water-fluoridation systems should be monitored and recorded regularly to prevent toxic effects of the element.

4.2.2 Fluoride-containing toothpaste

Fluoride toothpaste is the most widely used method of applying fluoride to teeth by so far. It is commonly used at home. It also has been using in community and school-based preventive programs. A recent systematic review concluded its beneficial use in preventing caries in children and adolescents, but only significantly for fluoride concentrations of 1000 ppm and above (Wong et al., 2011). Brushing teeth with fluoride containing toothpaste twice per day is recommended. The patients should brush before bed as the paste provides fluoride concentrations in saliva while the child is asleep. The effectiveness of fluoride toothpaste is concentration dependent. The relative caries preventive effects of fluoride toothpastes of different concentrations increase with higher fluoride concentration. The decision of what fluoride levels to use for children under 6 years should be balanced with the risk of fluorosis (Walsh et al., 2010). Studies have shown that use of fluoride toothpaste from an earl age is associated with higher levels of very mild fluorosis. The very mild grades are not aesthetically compromising, the use of fluoride toothpastes should continue to be promoted in communities, where or not they are served with fluoridated water or salt (WHO, 1994). However, in a recent study, it was indicated that there was weak unreliable evidence that starting the use of fluoride toothpaste in children aged <12 months may be associated with an increased risk of fluorosis. The evidence if use begins between the age of 12 and 24 months is equivocal. If the risk of fluorosis is of concern, the fluoride level of toothpaste for young children (under 6 years of age) is recommended to be lower than 1000 parts per million (ppm). More evidence from studies with low risk of bias is needed (Rasines, 2010). The author agrees with some other author's suggestion that children under 6 should use an adult-concentration paste (1000-1500 ppm fluoride), but a small pea-sized portion of it. The child should be encouraged to spit out excess paste and not swallow it. Children's pastes (500 ppm fluoride or less) could be recommended for children at low risk of caries living in an area where the water contains fluoride (Kidd, 2005). Some conclusions made by the WHO expert committee in 1994 are everyone should be encouraged to brush Daily with a fluoride toothpaste, every effort must be made to develop affordable fluoridated toothpastes for general use in developing countries, fluoridated toothpaste tubes should carry advice that for children under the age of 6 years brushing should be supervised and only a very small amount (less than 5 mm) should be placed on the brush or the chewing-stick (WHO, 1994).

4.2.3 Professionally applied fluoride (fluoride varnish in the pediatrician office)

It has been previously reported that fluoride varnish (a concentrated form of sodium fluoride) reduced caries in the primary dentition by 33% and in the permanent dentition by 46% when compared with placebo (Morinho et al., 2011). Therefore, their wider use is encouraged by WHO (1994). Visits to primary care physicians and pediatricians are the norm during children's first few years of life in many countries. Surveys of pediatric primary care providers suggest that they are willing to provide preventive dental care for their pediatric patients (Pierce et al., 2002). Lewis et al found that 74 % of US pediatricians expressed a willingness to apply fluoride varnish (Lewis et al., 2000). In promoting preventive dental health, pediatricians benefit all children and particularly the underserved. Therefore, pediatricians will require adequate training in oral health in medical school, residency, and in continuing education courses. It has been recently reported that *multiple applications of* fluoride *at the time of primary tooth emergence seem to be most beneficial to prevent dental caries formation.* Referrals to dentists for treatment of existing disease detected by physicians during regular visits limited the cumulative reductions in caries-related treatments, but also contributed to improved oral health (Pahel et al., 2011). Twice yearly application of fluoride varnish is indicated for the children over 6 years exposed to a greater cariogenic challenge or (in exceptional cases) when it is difficult to control caries in children under 6 years. Non-dental health care professionals should seek a professional advice from a pediatric dentist for appropriate application of the varnish.

4.2.4 Dietary fluoride supplements (tablets, drops, vitamins plus fluoride, lozenges)

The recent data on the value of fluorides administered during pregnancy fails to disclose any valid evidence to support such use even in non-fluoridated areas. *Fluoride ingestion by pregnant women does not benefit the teeth of their offspring, at least not the permanent teeth* (Sa Roriz Fonteles et al., 2005). In a recent panel by American Dental Association Council on Scientific Affairs, the following questions were addressed about the usage of fluoride supplements: When and for whom should the supplements be prescribed, and what should be the recommended dosage schedule for them?. The panel concluded that dietary fluoride supplements *should be prescribed only for children who are at high risk of developing caries and whose primary source of drinking water is deficient in* fluoride (Rozier et al., 2010). Supplements if indicated should be prescribed in accordance with the dosages recommended in Table 3 (AAPD, 2002). The natural (e.g. water) and cumulative (e.g. consumption amount of fluoride-rich foods, sources of drinking water) fluoride concentrations, should be determined and analyzed before fluoride prescripton. These clinical recommendations should be integrated with the practitioner's professional judgment and the patient's needs and preferences. Providers should carefully monitor the patient's adherence to the fluoride dosing schedule to maximize the potential therapeutic benefit.

Age	LESS than 0.3 ppm F*	0.3-0.6.ppm F*	MORE than 0.6 ppm F*
Birth-6 mos	0	0	0
6 mos-3 yrs	0.25 mg	0	0
3 yrs-6yrs	0.50 mg	0.25 mg	0
6 yrs up to at least 16 yrs	1.00 mg	0.50 mg	0

Table 3. Dietary fluoride supplementation schedule (*=drinking water fluoride concentration).

4.3 Sugar alcohols, casein phosphopeptides

Partial sugar substitution with polyols is an important dietary tool in the prevention of dental caries that should be used to enhance existing fluoride-based caries prevention programmes. Clinical studies have shown that xylitol, a natural, physiologic sugar alcohol of the pentitol type, can be used as a safe and effective caries-limiting sweetener. Habitual use of xylitol-containing food and oral hygiene adjuvants has been shown to reduce the growth of dental plaque, to interfere with the growth of caries-associated bacteria, to decrease the incidence of dental caries, and to be associated with remineralization of caries lesions. Other sugar alcohols that have been successfully used as sugar substitutes include D-glucitol (sorbitol), which, however, owing to its hexitol nature, normally has no strong effect on the mass and adhesiveness of bacterial plaque and on the growth of mutans streptococci. A tetritol-type alditol, erythritol, has shown potential as a non-cariogenic sugar substitute. Combinations of xylitol and erythritol may reduce the incidence of caries more effectively than either alditol alone (Makinen, 2011). Traditional delivering vehicles such as chewing-gums, hard candies and mints can only provide contact of the sugar substitutes with tooth surface for a few minute or even seconds. Therefore, novel delivery vehicles are still needed for the effective delivery of sugar substitutes before they can be considered as therapeutically effective.A group of peptides, known as casein phosphor peptide (CPP), have been shown to stabilize calcium and phosphate preserving them in an amorphous or soluble form known as amorphous calcium phosphate (ACP). Calcium and phosphate are essential components of enamel and dentine and form highly insoluble complexes, but in the presence of CPP they remain soluble and biologically available. This CPP-ACP complex applied to teeth by means of chewing-gum, toothpaste, lozenges, mouth rinses, or sprays is able to adhere to the dental biofilm and enamel hydroxyapatite providing bioavailable calcium and phosphate ions. When placed on the surface of a tooth with early carious lesions, pastes with CPP-ACP complexes can prevent tooth demineralization and improve enamel remineralization and enhance fluoride activity. Therefore, use of CPP-ACP based compounds offers a potential for use in the prevention of dental caries (Llena et al., 2009). Recently, probiotics have been investigating for dental caries prevention and inhibition. In caries, there are increases in acidogenic and acid-tolerating species such as mutans streptococci and lactobacilli, although other bacteria with similar properties can also be found and bifidobacteria, non-mutans streptococci, Actinomyces spp., Propionibacterium spp., Veillonella spp. and Atopobium spp. have also been implicated as significant in the aetiology of this disease (Aas et al., 2008). Therefore, to be able to develop probiotic or prebiotic interventions for applications in dental health care and to understand their mechanisms of action and potential risks, it is essential to have a clear understanding of the oral microbiota and their functions in dental/oral health and disease. However, some products have reached the market, there remains a paucity of clinical evidence to support the effectiveness of probiotics to prevent or treat caries (Meurman & Stomatova, 2007).

4.4 Counseling families on basic oral hygiene

The considerable potential of mothers should be a major focus of (oral) health professionals in developing oral health promotion programs for children and adolescents. Several maternal cognitive, behavioral, and psychosocial factors were associated with young children's brushing practices. Oral health-specific self-efficacy and knowledge measures are potentially modifiable cognitions and intervening on these factors could help foster healthy dental habits and increase children's brushing frequency early in life (Finlayson et al., 2007; Saied-Moallemi et al., 2008).

4.4.1 Feeding baby (Early Childhood Caries-ECC)

Early childhood caries (ECC) is defined as the presence of 1 or more decayed (noncavitated or cavitated lesions), missing (due to caries), or filled tooth surfaces in any primary tooth in a 71-month or younger child. In children younger than 3 years of age, any sign of tooth smooth surface caries is indicative of severe early childhood caries (S-ECC) (AAPD, 2003a). ECC has been found in general population but is more prevalent in low socioeconomic groups. It is 5 times more common than asthma, 7 times more common than hay fever, and 14 times more common than chronic bronchitis (Filstrup et al., 2003). The clinical appearance of the teeth in ECC is typical and follows a specific pattern: There is usually early and progressive carious lesions of the primary upper incisors in first years of age followed by the involvement of the upper and lower first primary molars, and the upper canines and sometimes lower canines (according to the sequence of eruption). The lower incisors are usually unaffected because of salivary flow from sub-lingual glands, and the contact of the tongue and lips at the time of feeding that covers the lower incisors. Therefore, milk and carbohydrates spread over all teeth except the lower incisors and prevent pudding or gathering of milk around these teeth (Tinanoff et al., 1998). The American Academy of Pediatric Dentistry (AAPD) has recognized the unique and virulant nature of ECC and accepted it as a serious public health problem. The presence of high levels of ECC, despite a reduction in permanent-dentition caries through fluoridation of water and use of fluoridated toothpastes, begs for a broader look at social and behavioral factors that correlate with this form of the disease. ECC not only affects teeth, but also may lead to more widespread health issues such as: chewing difficulty, malnutrition, gastrointestinal disorders, delayed or insufficient growth (especially in regard to the height and/or weight gain), poor speech articulation, low self-esteem and social ostracism. Additionally, repeated prescriptions of antibiotics, severe pain, sepsis and even death may also be observed. ECC is an infectious disease. Mutans Streptococci (streptococcus mutans and Streptococcus sobrinus species) are the most likely causes ECC and Lactobacilli participates in the development of the lesions and play role in lesion progression not its initiation (Parisotto et al., 2010). Bifidobacteria are asoosicated with S-ECC. S. mutans and S. sobrinus are also associated with lesion recurrence. Diet also plays an important role in the acquisition and clinical expression of the disease. Children with S-ECC, had higher scores of cariogenic bacteria for between-meal juice, solid retentive foods, and eating frequency than caries-free children. S. mutans positive children with ECC consume more cariogenic foods compared to caries-free children (Palmer et al., 2010). Acquisition may occur via vertical (from mother to child) or horizontal transmission (transmission of microbes between members of a group) (Berkowitz, 2006). Further details on vertical transmission of microorganisms will be presented in the following section. Risk factors for ECC are cariogenic bacteria, inappropriate feeding practices, social variables (education, lack of fluoride, access to healthcare, lack of health insurance, Treatment of ECC is generally problematic and costly because the cooperation of babies is low. Additionally within the first year after dental caries treatments, 40% recurrence rate has been reported around restored teeth and occurrence of new decays is common (Graves et al., 2004). Primary pediatric care providers are more likely to have earlier contact with children. Therefore, pediatricians as well as primary care health professionals will be responsible for the prevention of ECC. The diagnosis of impaired dentition and related prevention and outcomes should be included in their curricula. Primary prevention of ECC begins in the prenatal and perinatal periods (include pregnancy and first month of birth) and addresses the health of both mother and infant. Mother's or caregiver's teeth must be examined infants whose mothers have high levels of untreated dental caries are at greater risk of acquiring organisms. General approach which have been used to prevent ECC include training of mothers or caregivers to follow healthy dietary and feeding habits to prevent the development of ECC, early screening for signs of caries development (starting from about 7 to 8 month of age) to identify infants who are at risk developing ECC and assisting in providing information for parents about promoting oral health. Pediatricians can give the following recommendations for prevention of ECC to mothers and caregivers (AAPD, 2003b):

- Elimination of active dental caries lesions, gingival disease,
- Using fluoride and clorhexidine (Toothpaste, mouthwash, gel, varnish),
- Twice daily tooth brushing of the dentate infant (around 7th month of age),
- Oral health evaluation of the infant by a pediatric dentist before the first birthday,
- Infants should not be put to sleep with a bottle and nocturnal breastfeeding should be avoided after the first primary tooth begins to erupt,
- Mothers should be encouraged to have infants drink from a cup as they approach their first birthday,
- Infants should be weaned from the bottle at 12 to 14 months of age,
- An attempt should be made to assess and decrease the mother's/primary caregiver's mutans streptococci level to decrease the transmission of cariogenic bacteria,
- Stop saliva-sharing activities, such as tasting food before feeding and sharing toothbrushes.

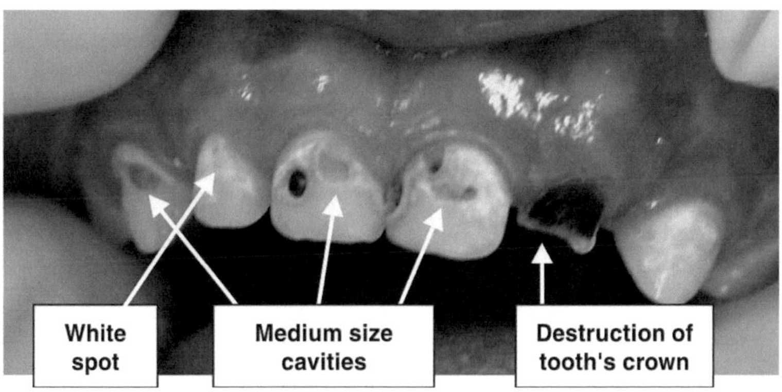

Fig. 4. Child's teeth with ECC. Observe the different phases of development (Quoted from Losso EM, Tavares MCR, da Silva JYB, Urban C (2009). Severe early childhood caries: an integral approach, *J Pediatr* 4, 295-300.

4.4.2 Initial acquisition of Mutans Streptococci (MS) by infants from their mothers

MS, consisting mainly of the species Streptococcus mutans and Streptococcus sobrinus, are commonly cultured from the mouths of infants, with prevalence of infection ranging from around 30 % in 3 month old predentate children to over 80 % in 24 month old children with primary teeth. MS is usually transmitted to children through their mothers. Domejean et al. (2010) indicated that MS can colonize horizontal as well as vertical transmission does occur.

The risk of transmission increases with high maternal salivary levels of MS and frequent inoculation. Köhler & Andreen (2010) reported that children colonised by MS at an early stage developed more caries than those colonised at a later stage and early maternal caries prevention is an efficient method to prevent early colonization of MS in their children. Factors that affect the colonization of MS may be divided into bacterial virulence, host-related and environmental factors. Complex interactions among these factors determine the success and timing of MS colonization in the child. As clinical studies have shown that caries risk is correlated with age at which initial MS colonization occurred, strategies for the prevention of dental caries should include timely control of colonization of the cariogenic bacteria in the mouths of young children.

4.4.3 Mechanical and chemical home oral hygiene (reduction of dental plaque and microorganisms)

Dentistry, particularly dentistry for children has come a long way toward reaching a ratio of 90% prevention to 10% treatment in many developed countries. At the core of this preventive approach is home oral hygiene and plaque control. The traditional focus of oral hygiene has been and will go on to be the control of the two most prevalent oral diseases, caries and periodontal disease. Although plaque control is essential for oral hygiene, it is important to realize that no clear relationship exists between plaque control and the prevention of caries (unlike with periodontal disease). As discussed previously in the section 2.1, the complex etiology of caries centers on the following factors: tooth susceptibility, bacterial plaque, refined carbohydrates, and time. Many other variables such as oral sugar clearance and salivary flow and pH, add to the complexity of the caries process. This complex etiology helps to explain the difficulty in demonstrating a relationship between oral hygiene practices and caries prevention. Despite this ambiguity, plaque control remains an essential element for oral health. In the absence of oral hygiene dental plaque accumulates leading to shifts in bacterial populations away from those associated with health. Plaque control efforts should be directed toward two goals: (1) limiting the numbers of mutans streptococci in plaque for prevention of caries by mechanical elimination of supragingival plaque (toothbrushing) and limitation of dietary sucrose, and (2) maintaining the predominantly gram-positive flora associated with gingival health by mechanical removal of plaque from the subgingival area (flossing) on a regular basis. Brushing twice daily with fluoride toothpaste has been advocated by the profession for many years, and this behavior is a routine part of many people's behavior. This daily brushing with fluoride toothpaste is believed to be the primary reason for the decline of caries observed in many populations since the 1970s. The behavior should not be taken for granted. Children should always be asked whether, and how often, they brush their teeth and what toothpaste they use. Most toothpastes contain fluoride, but not all, and it is important to check the fluoride concentration in toothpaste to administer proper dosage to the child. The use of chemotherapeutic agents, particularly chlorhexidine, can also play a role in maintenance of gingival health. The appropriateness and effectiveness of home oral hygiene procedures change throughout childhood. It is necessary to involve the parent at some level of the oral hygiene procedures. Age categories for specific home oral hygiene recommendations are prenatal period, infants (0-1 yrs), toddlers (1-3 yrs), preschoolers (3-6 yrs), school-aged children (6-12 yrs) and adolescents (12-19 yrs). The American academy of pediatric dentistry recommends that children have their first dental visit at approximately the time of eruption of the first tooth or, at the latest, by the age of 12 months (AAPD,

2003b). Therefore, pediatricians and primary health care providers must refer children to pediatric dentists in order to get them their regular dental visits. Objectives to be accomplished at the first visit: *Instruction of the parents in the use of oral hygiene procedures, infant dental examination and fluoride status review, dietary issues related to nursing and bottle caries.*

Mouthrinsing for the prevention of dental caries in children and adolescents was established as a mass prophylactic method in the 1960s and has shown average efficacy of caries reduction between 20-50%. Commonly, weekly or twice monthly rinsing procedures using neutral 0.2% NaF solutions have been used in schools or institutions in areas with low fluoride concentrations in the drinking water. Today, when dental caries has declined substantially in the western countries, and relatively few individuals are suffering from caries, the efficiency of large scale mouthrinsing is questioned and more individual approaches of caries prevention strategies are needed. Therefore in high risk patients, daily mouthrinses using 0.05% NaF can be recommended combined with other selective preventive measures such as sugar restriction, improved oral hygiene, antibacterial treatments, and so forth. Mouthrinsing solutions have therefore been combined with antiplaque agents like chlorhexidine and other agents which can improve the caries preventive effect in high caries risk patients. Other agents than sodium fluoride have been used, such as stannous and amine fluoride with proven clinical effects. However, although a series of new formulas of mouthrinses containing fluoride combined with different antiplaque agents have shown promising antibacterial and antiplaque efficacy, their long-term clinical effects are sparsely documented. Acute and chronic side effects from established and recommended mouthrinsing routines are extremely rare but ethanol containing products should not be recommended to children for long-term use. (FDI Commision, 2002).

5. Clinical assessment and management of the oral environment in a child patient receiving cancer treatment

5.1 The impact of cancer therapies on the oral cavity

The likelihood is high that aggressive cancer treatment will have toxic effects on normal cells as well as cancer cells. The gastrointestinal tract, including the mouth, is particularly prone to damage. This is true whether the treatment is radiation or chemotherapy. Most patients being treated for head and neck cancer will experience some oral complications, and while most of these are manageable, complications can sometimes become severe enough that treatment must be completely stopped. In addition, surgical solutions to tumor removal may lead to oral and nutritional problems as well. The most common oral problems occurring after radiation and chemotherapy are *mucositis* (an inflammation of the mucous membranes in the mouth), *infection, pain,* and *bleeding*. Other possible complications might include dehydration and malnutrition, commonly brought on by difficulties in swallowing (dysphagia). Radiation therapy to the head and neck may injure the glands that produce saliva (xerostomia), or damage the muscles and joints of the jaw and neck (trismus). These treatments may also cause hypovascularization (reduction in blood vessels and blood supply) of the bones of the maxilla or mandible (the bones of the mouth). In addition, treatments may affect other forms of dental disease (caries, or soft tissue complications), or even cause bone death (osteonecrosis). By identifying patients at risk for oral complications, health care providers are able to start preventive measures before cancer therapy begins, reducing the occurrence of problems brought about by different treatment modalities. *The most important risk factors leading to problems are oral or dental disease that already exists, and poor oral care during cancer therapy.* Other risk factors include the type of cancer, the chemotherapy type and schedule used, the area irradiated and how much radiation is given, how low blood counts are decreased and for how long, the patient's age, and the general condition of the patient's health pre-treatment. Pre-existing oral conditions may increase the risk of infection or other problems. Problems such as caries, calculus and tartar on the teeth, broken (fractured) teeth, the condition and quality of existing dental repairs such as crowns or fillings, periodontal disease, and appliances such as removable fixtures, or orthodontic brackets can make therapy more difficult later on. Bacteria and fungi can live in the mouth, and may develop into an infection when the immune system is not working well, or when white blood cell counts are low. Both of these factors can be caused by the treatment methods used. Where the gums (gingiva) or other soft tissues are irritated, tissues can thin and waste away, causing sores in the mouth. These complications can result in a significant reduction in the quality of life for the patient.

5.2 Oral mucositis

5.2.1 What is oral mucositis?

Mucositis is a common toxicity associated with both chemotherapy, and head and neck radiation used for the treatment of cancer (Scully et al., 2003, 2004). It is characterized by ulceration in the oro-oesophageal and gastrointestinal mucosae that results in pain, dysphagia, diarrhoea and dysfunction depending on the tissue affected (Sonis & Fey, 2002). Oral mucositis results in severe discomfort and impairs patients' ability to eat, swallow and talk. Concomitant therapy-induced myelosuppression places patients at significant risk of bacteraemia and sepsis from oral microorganisms resulting in increased days of fever, antibiotic use and hospitalization (Donnelly et al., 1995). Historically, mucositis has been associated with particular high-risk groups such as patients being irradiated for cancers of the head and neck, individuals receiving conditioning regimens for stem cell transplant that include total body irradiation or high dose melphalan and patients receiving specific induction protocols for acute leukaemia. Mucositis has been consistently reported to occur in at least 75% of treated patients in these groups. Radiation-induced mucositis occurs in almost all patients who are treated for cancers of the mouth, oropharynx and nasopharynx, and in approximately two-thirds of those treated for cancers of the hypopharynx or larynx. Mucositis risk and severity are determined by the treatment dose, radiation field size and fractionation schedules prescribed for individual patients. Hyperfractionated schedules and combination of radiation with chemotherapy increase the prevalence, severity and duration of mucositis. In patients receiving cancer chemotherapy, the frequency and severity of mucositis is mainly determined by the type(s) and dose of cancer chemotherapeutic agents used. five-fluorouracil (5-FU), cisplatin, etoposide and melphalan are particularly stomatotoxic (Chi et al., 1995; Pico et al., 1998) and mucositis is common with doxorubicin, vinblastine, taxanes and methotrexate, but uncommon with asparaginase and carmustine (Symonds, 1998). Finally, mucositis is seen in 75–99% of patients receiving conditioning regimens for haemopoietic stem cell transplantation (HSCT) particularly in those that combine total body irradiation (TBI) and chemotherapy (Blijlevens et al, 2000). Mucositis is the most common symptom and distressing complication of HSCT (Bellm et al., 2000), and some 30–50% of patients with HSCT complain that mucositis is their most significant toxicity. The only independent risk factor identified for mucositis is the conditioning regimen: high-dose melphalan (HDM) regimens exceed busulphan, busulphan-cyclophosphamide, cyclophosphamide–TBI, cyclophosphamide–carmustine (BCNU) and cyclophosphamide-etoposide–carmustine (Wardley et al., 2000).

5.2.2 Clinical diagnosis

Diagnosis of mucositis is clinical and based on the use of known stomatotoxic therapy, and the appearance, timing and location of oral lesions. Chemotherapy-induced mucositis occurs on the movable mucosae, rarely affecting the dorsum of the tongue, the hard palate or the gingiva. Radiation-induced mucositis also affects the movable mucosae and may involve the hard palate, albeit rarely. Infections and graft-versus-host disease (GVHD) are the most common differential diagnoses. Viral infections differ clinically from mucositis in that they are typically croppy, localized and involve keratinized mucosa of the hard palate, gingival and dorsal tongue and their onset often coincides with fever. Culture or exfoliative cytology at the time of lesion presentation is prudent. Graft-vs-host disease is limited to patients who have received allogeneic HSCT and develops following haematologic recovery (beyond 21 days after transplant) and typically results in dramatic oral lesions that are often lichenoid in character, sometimes also with xerostomia (Woo et al., 1997). Neutropenia, induced by chemotherapy, may be associated with necrotizing gingivitis.

The early clinical sign of mucositis is erythema presenting about 4–5 days following chemotherapy infusion or at cumulative doses of head and neck radiation of about 10 Gy. Patients also often complain of burning and intolerance of spicey foods at this stage. Seven to 10 days after chemotherapy or at cumulative radiation doses of 30 Gy, ulcers develop, resulting in marked discomfort, often requiring opioid intervention and in many cases causing patients to alter their diet. In the case of chemotherapy-induced mucositis, lesions are seen mostly on the movable mucosae of the buccal mucosae and lateral and ventral surfaces of the tongue. The hard palate and gingiva appear not susceptible to chemotherapy-induced mucositis. In contrast, radiation-induced mucositis may involve any radiation-exposed area, including the hard palate, albeit rarely. Chemotherapy-induced mucositis lasts approximately 1 week and generally heals spontaneously by 21 days after infusion. Radiation-induced mucositis stays at a peak for at least 2 weeks following the completion of radiotherapy (typically 60–70 Gy). As a result, it is not uncommon for patients receiving radiotherapy for cancers of the mouth and contiguous areas, to have severe ulcerative oral mucositis persisting for 5–7 weeks. Chronic mucositis following radiation therapy does occur, but rarely. A large number of mucositis scoring systems have been devised (summarized by Sonis et al, 2004) but most lack standardization or validation. The two most commonly used scoring tools to describe toxicity are the WHO and the National Cancer Institute (NCI) common terminology criteria for adverse events (Table 4).

Grade	Clinical features
0	-
1	Soreness/erythema
2	Erythema, ulcers but able to eat solids
3	Ulcers but requires liquid diet
4	Oral alimentation not possible

Table 4. WHO Mucositis scale (WHO, 1979).

5.2.3 Prevention and treatment options

There are a number of strategies adopted by oncologists to minimize the adverse effects of cancer therapy such as dose reduction, and other preventive treatment options. For example, leucovorin has been used for years to minimize the mucositis resulting from use of 5-FU (Lalla and Peterson, 2005). These are the province of oncologists and are not discussed further here. There has been a range of interventions developed for prophylaxis of oral mucositis but a more rational approach may be warranted. Indeed, there are very few randomized controlled double-blind trials (RCTs) assessing most of the interventions. A recent Cochrane review (Worthington, 2011) concluded that *cryotherapy (ice chips) and Keratinocyte Growth Factor (Palifermin ®) have shown some evidence of benefit in the prevention of mucositis. There is weaker less reliable evidence of a benefit associated with aloe vera, amifostine, intravenous glutamine supplementation, granulocyte-colony stimulating factor, honey, laser, polymixin/tobramycin/amphotericin (PTA) lozenges and sucralfate. There is no evidence that chlorhexidine is more effective that placebo and this intervention should not be used in the preventionofmucositis.*

The outcomes from studies testing GM-CSF, benzydamine hydrochloride or amifostine are mixed. (Mascarin et al, 1999; Tejedor et al, 2000). *Benzydamine HCl has been shown in single centre studies and in a multicentre double blind randomized placebo controlled trial in radiation therapy to reduce the intensity and duration of mucosal damage as well as to delay the need to use systemic pain-relievers including opioids* (Epstein et al., 1989, 2001). Benzydamine was not effective however, in patients receiving accelerated radiotherapy doses of more than 220 cGy. A preliminary study indicated that the severity of oral mucositis, both objective and subjective, in HSCT patients may be reduced by 0.1% topical tretinoin cream which has anti-inflammatory activity, administered daily from the beginning of the HCST conditioning until marrow engraftment (Cohen et al., 1997). Local antimicrobials containing amphotericin, polymixin and tobramycin may have some activity (Bondi et al., 1997). *Small single centre trials show that the incidence, severity and duration of radiochemotherapy-induced mucositis can be significantly reduced by oral rinsing with povidone iodine performed in addition to the standard prophylaxis scheme* (Adamietz et al. 1998). Mixed results have been seen with oral glutamine, which is involved in protein and nucleic acid synthesis: one group showed a decrease in the severity and duration of oropharyngeal mucositis in autologous HSCT patients but not in allogeneic HSCT patients. It is possibly because of interaction with methotrexate (Anderson et al., 1998a,b). While similar results were shown in a trial of intravenous glutamine in HSCT (MacBurney et al., 1994), and from an uptake-enhanced glutamine suspension used orally (Peterson, 2006), others have found no benefit (Schloerb & Skikne, 1999). Mucositis invariably requires systemic analgesics, adjunctive medications, physical therapy and psychologic therapy in addition to oral care. A recent Cochrane review (Worthington, 2004) concluded that there was *no evidence that patient controlled analgesia (PCA) is better than continuous infusion method for controlling pain, but less opiate was used per hour, and duration of pain was shorter, for PCA.* Only weak and unreliable evidence that allopurinol mouthwash, vitamin E, immunoglobulin or human placental extract improve or eradicate mucositis.

Pain from established mucositis can be reduced by systemic analgesics with non-steroidal agents and othernon-opiods used first, combined with opioids such as morphine and hydromorphone when pain is severe. In the in-patient setting, PCA provides the most effective pain control with lower total doses of opioid. Topical analgesics may combat pain and dysphagia when used prior to meals. Capsaicin may also provide analgesia (Berger et al., 1995). Cubukcu & Sevinir (2007) used debridement technique to promote healing of established mucositis and to alleviate symptom clusters in a group of children who were on induction chemotherapy. They concluded that debridement promoted resolution and decreased the severity of oral mucositis significantly. Thus, the subjects had less oral discomfort, pain, and nutritional difficulties. *In general, mucositis should be treated conservatively to avoid further tissue irritation and damaging the remaining cells from which the epithelium will regenerate. Plaque control and oral hygiene should be maintained with careful tooth brushing* (Borowski et al, 1994). *The potential benefit of prophylactic rinses with chlorhexidine may be to control plaque levels, gingivitis, reduce caries risk and oropharyngeal candidosis, rather than any direct effect upon oral mucositis. The patient should be advised to take a soft bland diet, avoiding irritants such as tobacco, alcohol or spices. Nutrition should be maintained.*

6. Conclusion

Tooth caries (decay) remains a substantial problem in young children and is made worse by existing barriers that prevent them from obtaining dental care. Because most children are exposed to medical care but not dental care at an early age, pediatricians have the opportunity to play an important role in helping children and their families gain access to dental care. Instructional efforts to increase pediatricians' dental knowledge or opinions of the importance of oral diseases are unlikely to be effective in increasing dental referral unless they include methods to increase confidence in providers' ability to identify and appropriately refer children with disease. Pediatricians can provide oral health promotion and disease prevention activities, thereby eliminating or delaying dental disease and the need for treatment at a very young age.

7. References

Aas JA, Griffen AL, Dardis SR, Lee AM, Olsen I (2008). Bacteria of dental caries in primary and permanent teeth in children and young adults. *J Clin Microbiol* 46, 4 (Jan 2008), 1407-1417, ISSN 0095-1137.

Adamietz IA, Rahn R, Bottcher HD, Schafer V, Reimer K, Fleischer W (1998). Prophylaxis with povidone-iodine against induction of oral mucositis by radiochemotherapy. *Support Care Cancer* 6, 4 (Jul 1998), 373-377, ISSN 0941-4355.

Ahola AJ, Yli-Knuuttila H, Suomalainen T, Poussa T, Ahlström A, Meurman JH, Korpela R (2002). Short-term consumption of probiotic-containing cheese and its effect on dental caries risk factors. *Arch Oral Biol* 47, 11 (Nov 2002), 799-804, ISSN 0003-9969.

Alaluusa S, Kiviranta H, Leppanilmi A (2002). Natal and neonatal teeth in relation to environmental toxicants. *Pediatr Res* 52, 5 (Nov 2002), 652-655, ISSN 0031-3998.

Almonaitiene R, Balciuniene I, Tutkuviene J (2010). Factors influencing permanent teeth eruption. Part One-general factors. *Stomatologija* 12, 3, 67-72, ISSN 1392-8589.

AlQahtani SJ, Hector MP, Liversidge HM (2010). Brief communication: The London atlas of human dental development and eruption. *Am J Phys Anthropol* 142, 3 (Jul 2010), 481-490, ISSN 0002-9483.

American Academy of Pediatric Dentistry (2003b). Clinical guidelines on infant oral healthcare, accessed 3/29/2010, avaliable from: http://www.aapd.org/media/Policies_Guidelines/G_InfantOralHealthCare.pdf.

American Academy of Pediatric Dentistry, Originating Group and Review Council (2003a). Policy on ECC: Classification, consequences, and preventive strategies. *Pediatr Dent* 25, 24-28, ISSN 0164-1263.

American Academy of Pediatric Dentistry: Guidelines on infant oral health care (2002). *Pediatr Dent* (supplemental issue: reference manual 2002-2003) 24,47, ISSN 0164-1263.

Anderson PM, Schoreder G, Skubitz KM (1998). Oral glutamine reduces the duration and severity of stomatitis after cytotoxic cancer chemotherapy. *Cancer* 83, 1433-1439, ISSN 0008-543X.

Bellm LA, Epstein JB, Rose-Ped A, Martin P, Fuchs HJ (2000). Patient reports of complications of bone marrow transplantation. *Support Care Cancer* 8, 1 (Jan 2000), 33-39, ISSN 0941-4355.

Berger A, Henderson M, Nadoolman W, Duffy V, Cooper D, Saberski L, Bartoshuk L (1995). Oral capsaicin provides temporary relief for oral mucositis pain secondary to chemotherapy/radiation therapy. *J Pain Symptom Manage* 11, 5 (May 1995), 331, ISSN 0885-3924.

Berkowitz RJ (2006). Mutans streptococci: Acquisition and transmission. *Pediatr Dent* 28, 2 (Mar-Apr 2006), 106-109, ISSN 0164-1263.

Blijlevens NM, Donnely JP, De Pauw BE (2000). Mucosal barrier injury: biology, pathology, clinical counterparts and consequences of intensive treatment for hematological malignancy: an overview. *Bone Marrow Transplant* 25, 12 (Jun 2000), 1269-1278, ISSN 0268-3369.

Bondi E, Baroni C, Prete A, Gatti M, Carrassi A, Lodi G, Porter SR (1997). Local antimicrobial therapy of oral mucositis in pediatric patients undergoing bone marrow transplantation. *Oral Oncol* 33, 5 (Sep 1997), 322-326, ISSN 1368-8375.

Borowski B, Benhamou E, Pico JL, Laplanche A, Margainaud JP, Hayat M (1994). Prevention of oral mucositis in patients treated with high-dose chemotherapy and bone marrow transplantation: a randomised controlled trial comparing two protocols of dental care. *Eur J Cancer B Oral Oncol* 30B, 2:93-7, ISSN 0964-1955.

Buzalaf MA, Levy SM. Fluoride intake of children. *Monogr Oral Sci* 22, (Jun 2011), 1-19, ISSN 0077-0892.

Carlstedt K, Krekmanova L, Dahllöf G, Ericsson B, Braathen G, Modéer T (1996). Oral carriage of Candida species in children and adolescents with Down's syndrome. *Int J Paediatr Dent* 6,2 (Jun 1996), 95-100, ISSN 0960-7439.

Cetinkaya M, Oz FT, Orhan AI, Orhan K, Karabulut B, Ilk O (2011). Prevalence of oral abnormalities in a Turkish newborn population. *Int Dent J* 61,2 (Apr 2011), 90-100, ISSN 0020-6539.

Chi KH, Chen CH, Chan WK (1995). Effect of granulocyte-macrophage colony stimulating factor on oral mucositis in head and neck cancer patients after cisplatin, fluoruracil, and leucovorin chemotherapy. *J Clin Oncol* 13, 10 (Oct 1995), 2620-2628, ISSN 0732-183X.

Cichon P, Crawford L, Grimm WD (1998). Early-onset periodontitis associated with Down's syndrome: clinical interventional study. *Ann Periodontol* 3,1 (Jul 1998), 370-380, ISSN 1553-0841.

Cohen G, Elad S, Or R, Galili D, Garfunkel AA (1997). The use of tretonin as oral mucositis prophlaxis in bone marrow transplantation patients: a preliminary study. *Oral Dis* 3, 4 (Dec 1997), 243-246, ISSN 1354-523X.

Conley H, Steflik DE, Singh B, Hoffman WH (1990). Clinical and histological findings of the dentition in a hypopituitary patient: report of case. *ASDC J Dent Child* 57,5 (Sept-Oct 1990), 376-379, ISSN 1945-1954.

Cubukcu CE, Sevinir B (2007). Debridement could be a solution to promote healing of established oral mucositis in children. *Eur Arch Paediatr Dent* 8, 2 (Jun 2007), 105-12, ISSN 1818-6300.

Cunha RF, Boer FA, Torriani DD, Frossard WT (2001). Natal and neonatal teeth: review of the literature. *Pediatr Dent* 23,2 (Marc-Apr 2001), 158-162, ISSN 0164-1263.

Dally A (1996). The lancet and the gum-lancet: 400 years of teething babies. *Lancet* 348, 9043 (Dec 1996), 1710-1711, ISSN 0140-6736.

Davidovich E, Aframian DJ, Shapira J, Peretz B (2010). A comparison of sialochemistry, oral Ph, and oral health status of Down syndrome children to healthy children. *Int J Paediatr Dent* 20, 4 (Jul 2010), 235-241, ISSN 0960-7439.

Demirjian A, Levesque GY, (1980). Sexual differences in dental development and prediction of emergence. *J Dent Res* 59, 7, 1110-1122, ISSN 0022-0345.

Doméjean S, Zhan L, DenBesten PK, Stamper J, Boyce WT, Featherstone JD (2010). Horizontal transmission of mutans streptococci in children. *J Dent Res* 89, 1 (Jan 2010), 51-55, ISSN 0022-0345.

Donelly JP, Dompeling EC, Meis JF, De Pauw BE (1995). Bacteriemia due to oral viridans streptococci in neutropenic patients with cancer: Cytostatics are a more important risk factor than antibacterial prohylaxis. *Clin Infect Dis* 20, 2 (Feb 1995), 469-470, ISSN 1058-4838.

Epstein JB, Silverman S Jr, Paggiarino DA, Crockett S, Schubert MM, Senzer NN, Lockhart PB, Gallagher MJ, Peterson DE, Leveque FG (2001). Benzydamine HCl for prophylaxis of radiation-induced oral mucositis: results from a multicenter, randomized, double-blind, placebo-controlled trial. *Cancer* 92, 4 (Aug 2001), 875-885, ISSN 0008-543X.

Epstein JB, Stevenson-Moore P, Jackson S, Mohamed JH, Spinelli JJ (1989). Prevention of oral mucositis in radiation therapy: a controlled study with benzydamine hydrochloride rinse. *Int J Radiat Oncol Biol Phys* 16, 6 (jun 1989), 1571-1575, ISSN 0360-3016.

Ertugrul F, Tuncer AV, Sezer B (2002). Infraocclusion of primary molars: a review and report of a case. *ASDC Dent Child* 69, 2 (May-Aug 2002), 166-171, ISSN 1945-1954.

FDI Commision (2002). Mouthrinses and dental caries. *Int Dent J* 52, 5 (Oct 2002), 337-345, ISSN 0020-6539.

Fejerskov O, Kidd EAM (2003). The role of dietary carbohydrate, In: *Essentials of Dental Caries-the disease and its management*. Kidd EAM, pp.7-8, Oxford University Press, ISBN 0198529783, New York.

Feldens CA, Faracol M, Ottoni AB, Feldens EG, Vitolo MR (2010). Teeting symptoms in the first year of life and associated factors: a cohort study. *J Clin Pediatr Dent* 34, 3 (Spring 2010), 201-206, ISSN 1053-4628.

Filstrup SL, Briskie D, Fonseca M, Lawrence L, Wandera A, Ingleheart MR (2003). ECC and quality of life: child and parent perspectives. *Pediatr Dent* 25, 5 (Sept-Oct 2003), 431-440, ISSN 0164-1263.

Finlayson TL, Siefert K, Ismail AI, Sohn W (2007). Maternal self-efficacy and 1-5-year-old children's brushing habits. *Community Dent Oral Epidemiol* 35, 4 (Aug 2007), 272-81, ISSN 0301-5661.
Fromm A (1967). Epstein's pearls, Bohn's nodules and inclusion cysts of the oral cavity. *J Dent Child* 34, 4 (Jul 1967), 275-287, ISSN 0022-0353.
Gladen BC, Taylor JS, Wu YC, Ragan NB, Rogan WJ, Hsu CC (1990). Dermatological findings in children exposed transplacentally to heat-degredated polychlorinated biphenyls in Taiwan. *Br J Dermatol* 122, 6 (Jun 1990), 799-808, ISSN 0007-0963.
Graves CE, Berkowitz RJ, Proskin HM, Chase I, Weinstein P, Billings R (2004). Clinical outcomes for ECC : Influence of aggresive dental surgery. *J Dent Child* 71, 2 (May-Aug 2004), 114-117, ISSN 1551-8949.
Gupta SK, Saxena P, Jain S, Jain D (2011). Prevalence and distribution of selected developmental dental anomalies in an Indian population. *J Oral Sci* 53 ,2, 231-238, ISSN 1343-4934.
Huston J, Wood AJ (2009). Sharing early preventive oral health with medical colleagues: a dental pain prevention strategy. *J Calif Dent Asssoc* 37, 10 (Oct 2009), 723-34, ISSN 1343-4934.
Jara L, Ondarza A, Blanco R, Valenzuela C (1993). The sequence of eruption of the permanent dentition in a children sample with Down's syndrome. *Arch Oral Biol* 38, 1 (Jan 1993), 85-89, ISSN 0003-9969.
Jimènèz- Farfan MD, Hernandez-Guerrero JC, Juarez-Lopez LA, Jacinto-Aleman LF, de la Fuente-Hernandez J (2011). Fluoride consumption and its impact on oral health. *Int J Environ Res Public Health* 8, 1 (Jan 2011), 148-160, ISSN 1660-4601.
Kidd, EAM (2005). Classification of dental caries, In: *Essentials of dental caries: the disease and its management.* Kidd EAM pp.13 and 118, Oxford University Press, ISBN 0198529783, New York.
Köhler B, Andreen I (2010). Mutans streprococci and caries prevalence in children after early maternal caries prevention: a follow-up at eleven and fifteen years of age. *Caries Res* 44, 5 (Sept 2010), 453-458, ISSN 0008-6568.
Lalla RV, Peterson DE (2005). Oral mucositis. *Dent Clin North Am* 49, 1 (Jan 2005), 167-184, ISSN 0011-8532.
Leung AK (1989). Teething. *Am Fam Physician* 39, 2 (Feb 1989), 131-134, ISSN 0002-838X.
Lewis CW, Grosman DC, Domoto PK, Deyo RA (2000). The role of the pediatrician in the oral health of children: A national survey. *Pediatrics* 106, 6 (Dec 2000), 84, ISSN 1098-4275.
Llena C, Forner L, Baca P (2009). Anticariogenicity of casein phoshopeptide amorphous calcium phospate: a review of the literature. *J Contemp Dent Pract* 10, 3 (May 2009), 1-9, ISSN 1526-3711.
Losso EM, Tavares MCR, da Silva JYB, Urban C deA (2009). Severe early childhood caries: an integral approach, *J Pediatr (Rio J)* 85, 4 (Jul-Aug 2009), 295-300, ISSN 1678-4782.
MacBurney M, Young LS, Ziegler TR, Wilmore DW (1994). A cost-evaluation of glutamine-supplemented parental nutrition in adult bone marrow transplant patients. *J Am Diet Assoc* 94, 11 (Nov 1994), 1263-1266, ISSN 0002-8223.
Macknin ML, Piedmonte M, Jacobs J, Skibinski C (2000). Symptoms associated with infant teething: a retrospective study. *Pediatrics* 105, 4 (Apr 2000), 747-752, ISSN 0031-4005.

Makinen KK (2011). Sugar alcohol sweeteners as alternatives to sugar with special consideration of xylitol. *Med Princ Pract* 20, 4 (May 2011), 303-320, ISSN 1011-7571.

Marakoglu K, Percin EF, Marakoglu I, Gursoy UK, Goze F (2004). Anencephalic infant with cleft palate and natal teeth: a case report. *Cleft Palate Craniofac J* 41, 4 (Jul 2004), 456-458, ISSN 1055-6656.

Marinho VCC, Higgins JPT, Logan S, Sheiham A (2002). Fluoride varnishes for preventing dental caries in children and adolescents (Review). *Cochrane Database Syst Rev* 1, CD002284.

Marks SC Jr., Schroeder HE (1996). Tooth eruption: theories and facts. *Anat Rev* 245, 2 (June 1996), 374-393, ISSN 0003-276X.

Masatomi Y, Abe K, Ooshima T (1991). Unusual multiple natal teeth: case report. *Pediatr Dent* 13, 3 (May-June 1991), 170-172, ISSN 0164-1263.

Mascarin M, Franchin G, Minatel E, Gobitti C, Talamini R, De Maria D, Trovò MG (1999). The effect of granulocyte colony-stimulating factor on oral mucositis in head and neck cancer patients treated with hyper fractionated radiotherapy. *Oral Oncol* 35, 2 (Mar 1999), 203-208, ISSN 1368-8375.

McDonagh MS, Whiting PF, Wilson PM, Sutton AJ, Chestnutt I, Cooper J, Misso K, Bradley M, Treasure E, Kleijnen J (2000). Systematic review of water fluoridation. *BMJ* 321, 7265 (Oct 2000) :855-859, ISSN 0959-8138.

Meurman JH, Stamatova I (2007). Probiotics: contributions to oral health. *Oral Dis* 13, 5 (Sept 2007), 443-445, ISSN 1354-523X.

Mg'ang'a PM, Chindia ML (1990). Dental and skeletal changes in juvenile hypothyroidism following treatment: case report *Odontostomatol Trop* 13, 1 (Jan 1990), 25-27, ISSN 0251-172X.

Moore PA, Guggenheimer J (2008). Medication-induced hyposalivation: etiology, diagnosis and treatment. *Compend Contin Educ Dent* 29, 1 (Jan-Feb 2008), 50-55, ISSN 1548-8578.

Morinushi T, Lopatin DE, Van Poperin N (1997). The relationship between gingivitis and the serum antibodies to the microbiota associated with periodontal disease in children with Down's syndrome. *J Periodontol* 68, 7 (Jul 1997), 626-631, ISSN 0022-3492.

Moynihan PJ (2002). Dietary advice in dental practice. *Br Dent J* 193, 10 (Nov 2002), 563-568, ISSN 0007-0610.

Ondarza A, Jara L, Muñoz P, Blanco R (1997). Sequence of eruption of deciduous dentition in a Chilean sample with Down's syndrome. *Arch Oral Biol* 42, 5 (May 1997), 401-406, ISSN 0003-9969.

Padmanabhan MY, Pandey RK, Aparna R, Radhakrishnan V (2010). Neonatal sublingual traumatic ulceration - case report & review of the literature. *Dent Traumatol* 26, 6 (Dec 2010), 490-5, ISSN 1600-9657.

Pahel BT, Rozier RG, Stearns SC, Quinonez RB (2011). Effectiveness of preventive dental treatments by physicians for young medicaid enrollees. *Pediatrics* 127, 3 (Feb 2011), 682-689, ISSN 0031-4005.

Palmer CA, Kent R Jr, Loo CY, Hughes CV, Stutius E, Pradhan N, Dahlan M, Kanasi E, Arevalo Vasquez SS, Tanner AC (2010). Diet and caries-associated bacteria in severe early childhood caries. *J Dent Res* 89, 11 (Sept 2010), 1224-1229, ISSN 0022-0345.

Parisotto TM, Steiner-Oliveira C, Silva CM, Rodrigues LK, Nobre-dos-Santos M. (2010). Early childhood caries and mutans streptococci: a systematic review. *Oral Health Prev Dent* 8, 1, 59-70, ISSN 1602-1622.

Petersen PE. (2003). The world oral health report: Continuous improvement of oral health in the 21st century--the approach of the WHO Global Oral Health Programme. *Community Dent Oral Epidemiol* 31, 1 (Dec 2003), 3-24, ISSN 0301-5661.

Peterson DE (2006). New strategies for management of oral mucositis in cancer patients. *J Support Oncol* 4, 2 (Feb 2006), 9-13, ISSN 1544-6794.

Philbrick WM, Dreyer BE, Nakchbandi IA, Karaplis AC (1998). Parathyroid hormone-related protein is required for tooth eruption. *Proc Natl Acad Sci USA* 95, 20 (Sep 1998), 11846-11851, ISSN 0027-8424.

Pico JL, Avila-Garavito A, Naccache P (1998). Mucositis: its occurence, consequences, and treatment in the oncology setting. *Oncologist* 3, 6, 446-451, ISSN 1549-490X.

Pierce KM, Rozier G, Vann WF Jr. (2002). Accuracy of pediatric primary care providers' screening and referral early childhood caries. *Pediatrics* 109, 5 (May 2002), 82, ISSN 1098-4275.

Pridds RW, Price C (1984). The so-called eruption sequestrum. *Oral Surg* 58, 3 (sep 1984), 321-326, ISSN 0030-4220.

Profit WR, Fraizer-Bowers SA (2009). Mechanisms and control of tooth eruption: overview and clinical implications. *Orthod Craniofac Res* 12, 2 (May 2009), 59-66, ISSN 1601-6343.

Rasines G (2010). Using a fluoridated supplement with a high fluoride concentration in children aged under 6 years may increase the risk of fluorosis. *Evid Based Dent* 11, 1, 8-9, ISSN 1476-5446.

Richardsson A, Deussen FF (1994). Facial and dental anomalies in cleidocranial dysplasia: a study of 17 cases. *Int J Paediatr Dent* 4, 4 (Dec 1994), 225-231, ISSN 0960-7439.

Rozier RG, Adair S, Graham F, Iafolla T, Kingman A, Kohn W, Krol D, Levy S, Pollick H, Whitford G, Strock S, Frantsve-Hawley J, Aravamudhan K, Meyer DM (2010). Evidence based clinical recommendations on the prescription of dietary fluoride supplements for caries prevention: a report of the ADA council on scientific affairs. *J Am Dent Assoc* 141, 12 (Dec 2010), 1480-1489, ISSN 1943-4723.

Sa Roriz Fonteles C, Zero DT, Moss ME, Fu J (2005). Fluoride concentrations in enamel and dentin of primary teeth after pre- and postnatal fluoride exposure. *Caries Res* 39, 6 (Nov-Dec 2005), 505-508, ISSN 0008-6568.

Saied-Moallemi Z, Virtanen JI, Ghofranipour F, Murtomaa H (2008). Influence of mothers' oral health knowledge and attitudes on therir children's dental health. *Eur Arch Paediatr Dent* 9, 2 (Jun 2008), 79-83, ISSN 1818-6300.

Sampaio FC, Levy SM (2011). Systemic fluoride. *Monogr Oral Sci* 22 (Jun 2011), 133-45, ISSN 0077-0892.

Schloerb PR, Skikne BS (1999). Oral and parental glutamine in bone marrow transplantation: a randomized, double blind study. *JPEN J Parenter Enteral Nut*r 23, 3 (May-June 1999), 117-122, ISSN 0148-6071.

Scully C, Epstein J, Sonis S (2003). Oral mucositis: a challenging complication of radiotherapy, chemotherapy, and radiochemotherapy. Part 1, pathogenesis and prophylaxis of mucositis. *Head Neck* 25, 12 (Dec 2003), 1057-1070, ISSN 1043-3074.

Scully C, Epstein J, Sonis S (2004). Oral mucositis: a challenging complication of radiotherapy, chemotherapy, and radiochemotherapy. Part 2, diagnosis and management of mucositis. *Head Neck* 26, 1 (Jan 2004), 77-84, ISSN 1043-3074.

Seminario AL, Ivancakova R (2004). Natal and neonatal teeth. *Acta Medica* 47, 4, 229-233, ISSN 1211-4286.

Sonis ST (2002). The biological role of nuclear factor-κβ in disease and its potential involvement in mucosal injury associated with antineoplastic therapy. *Crit Rev Oral Biol Med* 13, 5, 300-309, ISSN 1045-4411.

Sonis ST, Elting LS, Keefe D, Peterson DE, Schubert M, Hauer-Jensen M, Bekele BN, Raber-Durlacher J, Donnelly JP, Rubenstein EB; Mucositis Study Section of the Multinational Association for Supportive Care in Cancer; International Society for Oral Oncology (2004). Perspectives on cancer therapy-induced mucosal injury: pathogenesis, measurement, epidemiology, and consequences for patients. *Cancer* 100, 9 (May 2004), 1995-2025, ISSN 0008-543X.

Sood S, Sood M (2010). Teething: myths and facts. *J Clin Pediatr Dent* 35, 1 (Fall 2010), 9-13, ISSN 1053-4628.

Spouge JD, Feasby WH (1966). Erupted teeth in the newborn. *Oral Surg* 22,198-208.

Starkey PE, Shafer WG (1963). Eruption sequestra in children. *J Dent Child* 30, 4-86.

Symonds RP (1998). Treatment-induced mucositis: an old problem with new remedies. *Br J Cancer* 77, 10 (May 1998), 1689-1695, ISSN 0007-0920.

Tasanen A (1968). General and local effects of the eruption of deciduous teeth. *Ann Paediatr Fenn* 14,1-40.

Tejedor M, Valerdi JJ, Arias F, Dominguez MA, Pruja E, Mendez L, Illarramendi JJ (2000). Hyper fractionated radiotherapy concomitant with cisplatin and granulocyte macrophage colony-stimulating factor (Filgrastim) for laryngeal carcinomas. *Cytokines Cell Mol Ther* 6, 1 (Mar 2000), 35-39, ISSN 1368-4736.

Tinanoff N (1998). Introduction to the early childhood caries conference: Initial description and current understanding. *Community Dent Oral Epidemiol* 26,1, 5-7, ISSN 0301-5661.

Tsiklakis K, Patsakas A (1989). Differential diagnosis of bluish and pigmented lesions of the oral mucosa. *Hell Stomatol Chron* 33, 2 (Apr-Jun 1989), 113-20, ISSN 1011-4181.

Uzamis M, Olmez S, Ozturk H, Celik H (1999). Clinical and ultrastructural study of natal and neonatal teeth. *J Clin Pediatr Dent* 23, 3 (spring 1999), 173-177, ISSN 1053-4628.

Vadiakas G (2008). Case definition, aetiology and risk assessment of early childhood caries (ECC): a revisited review. *Eur Arch Paediatr Dent* 9, 3 (sep 2008), 114-125, ISSN 1818-6300.

Walsh T, Worthington HV, Glenny AM, Appelbe P, Morinho VC, Shi X (2010). Fluoride toothpastes of different concentrations for preventing dental caries in children and adolescents. *Evid Based Dent* 20, 1 (Jan 2010), 6-7, ISSN 1469-493X.

Wardley AM, Jayson GC, Swindell R, Morgenstern GR, Chang J, Bloor R, Fraser CJ, Scarffe JH (2000). Prospective evaluation of oral mucositis in patients receiving myeloablative conditioning regimens and haemapoietic progenitor rescue. *Br J Haematol* 110, 2 (Aug 2000), 292-299, ISSN 0007-1048.

Watkins JJ (1975). An unusual eruption sequestrum. *Br Dent J* 138, 10 (May 1975), 395-396, ISSN 0007-0610.

Wise G. et al. (2002). Cellular, molecular, and genetic determinants of tooth eruption. *Crit Rev Oral Biol Med* 13, 4, 323-335, ISSN 1045-4411.

Wong MC, Clarkson J, Glenny AM, Lo EC, Marinho VC, Tsang BW, Walsh T, Worthington HV (2011). Cochrane reviews on the benefits/risks of fluoride toothpastes. *J Dent Res* 90, 5 (May 2011), 573-579, ISSN 1544-0591.

Woo SB, Lee SJ, Schubert MM (1997). Graft-vs.-host disease. *Crit Rev Oral Biol Med* 8, 2, 201-216, ISSN 1045-4411.

World Health Organization (WHO) oral health country / area profile (2011). Geneva: WHO; available at: URL:http://www.mah.se/CAAP/methods-and-indices.html.

World Health Organization (WHO) technical report series (1994). Fluorides and oral health. *WHO expert committee on oral health status and fluoride use.* Geneva, 846, 118, ISSN 05123054.

World Health Organization (WHO) Technical Report Series (2003). Diet, nutrition and the prevention of chronic diseases, *WHO Expert Committee.* Geneva, 196 (Jan-Feb 2002), 797, ISBN 92 4 120916 X.

Worthington HE, Clarkson JE, Eden OB (2004). Interventions for treating oral mucositis for patients with cancer receiving treatment. *Cochrane Database Syst Rev* 2, CD001973, ISSN 1469-493X.

Worthington HV, Clarkson JE, Bryan G, Furness S, Glenny AM, Littlewood A (2011). Interventions for preventing oral mucositis for patients with cancer receiving treatment. *Cochrane Database Syst Rev.* 13, 4 (Apr 2011), CD000978, ISSN 1469-493X.

Zhu J, King D (1995). Natal and neonatal teeth. *ASDC J Dent Child* 62, 2 (Mar-Apr 1995), 123-128, ISSN 1945-1954.

9

Interdisciplinary Model of Attention for Children Undergoing Hospitalized Surgical Procedures

Renata Panico Gorayeb[1], Maria de Fátima Galli Sorita Tazima[2], Flávio de Oliveira Pileggi[2], Maria Angela Marchini Gorayeb[1], Ricardo Gorayeb[1] and Yvone A.M.V. Vicente[2]

[1]Psychology, Department of Neurology, Psychiatry and Medical Psychology, School of Medicine of Riberao Preto, University of Sao Paulo,
[2]Pediatric Surgery, Department of Surgery and Anatomy, School of Medicine of Riberao Preto, University of Sao Paulo
Brazil

1. Introduction

In this chapter we aim to present a model of comprehensive care for hospitalized children in a public Brazilian university hospital. This service is provided by a team of pediatric surgeons, psychologists, nurses and social workers, all of who specialize either in pediatrics or in the surgical procedures of the pediatric surgical clinic.

As part of their continuing education, these professionals regularly participate in conferences and courses specific to developments in maternal/pediatric care, therapeutic coping techniques in the realm of maternal/pediatric care, and the major diseases that affect children in this age group.

The team is responsible for the care of children and adolescents aged 0-18 years, of both sexes, who require either outpatient or inpatient medical and surgical care. In this chapter we will discuss the provided surgical care and the specific details of its treatment, care, and guidance, for both the child and the child's family, in bio-psycho-social aspects.

The interdisciplinary approach has been emphasized in recent years by promoting a broader understanding of the patient, his or her medical condition, and its context, demonstrating that this joint service improves the diagnosis, prognosis and quality of life of the patient.

The main objectives of this interdisciplinary model of care are:

- To wholly assist the patient and his or her family, caring for their bio-psycho-social needs
- To assist the patient and his or her family in acquiring a better understanding of the diagnosis and prognosis of each condition

- To promote the understanding, development and acceptance of invasive procedures and hospitalization
- To help understand the cognitive and affective aspects of disease perception and their influences on the quality of life of patients and their families, supporting the diagnosis and treatment compliance, thus providing greater progression

Based on these objectives, the Pediatric Surgery Team of the University Hospital of the Faculty of Medicine of Ribeirão Preto of the University of São Paulo (HCFMRPUSP) developed a protocol of integrated care for patients and their families. Through this protocol, all children and families who will experience a surgical procedure are treated in consultation with an interdisciplinary team composed of surgeons and psychologists in order to provide guidance and explanation of the possible conflicts related to the surgery for both the child and the family.

This model was developed from concepts described in several papers cited in the international literature, especially Canada, USA, France and China, which aimed specifically at the orientation of these patients for the procedures they will be undergoing, desensitization to invasive procedures, child-parent coping strategies, treatment and prognosis, as well as interdisciplinary interaction.

2. How pediatric illness can interfere with the family dynamic

Illness represents a modification of the bio-psycho-social scheme in a very particular and individual way, known in healthcare literature as one of the main factors that affect anxiety levels, quality of life, and individual behavior.

In the case of children, it is emphasized that they are in the process of building their own representations of reality and they do so through the summation of all their experiences.

Within the many objective and subjective lived experiences in the developing child's life, the importance of the relative and reactive models provided by adults during the child's early social environment stands out. The younger the child, therefore, the greater the influence of the behavioral patterns and coping mechanisms displayed by the child's adult references.

In the case of illness, which is not represented by any distinctive cognitive or affective form, the child is strongly influenced by the actions of those individuals who provide it with emotional support because these adults are significant role models who will utilize their own prior associations to deal with the new reality of their child's health.

The manner in which children therefore deal with this new reality is oftentimes reflective of their parents' coping mechanisms and the way their parents deal with the anxiety that stems from fear and uncertainty about their child's diagnosis/prognoses.

The new reality creates uncertainty about how, and if, these adults will or will not be capable of reasonably and appropriately recoding the experience of surgery and/or hospitalization for their children to understand.

For parents, the expectation surrounding the responsibility they feel to maintain the health and wellbeing of their children transforms the surgical procedure into a trigger of extreme anxiety.

The child's exposure to the risks of a hospitalization or surgery may induce negative fantasies and fearful reactions in both the parents and the child, exacerbating a natural reaction of anxiety and possibly causing a dysfunctional or pathological reaction of anxiety, and consequently a possible behavioral disruption.

The difficulty in understanding the procedure to be performed on the child, or even the hospital context to which the child will be exposed, the possibility of injury, loss or separation from the child, the anesthetic risk, and especially the fear of prognosis are some of the reasons these parental feelings are evoked.

For the infant, who is still in full development of its impressions, the principal sentiment is fear of the unknown, the pain, and the risk of separation from its attached adults, such as the mother.

Upon admission, everything surrounding the child is new and often scary. The child finds itself in a new routine with environmental and social restrictions and is often exposed to procedures that cause pain and/or discomfort.

These potentially anxiety-inducing changes are more intense during hospitalization due to the environmental restrictions, the hospital routine, and the prognosis, among other factors.

However, the process becomes more complex during surgery. There will also be an invasive intervention that includes anesthetic procedures, being that various studies show that surgery, and anesthesia in particular, are stimuli that trigger stress and anxiety because they can be symbolically associated with the fear of loss.

These factors may lead to behavioral changes in the child during and after hospitalization, such changes being more frequent in children who have not constructively addressed and coped with the stress they experienced.

In pediatric surgery, anxiety can be observed both in the child and in the parents, so that parental coping techniques, the representation of their anxiety and consequently the manner in which they deal with the child, can help or hinder the team's work and the child's recovery.

Very anxious parents exacerbate their child's inappropriate behavior, often hampering treatment and even the child's prognosis. For this group, with greater difficulty in coping with fear and anxiety, the child's behavior often changes during and after hospitalization, encouraging behaviors that are disturbing, such as nail biting and enuresis, and emotional, such as tantrums and night terrors. The same changes can also occur in the parents.

Note that empowering both children and adults to face and cope with the illness and proposed surgical procedure provides a way to deal with the information and can reduce fears and the implicit risks of a hospitalization. It is known that the quantity and quality of information received by the family and by the patient influence their trust in the team and consequently reduce anxiety and behavioral changes, which improves adherence to treatment.

In this way, we emphasize the idea that when information and psycho-emotional support are provided to patients and their families there is often an improvement in the acceptance of the proposed procedures and, especially, an increased confidence in the team.

This work is done in order to allow patients and their parents to understand the context of their clinical situation with detailed quantitative and qualitative information about the treatments and proposed procedures.

Therefore, when the whole family can be prepared and supported by a psychological intervention, damage to the child's behavior and the family's anxiety can be reduced.

This procedure is done by encouraging better a better compliance with the treatment as a whole, which shows that parental anxiety and pediatric behavioral changes, recognized in literature as the main factors that influence a child's health during the post-operative recovery, can be managed.

The work of this team, carried out by a clinical psychology specialist professional in conjunction with surgeon colleagues, all looking for a better pediatric recovery, confirms and reinforces the literature about the importance of interdisciplinary work in planning a pre-operative preparation for the child and family before a medical intervention.

Thus, we present the protocol that is necessary for providing comprehensive interdisciplinary care to the hospitalized child, especially in the case of a surgery. This work is done as much for the children as for their caregivers.

3. Interdisciplinary care protocol for pediatric surgery at HCFMRPUSP

This protocol was structured on a 2002 survey that aimed specifically to evaluate parents' understanding of their child's illness and the surgical procedures to be performed. We sought to investigate what were the principal doubts, fears, fantasies, and anxieties experienced by parents with regard to the risks and the diagnosis, as well as the hospitalization itself.

This work was carried out in order to understand what were the preconceived notions of the general population and also to assess the level of understanding and anxiety in the parents, before and after hospitalization of the child. In children, we analyzed changes in behavior before and after hospitalization, assembling comparative measurements.

The results of this study show data that compare to the related literature, where one can observe, through research tools, that:

- Maternal anxiety was significantly reduced, by around 30% on average, one month after the surgery when the mother received psycho-affective care and guidance before and during the surgical procedure of her child. Mothers without this care and guidance display an average reduction of 8% in levels of anxiety. These data point to a conclusion that psychological intervention leads to a better adjustment in the way that the mother/caretaker represents and copes with the illness, which she consequently passes on to the child.
- The mothers' levels of informed understanding, measured by correct information about the diagnosis, prognosis, and care for the child, before and after the surgery, were much more comprehensive in the group receiving psychological treatment, at 80% about activity restrictions after surgery and 100% about home care, while these figures respectively, were 50% and 40% in the group of mothers who did not receive guidance.

Further, the adequacy and retention of the information relayed by the pediatric surgeons, of a total of 40 general questions about the treatment, displayed a 67.5% satisfactory response rate in the group that was treated with psychological intervention, whereas the group that only received the usual guidance displayed a 30% satisfactory response rate. The same was true for the unsatisfactory response rate, where the control group who received no further guidance answered 22.5% of questions unsatisfactorily, demonstrating inadequacy in the care of the children, while the psychologically guided group did not offer any inadequate responses. Attention should be paid to the potential risks in the post-operative home-care of children whose families were not cared for and guided in an interdisciplinary manner.

- The frequency of unwanted children's behavior such as bedwetting, nail biting, insomnia, night terrors, and overuse or re-attachment of comfort objects (pacifier, bottle) was also lower in the group of children who were given therapeutic space to express their concerns and be guided in a more appropriate coping mechanism to deal with the fear of hospitalization and possible separation from their protective parental figures.

In this way, it was determined that the reception and guidance of the caregivers and the children is beneficial for the family, which produces a more relaxing work environment for the professional, which in turn also provides for fewer minor complications, due to the parents' better understanding of appropriate post-operative homecare and of the measures to be taken in the hospital itself.

Therefore, since 2002, this model protocol has been used by the interdisciplinary pediatric surgery team at HCFMRPUSP, with constant improvements made with respect to the integration of the group for the best possible care for the child and family and seeking to promote a less aversive process for those involved in pediatric surgery.

In this model of care, all children entering the Department of Pediatric Surgery at HCFMRPUSP after a medical screening to assess their clinical needs are referred for a psychological evaluation so that their psycho-emotional and social needs can be perceived in a more global way.

The first meeting assesses the parents' and the child's previous understanding of the health issue and the need for clinical or surgical treatment. Also assessed are the psycho-emotional resources for coping with clinical questions and hospital situations to which they will be submitted.

When the child's visit to the hospital requires only clinical, and not surgical, procedures, the child and its family are evaluated by a psychologist in their understanding of the diagnosis, treatment, and prognosis, as well as their methods of coping with the particular situation.

During this assessment, the family group receives additional information about ways to manage the child's behavior in order to favor the treatment and are offered, when necessary, invitations to join support groups for chronic illnesses or individual counseling when the child and/or parents present difficulties in accepting the course of action proposed by the professionals.

Following the chapter is an outline of the protocol for psychological preparation of the pre-surgery child that is used at HCFMRPUSP.

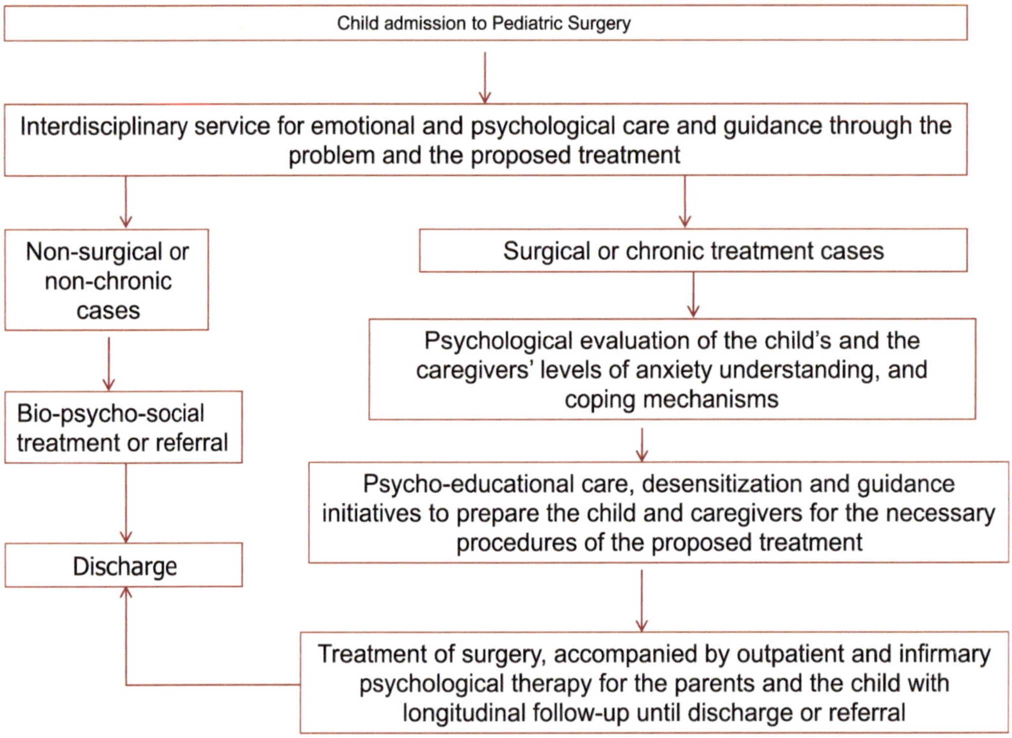

Table 1. Protocol for psychological preparation of the pre-surgery child - HCFMRPUSP

Also assessed during this meeting are the issues of the child's global development, and necessary referrals are made to ensure the best possible neuro-psycho-motor development. Only after all these issues have been met and forwarded to the appropriate clinical follow-up services can the child be discharged from the Pediatric Surgery Interdisciplinary Team.

When the child has an organic impairment that requires surgical treatment, the care of the team, in addition to that which is listed above, also includes an interdisciplinary reception and guidance where the illness, procedures, processes, treatments and invasive interventions are clarified in simple and didactic terms, first by the medical team and later by the psychological team.

In this context, parents/caregivers and children are guided through questions about the child's health, the treatment processes, and the hospitalization. During this first meeting of the child to be operated on, a psycho-emotional assessment of the parents and the child about the diagnosis, the pre-operative, operative, and post-operative procedures, and the hospitalization is performed in order to explain and reduce any doubts or possible negative fantasies regarding the experience.

It is often the case that this work is not concluded after only one session, and returns become necessary so that the staff, the child, and the parents are all aware, accepting, and comfortable with the procedures and its possible risks and benefits.

The process of Psychological Intervention is applied to the child and its parents through psycho-educational guidelines, or information for caregivers and children.

For these sessions, verbal instructions, didactic play materials, such as teaching material understandable to laypeople or hospital toys, and real hospital equipment are used as technical resources that may promote desensitization to procedures that may occur during the doctor visits and on the day of the surgery.

The handling of these materials is stimulated so that the real medical procedures will have been previously simulated in a play environment, seeking to promote desensitization of potentially anxiety-inducing situations that parents and children will experience.

Also provided are clarifications of the doubts and eventually presented inappropriate illusions. As part of the psychological intervention process, the most anxious parents and children visit the pediatric pre-anesthesia room of the surgery center and also the recovery room, where they receive a demonstration and explanation of the procedures that will occur there, which are presented by the team's psychologist.

If the child experiences any difficulty in interacting with the medical staff, returns are scheduled weekly or biweekly, except in the case of an emergency surgery, until the child is able to recover from its fear and illusions and interacts appropriately with the team during its evaluations and clinical procedures, which are often invasive.

What occurs, therefore, is an adaptation of the child to the members of the team and to the hospital equipment through successive exposure, as well as a systematic desensitization by reciprocal inhibition, through relaxation technique training, in the cases where the child exhibits resistance to being examined or to remaining calm in the hospital environment.

When an emergency or urgent surgery is required, the child is hospitalized and this procedure of desensitization to the team and the treatment is performed intensively in the infirmary.

4. The psychological focus on interdisciplinary care in pediatric surgery

The psychologist works together with the interdisciplinary team, both on an outpatient basis and in the infirmary.

The following take place in the clinic:

- Pre-operative group therapy that guides and prepares patients and parents for surgery;
- Therapy for families and patients suffering from syndromes and malformations;
- Orientation and guidance for children and parents with difficulty accepting or understanding processes, procedures, diagnoses and/or prognoses;
- Clinical therapy for children and adolescents who complain of daytime and nocturnal enuresis, encopresis, chronic constipation, and colon management;
- Guidelines for parents for the management of their children's behavior.

The specific objectives of the orientation and psychological counseling are:

- To guide and inform parents and patients about the disease and the procedures to be performed during the surgery and hospitalization;
- To promote desensitization to the procedures and to the hospital setting;
- To create awareness of the emotional family aspects that can interfere with adherence to pediatric treatment and to improve the quality of life of the patient and the family.

The following are used as educational materials for working with children and families:

- Playful/didactic hospital supplies that replicate those actually used in real procedures;
- Life-size cloth dolls of that represent a child of approximately one (1) meter in height with internal organs that replicate the human body;
- Real hospital equipment

The orientation and guidance therapy is performed primarily in groups, optimizing in this way the care offered to patients despite the high demand of the clinic. This form of care matches the data published in literature that demonstrates that group activities, beyond permitting a greater comprehensiveness of care, assists the patient in identifying with other people with the same needs, providing a space for clarification of doubts and exchange about similar situations between families.

For these pre-operative guidance and orientation groups, three meetings are generally held, following the procedures described below.

- **1st Meeting** - Parents (Informational meeting)

Informational meeting with the parents about the illness, hospitalization, and surgery of their children, as well as the goals of the group meetings with the children. The objective of this first meeting is for the parents to have a better understanding of their children's illness and the procedures that will be performed by the team, at the same time becoming aware that their children are not the only ones affected by the problem, so that they may thus act more appropriately toward the children's doubts.

- **2nd Meeting** - Children

This meeting is aimed at assessing the children's level of anxiety and understanding, as well as the children's own awareness of their health problem, the proposed treatment, and finally their reaction to the hospital. The order of activities is:

- Introductions and meeting of the children and staff;
- Evaluation of the knowledge and understanding of the children of their own disease;
- Creating awareness that other children are suffering from the same problem;
- Fun activities with hospital toys that promote desensitization to hospitalization;
- Investigation into the expectations of hospitalization and surgery;
- Explanation in a playful and didactic manner, provided by the doctor with the aid of mannequins, about the procedures which the children will go through during hospitalization (pre-anesthetic fasting, venous access, surgery, dressings, care and post-operative changes);
- Orientation about the sequence of surgery, return visits, and discharge;
- Final fun activity where the children simulate hospitalization.

- **3rd Meeting** - Parents and Children

The goal of this meeting is to evaluate the degree of comprehension of information received and to visit the hospital, in the following order:

- Investigation into the absorbed information and, when necessary, more illustrative repetition of anything not understood;
- Explanation in a fun and didactic manner, provided by the nurse in charge of pediatric surgery, with mannequins and hospital equipment, about the procedures and stay in the infirmary;

- Familiarization with the hospital accommodations (bedroom, infirmary playroom, outdoor playground, pre-anesthetic room and recovery room) where the doctor and nurse discuss what happens in each environment; Interactive activities that provide information about the affinity between pairs of children, so that staff can properly select pairs that should be roomed together;
- Closing play with the staff.

In the infirmary, follow-up care and treatment of patients seen in preoperative groups or individually in the clinic is continued, and also, when necessary new treatments are initiated, using the same criteria from the clinic for patients that begin their treatment through a transfer from another center.

5. Importance of interdisciplinary care in pediatric surgery

Over 13 years of work (1998-2011) improvements has been observed, with the procedures that were adopted, both for pre-operative preparation and for the treatment of chronic patients.

For out-patient follow-ups and in the infirmary, the improvements were in the affective development of emotional conflicts, fears, illusions, prejudices against the disease; facilitation of desensitization to procedures and to the hospital setting; lower levels of anxiety in both patients and parents, who demonstrated awareness and comfortableness regarding the procedures; hospitalizations with fewer complications and faster recoveries.

This data shows the importance of the performance of an interdisciplinary staff in the treatment of a pediatric surgery patient and his/her family.

The importance of intervention procedures aimed at the pre-operative preparation of children and their families is increasingly recognized. We should stress the need for this process to be carried out by a specialist in psychology who does not only stop to provide information about clinical procedures.

It is necessary that intervention programs provide conditions in which the parents and children can express their fears and anxieties about the situation that they are experiencing so that they can understand it more effectively.

Psychological Intervention, performed by a professional who is qualified to identify the emotional characteristics of parents and children in a systematic manner and with interdisciplinary support, can reduce the harmful effects to the child-family-professional bonds and can also reduce the undesirable aspects of hospitalization and surgery and consequently support the healthy development of the child.

The presence of a psychology professional together with the surgical team is fundamental when attempting to provide effective treatment to pediatric patients and their families, providing them with an effective understanding of procedures, better interaction with the staff, greater adherence to treatment, and consequently fewer risks to the emotional development of the child as a result of hospitalization.

This team believes that the interdisciplinary treatment in pediatric surgery is of utmost importance, because surgery is a time of crisis for parents and children, during which they are frightened and concerned about the necessity of a surgical intervention.

While the child is afraid of the unknown, of pain and of separation from their loved ones, the adults, in turn, fear the inherent risks of the invasive procedures, illness, and the possible poor prognosis and the treatments to which the child may be submitted.

Therefore, we believe that a staff trained in the care of both children and caregivers, and able to deal with the children's and adults' fears and illusions about their reality, is very important for the proper development of the measures taken and actions necessary in each case.

Our experience supports the national and international published literature that is very rich in articles about the importance of humanizing clinical care with a child and family during illness, especially with those that require hospitalization and who are submitted to invasive procedures, aimed specifically at the preparation of these patients for the procedures they will be undergoing. Here can be mentioned the studies of desensitization to invasive procedures, child-parent coping strategies, treatment and prognosis, as well as interdisciplinary interaction.

From these considerations the importance of guidance and counseling programs for children, when subjected to surgery, as well as for parents, can be emphasized, for both the literature and the real experience reported here show that these interventions are effective in the reduction of anxiety in mothers and children, providing better conditions for confronting stressful situations, and lower rates of behavioral changes in children after surgical procedures.

6. References

Altshuler, J.L.; Genevro, J.L.; Ruble, D.N.; Bornstein, M.H. *Children's Knowledge And Use Of Coping Strategies During Hospitalization For Elective Surgery.* Journal Of Applied Developmental Psychology. 1995 Jan-Mar, Vol 16 (1), P 53-76

Bevan Jc, Johnston C, Haig Mj, Tousignant G, Lucy S, Kirnon V, Assimes Ik, Carranza R. *Preoperative Parental Anxiety Predicts Behavioural And Emotional Responses To Induction Of Anaesthesia In Children.* Can J Anaesth. 1990 Mar;37(2):177-82 Pmid: 2311148

Blount Rl, Cohen Ll, Frank Nc, Bachanas Pj, Smith Aj, Manimala Mr, Pate Jt. *The Child-Adult Medical Procedure Interaction Scale-Revised: An Assessment Of Validity.* J Pediatr Psychol. 1997 Feb;22(1):73-88

Brewer S, Gleditsch Sl, Syblik D, Tietjens Me, Vacik Hw. Pediatric Anxiety: Child Life Intervention In Day Surgery. J Pediatr Nurs. 2006 Feb;21(1):13-22.

Caldwell-Andrews Aa, Blount Rl, Mayes Lc, Kain Zn. Behavioral Interactions In The Perioperative Environment: A New Conceptual Framework And The Development Of The Perioperative Child-Adult Medical Procedure Interaction Scale. Anesthesiology. 2005 Dec;103(6):1130-5. Pmid: 16306723

Christiano, B.; Russ, S.W. Response: Developing Preparatory Interventions For Use In Pediatric Settings. Journal Of Pediatric Psychology. 1998, Vol 23 (1), P 31-32

Clewes, J.L.; Endler, N.S. State Trait Anxiet And The Experience Of Elective Surgery In Children. Canadian Journal Of Behavioural Science. 1994 Apr, Vol 26 (2), P 183-198

Crepaldi, M.A. Hospitalização Na Infância - Representações Sociais Da Família Sobre A Doença E A Hospitalização De Seus Filhos. Cabral Editora Universitária- São Paulo, 1999

Dreger Va, Tremback Tf. Management Of Preoperative Anxiety In Children. Aorn J. 2006 Nov;84(5):778-80, 782-6, 788-90 Passim; Quiz 805-8.

Ellerton Ml, Merriam C. Preparing Children And Families Psychologically For Day Surgery: An Evaluation. J Adv Nurs. 1994 Jun;19(6):1057-62.

Fortier Ma, Martin Sr, Maclaren Chorney J, Mayes Lc, Kain Zn. Preoperative Anxiety In Adolescents Undergoing Surgery: A Pilot Study. Paediatr Anaesth. 2011 Sep;21(9):969-73. Doi: 10.1111/J.1460-9592.2011.03593.X. Epub 2011 Apr 25.

Frank, N.C.; Blount, R.L.; Smith, A.J.; Manimala, M.R.; Martin, J.K. Parent And Staff Behavior, Previous Child Medical Experience, And Maternal Anxiety As They Relate To Child Procedural Distress And Coping. Journal Of Pediatric Psychology. 1995, Vol 20 (3), P 277-289

Frisch Am, Johnson A, Timmons S, Weatherford C.Nurse Practitioner Role In Preparing Families For Pediatric Outpatient Surgery. Pediatr Nurs. 2010 Jan-Feb;36(1):41-7.

Gabrielle Pagé M, Campbell F, Isaac L, Stinson J, Martin-Pichora Al, Katz J. Reliability And Validity Of The Child Pain Anxiety Symptoms Scale (Cpass) In A Clinical Sample Of Children And Adolescents With Acute Postsurgical Pain. Pain. 2011 Sep;152(9):1958-65. Epub 2011 Apr 12.

Gorayeb, RP & Petean, EB, *Intervenção Psicológica Realizada Em Crianças Submetidas A Cirurgias Eletivas E Suas Mães* - Dissertação De Mestrado Apresentada A FFCLRP-USP em 2002

Gorayeb, RP ; Petean, EBL ; Pileggi FO; Tazima, MFGS; Vicente, YAMVA ; Gorayeb, R. *Importance of psychological intervention for the recovery of children submitted to elective surgery.* Journal of Pediatric Surgery (Print), v. 44, p. 1390-1395, 2009.

Guaratini, A.A.; Marcolino, J.A.M.; Teixeira, A.B.; Bernardis, R.C.; Passarelli, M.L.B.; Mathias, L.A.S.T. Estudo Transversal De Ansiedade Pré-Operatória Em Crianças: Utilização Da Escala De Yale Modificad. Revista Brasileira De Anestesiologia. 2006 Nov/Dez V.56 N.6

Justus R, Wyles D, Wilson J, Rode D, Walther V, Lim-Sulit N. Preparing Children And Families For Surgery: Mount Sinai's Multidisciplinary Perspective. Pediatr Nurs. 2006 Jan-Feb;32(1):35-43.

Kain Zn, Caldwell-Andrews A, Wang Sm. *Psychological Preparation Of The Parent And Pediatric Surgical Patient.* Anesthesiol Clin North America. 2002 Mar;20(1):29-44.

Kain Zn, Caldwell-Andrews Aa, Mayes Lc, Weinberg Me, Wang Sm, Maclaren Je, Blount Rl. *Family-Centered Preparation For Surgery Improves Perioperative Outcomes In Children: A Randomized Controlled Trial.* Anesthesiology. 2007 Jan;106(1):65-74.

Kain Zn, Caldwell-Andrews Aa. *Preoperative Psychological Preparation Of The Child For Surgery: An Update.* Anesthesiol Clin North America. 2005 Dec;23(4):597-614, Vii. Pmid: 16310653

Kain Zn, Mayes Lc, Caldwell-Andrews Aa, Karas De, Mcclain Bc. *Preoperative Anxiety, Postoperative Pain, And Behavioral Recovery In Young Children Undergoing Surgery.* Pediatrics. 2006 Aug;118(2):651-8

Li Hc, Lopez V, Lee Tl. *Psychoeducational Preparation Of Children For Surgery: The Importance Of Parental Involvement.* Patient Educ Couns. 2007 Jan;65(1):34-41. Epub 2006 Jul 26.

Li Hc, Lopez V. *Effectiveness And Appropriateness Of Therapeutic Play Intervention In Preparing Children For Surgery: A Randomized Controlled Trial Study.* J Spec Pediatr Nurs. 2008 Apr;13(2):63-73.

Li Hc, Lopez V.2008. *Effectiveness And Appropriateness Of Therapeutic Play Intervention In Preparing Children For Surgery: A Randomized Controlled Trial Study.* J Spec Pediatr Nurs. Apr;13(2):63-73.

Lumley, M.A.; Melamed, B.G.; Abeles, L.A. - *Predicting Children's Presurgical Anxiety And Subsequent Behavior Changes.* Journal Of Pediatric Psychology. 1993 Aug, Vol 18 (4), P 481-497

Lumley, M.A.; Melamed, B.G.; Abeles, L.A. *Predicting Children's Presurgical Anxiety And Subsequent Behavior Change*. Journal Of Pediatric Psychology. 1993 Aug, Vol 18 (4), P 481-497

Lynch M. *Preparing Children For Day Surgery*. Child Health Care. 1994 Spring;23(2):75-85.

Marcolino, J.A.M.; Suzuki, F.M.; Alli, L.A.C.; Gozzani, J.L.;Mathias, L.A.S. *Medida Da Ansiedade E Da Depressão Em Pacientes No Pré-Operatório. Estudo Comparativo*. Revista Brasileira De Anestesiologia. 2007 Mar/Abr V.57 N.2

Margolis, J.O.; Ginsberg, B.; Dear, G.L.; Ross, A.K.; Goral, J.E.; Bailey, A.G. *Peadiatric Preoperative Teaching: Effects At Induction And Postoperatively*. Paediatr Anaesth.1998, Vol 8(1), P17-23

Martin Sr, Chorney Jm, Tan Et, Fortier Ma, Blount Rl, Wald Sh, Shapiro Nl, Strom Sl, Patel S, Kain Zn. 2011. *Changing Healthcare Providers' Behavior During Pediatric Inductions With An Empirically Based Intervention*. Anesthesiology. Jul;115(1):18-27.

Martin Sr, Chorney Jm, Tan Et, Fortier Ma, Blount Rl, Wald Sh, Shapiro Nl, Strom Sl, Patel S, Kain Zn. *Changing Healthcare Providers' Behavior During Pediatric Inductions With An Empirically Based Intervention*. Anesthesiology. 2011 Jul;115(1):18-27.

Martin Sr, Fortier Ma, Kain Di, Tan Et, Huszti H, Wahi A. 2011. *Desire For Perioperative Information And Parental Ethnicity*. Paediatr Anaesth. May 9.

Matsumoto H, Vitale Mg, Hyman Je, Roye Dp Jr. 2001. *Can Parents Rate Their Children's Quality Of Life? Perspectives On Pediatric Orthopedic Outcomes*. J Pediatr Orthop B. May;20(3):184-90.

Messeri A, Caprilli S, Busoni P. *Anaesthesia Induction In Children: A Psychological Evaluation Of The Efficiency Of Parents' Presence*. Paediatr Anaesth. 2004 Jul;14(7):551-6. Pmid: 15200651

Michielsen A, Van Wijk I, Ketelaar M. *Participation And Quality Of Life In Children And Adolescents With Congenital Limb Deficiencies: A Narrative Review*. Prosthet Orthot Int. 2010 Dec;34(4):351-61. Epub 2010 Aug 13.

Moro, E.T.; Módoto, N.S.P. *Ansiedade, A Criança E Os Pais*. Revista Brasileira De Anestesiologia. 2006 Set/Out V.54 N.5

Murphy-Taylor C. *The Benefits Of Preparing Children And Parents For Day Surgery*. Doncaster Children's Hospital. Br J Nurs. 1999 Jun 24-Jul 7;8(12):801-4.

Palermo, T.M.; Drotar, D. *Prediction Of Children's Postoperative Pain: The Role Of Presurgical Expectations And Anticipatory Emotions*. Journal Of Pediatric Psychology. 1996, Vol 21 (5), P 683-698

Piira T, Sugiura T, Champion Gd, Donnelly N, Cole As.*The Role Of Parental Presence In The Context Of Children's Medical Procedures: A Systematic Review*. Child Care Health Dev. 2005 Mar;31(2):233-43.

Sadhasivam S, Cohen Ll, Szabova A, Varughese A, Kurth Cd, Willging P, Wang Y, Nick Tg, Gunter J. *Real-Time Assessment Of Perioperative Behaviors And Prediction Of Perioperative Outcomes*. Anesth Analg. 2009 Mar;108(3):822-6.

Thompson, R.H.; Vernon, D.T. *Research On Children's Behavior After Hospitalization: A Review And Synthesis*. Journal Of Developmental And Behavioral Pediatrics. 1993 Feb, Vol 14 (1), P 28-35

Van Der Bruggen Co, Stams Gj, Bögels Sm. *Research Review: The Relation Between Child And Parent Anxiety And Parental Control: A Meta-Analytic Review*. J Child Psychol Psychiatry. 2008 Dec;49(12):1257-69. Epub 2008 Mar 17.

William Li Hc, Lopez V, Lee T. *Effects Of Preoperative Therapeutic Play On Outcomes Of School-Age Children Undergoing Day Surgery*. Res Nurs Health. 2007 Jun;30(3):320-32

Zuckerberg Al. *Perioperative Approach To Children*. Pediatr Clin North Am. 1994 Feb;41(1):15-29.

Part 4

Psychosocial Issues

10

Adolescent Psychosocial Development and Evaluation: Global Perspectives

Fadia AlBuhairan[1], Rosawan Areemit[2],
Abigail Harrison[3] and Miriam Kaufman[4]
[1]*Department of Pediatrics, King Abdulaziz Medical City and King Saud bin Abdulaziz University for Health Sciences, Riyadh,*
[2]*Division of Ambulatory Pediatrics, Department of Pediatrics, Faculty of Medicine, Khon Kaen University, Khon Kaen,*
[3]*Department of Child Health, University of the West Indies, Mona,*
[4]*Division of Adolescent Medicine, Department of Pediatrics, The Hospital for Sick Children and University of Toronto,*
[1]*Saudi Arabia*
[2]*Thailand*
[3]*Jamaica*
[4]*Canada*

1. Introduction

Adolescence is a product of the modern world. It has developed into a distinct stage of life as a result of a shift in many societies requiring a highly trained work force. When this is not needed, young people usually acquire skills needed to work as they grow up. As they go through puberty, they acquire additional responsibilities, usually with the oversight of parents or in apprenticeship to others outside of the family. Young women usually marry close to the time of the onset of fertility. However, with increasing education needs, there is an increasing gap between physical maturation and the ability to take on adult responsibilities. Young people who join the workforce early can be at a disadvantage compared to those who can complete more education. Young women have increasing control over their fertility in these societies, which also gives them these extra years to become more educated.

These factors lead to a cohort of young people who have adult bodies without having adult responsibilities. They have the luxury of time to contemplate, to take risks, and to define themselves in new ways. All of this has led to the phenomenon of adolescence, which encompasses and goes beyond the physical changes of puberty.

This is not to say that adolescent development has not previously existed; it is rather that societies' awareness of this developmental stage of life has only recently emerged or been modified because of the societal changes that have occurred and the effects of globalization.

As a definable period of adolescence is created in a society, it is accompanied by new societal issues—children separating emotionally from their parents while still being reliant on them, experimentation with drugs and alcohol, sexual expression outside of traditional marriage, body image issues, and others. Healthcare practitioners can provide anticipatory guidance to parents and their adolescents, gathering data with sensitive, non-judgmental questioning. All of this must be based on an understanding of adolescent development.

2. Global trends in adolescent demographics

In many parts of the world, only childhood and adulthood are seen as distinct phases of life. Adolescents, as defined by the World Health Organization and United Nations, are those individuals aged 10-19 years (United Nations Children's Fund [UNICEF], 2011). Though different healthcare organizations and societies may define adolescents differently because of societal, cultural, and economic conditions, the term adolescent in this chapter will refer to the above-mentioned age group.

There are currently 1.2 billion adolescents in the world, making up 18% of the world's population. Eighty-eight percent of adolescents live in the developing world, and more than half of the world's adolescents live in South Asia or East Asia and Pacific region (UNICEF, 2011) (Figure 1). Previously, much focus was given to preventing communicable diseases of childhood. Significant improvement in that regard has come about, and now leaders globally are recognizing the need to address and focus on the second decade of life, adolescence, in order to sustain and consolidate the achievements made during the first decade of children's lives (UNICEF, 2011).

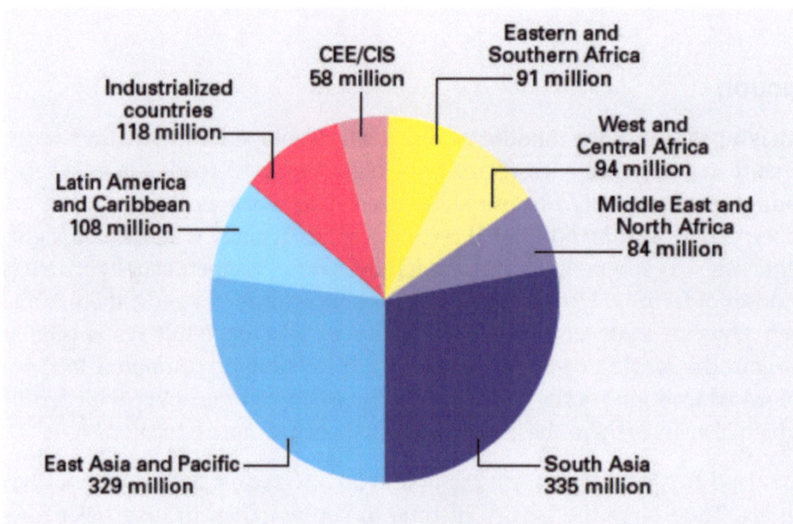

Source: UNICEF, *The State of the World's Children 2011: Adolescence an age of Opportunity* (2011), as cited in United Nations, Department of Economic and Social Affairs, Population Division. *World Population Prospects: The 2008 Revision*, www.esa.un.org/undp/wpp2008/index.htm, accessed October 2010.

Fig. 1. Adolescent population (10-19 years) by region, 2009

There are some clear demographic differences throughout the world. This may be explained by the differences in initiation of decline in fertility and mortality rates. Those countries, many of which are in North America and Europe, that had the earliest initiation of decline in fertility and mortality rates, now have low growth rates and an aging population. Countries that had a later initiation of decline in fertility and mortality rates, such as those in Latin America, the Caribbean, East Asia, and some parts of the Middle East and South Asia, continue to have moderate population growth. In most of Sub-Saharan Africa and some parts of the Middle East and South Asia, there has not yet been a decline in fertility and mortality rates, and so in these parts of the world, young and youthful populations are seen (Brown et al., 2002). These differences result in a contrast in the age structure and age-dependency ratios of individual countries and impact the economic and social structure of a country in varying ways (Assaad & Roudi-Fahimi, 2007; Brown et al., 2002).

When it comes to health care, pediatricians in developed countries have been given the responsibility to care for adolescents (American Academy of Pediatrics, 1978). This is largely due to the fact that adolescents continue to grow and develop, a hallmark of pediatrics. Although the physical development is the first and earliest to be completed, adolescents continue to undergo cognitive and emotional development well into their 20's. The age limit of Pediatrics varies across the world. Many developed countries have extended the age limit to 18 or even 21 years, while other countries, mostly developing countries, have lower age limits.

Adolescents are generally the healthiest of the population, with their leading causes of death being accidents, homicide, and suicide (Brown et al., 2002). HIV/AIDS is the leading cause of death in some parts of the world (Brown et al., 2002). All of these causes are preventable, and so when it comes to adolescent health, an adolescent's contact with a healthcare provider, for whatever reason, can be seen as an opportunistic time to address these matters. Risk-taking behaviors exacerbate the problems that may be faced during adolescence, and in some developing countries, work-related disability and mortality is an additional problem (Brown et al., 2002). When discussing adolescent health, much attention is frequently given to the problems that may be encountered such as risky behaviors. It is important to note, however, that it is only a minority of adolescents who are involved with serious problems as substance use, teenage pregnancy, and acts of violence (United Nations [UN], n.d.). Most adolescents actually go through this stage of life without much turbulence. It is a time when many adolescents gain personal growth, development, and independence and attain certain skills. Adolescence can and should be viewed as a time of opportunity.

Some of the problems that face adolescents differ depending on where they live. For example, substance use, eating disorders, and lack of exercise are more prevalent in developed countries. There are gender gaps when it comes to education, with generally more males attending secondary school in comparison to females. In fact, two thirds of children who never went to school or dropped out are girls. In South Asia, for example, 52% of boys but only 33% of girls are enrolled in secondary school. In contrast, girls in Latin America and the Caribbean have higher secondary school enrollment rates than boys, 56% and 52% respectively (UN, n.d.). This is important to address because the more education a girl receives, the more likely she is to postpone marriage and motherhood (UNICEF, 2011). It has also been found that knowledge and skills obtained through formal education is less advanced in students coming from developing countries in comparison to those students from developed countries (Nugent, 2005).

Reproductive health also varies across regions. Adolescent females are less likely to use contraceptives than adult women, and adolescent mothers are more at risk of developing complications related to pregnancy than adult mothers (Nugent, 2005). An adolescent mother is also more likely to drop out of school and be less educated than an adolescent female who has not become pregnant. Marital age has increased in many parts of the world, yet in some regions, child marriage (marriage by 18 years) continues to occur and is largely driven by 'poverty, parental concerns about premarital sex and pregnancy, and other economic and cultural reasons' (Nugent, 2005).

Because of these differences, a pediatrician's approach to the psychosocial history of an adolescent needs to be tailored to meet the needs of different regions/countries. Although we recognize each country, and sometimes different parts within the same country, may have their own unique issues, it is impossible to address matters of every single country. For this reason, in this chapter, we have decided to focus on some regions of the world and give an example of one country per region, though keeping in mind that this may not apply to every single country within the same region.

3. Developmental changes that occur during adolescence

Many changes occur during adolescence, the most obvious being the physical ones. Pediatric and other medical references tend to focus on these physical changes, and this information is readily available. For this reason, the physical changes that occur during puberty and adolescence will not be discussed here. Rather, the focus will be on the other developmental changes that occur: the cognitive and emotional changes. These develop more insidiously and health care providers may be less familiar with them. In addition, healthcare providers may be deceived by the physical appearances of adolescents which are not necessarily proportionate to their cognitive and/or emotional development.

3.1 Cognitive development

Adolescence is a sensitive and critical period for both normal and maladaptive patterns of development. This period was formerly described as the time of transition from concrete operational thinking to formal logical (abstract) thinking, including development in reasoning and judgment.

New perspectives emphasize that adolescent thinking is a function of social, emotional, and cognitive processes (Steinberg, 2005). There is growing evidence that the brain continues to mature throughout adolescence and into early adulthood (Gogtay et al., 2004). During this period, brain, behavioral, and cognitive development systems mature at different rates, causing adolescence to be a period of increased vulnerability and adjustment.

Two issues are especially relevant to understanding adolescent psychological development. First, brain development in this period is mostly in regions that have an important role in regulation of behavior and emotion and to the perception and evaluation of risk and reward. Significant changes include myelination and synaptic pruning, which increase the efficiency of information processing and enhance transmission of brain messages (Paus, 2005). Areas associated with more basic functions, including the motor and sensory areas, mature in the early teen years, while the prefrontal cortex, the reasoning area of the brain and an important area for controlling impulses, emotions and executive functioning, appears to reach adult dimension in the early 20s, with girls developing earlier than boys (Geidd et al., 1999; Gogtay et al., 2004; Luna et al., 2010). Executive functions include the ability to inhibit impulses, weigh consequences of decisions, prioritize, strategize, long-term planning, decision-making, self-evaluation, self-regulation, and the coordination of affect and cognition. Second, changes in arousal and motivation brought on by pubertal maturation precede the development of regulatory competence (Blakemore et al., 2010). The brain's reward center, the ventral striatum, also is more active during adolescence than in adulthood.

This creates a gap between the adolescent's affective experience and the ability to regulate arousal and motivation. While the adolescent brain continues to strengthen its connections between reasoning and emotion related regions, each adolescent progresses at varying rates in developing their ability to think and their own view of the world.

Adolescent thinking becomes more multidimensional and they are better to contemplate hypothetical situations and the relationship between varied actions or decisions and outcomes, but decision-making remains susceptible to emotions.

Adolescent cognitive development can be characterized into 3 stages: early, middle, and late (Cromer, 2011; Radzik et al., 2007).

In early adolescence, the use of formal logical operations is mainly focused on schoolwork and in home environments. This includes questioning authority and societal standards. There is development of enhanced ability to verbalize thoughts and views, starting with those related to their life. These include choices regarding engaging in sports, peer groups, dress, and parental rules that adolescents think should be changed. At this stage, they may be unable to perceive long-term outcomes of current decision-making.

In middle adolescence, more complex thinking processes are used. The focus expands to include more philosophical and futuristic concerns. Middle adolescents tend to question and analyze more extensively in order to form their own code of ethics, identity, and possible future goals, which may begin to influence relationships with others. They may perceive future implications, but may not apply it in decision-making.

In late adolescence, complex thinking processes are used to focus on less self-centered concepts as well as personal decision-making. Adolescents may think about more global concepts such as justice, history, politics, and patriotism. They develop idealistic views on specific topics or concerns and may debate and develop intolerance of opposing views. They tend to focus on making career decisions and think about their emerging role in society. At this stage, they are able to think things through independently and weigh consequences before making decisions. Table 1 summarizes the cognitive changes that occur during adolescence.

Understanding cognitive development during this period is helpful in understanding age differences in judgment and decision-making, risk-taking, sensation-seeking, and also why adolescence can be a time of increased risk for the onset of a wide range of emotional and behavioral problems, including depression, violent delinquency, and substance abuse.

	Early adolescence	Middle adolescence	Late adolescence
Cognitive development	Emergence of formal logical operations	More complex thinking processes used	Complex thinking processes used
	Focus on personal decisions, demonstrated in schoolwork and home environments	Focus expands to include more philosophical and futuristic concerns	Focus on less self-centered concepts as well as personal decision-making
	May be unable to perceive long-term outcomes of current decision-making	May perceive future implications of actions, but may not apply it in decision-making	Able to think things through independently and weigh consequences before making decisions
Emotional development	Peers are an increasingly important source of support	Increased conflict with parents as peer group interest peaks	Adolescent - parent communication improves
	Increased closeness of same sex interaction	Increased experience of a wide range of emotions	Increased autonomy from parents
	Increased need for privacy with increased interest in personal physical appearance and body image	Cognitive control over emotional responses limited	Increased confidence in personal beliefs and ability to express them
	Increasing awareness of a wider range of emotions begins	Sensation seeking at its peak with increased risk taking behavior Increased sexual arousal with increased sexual activity and experimentation	Improved cognitive control over emotional responses

Table 1. Cognitive and emotional developmental changes that occur during adolescence

3.2 Emotional development

Adolescence has been quaintly described as "that awkward period between sexual maturation and the attainment of adult roles and responsibilities"(Dahl, 2004). It is a time of great change with concurrent but asynchronous physical, cognitive, and emotional development. Although most adolescents progress through this phase unscathed with gradual, appropriate changes, some may experience significant challenges. Adolescents experience many changes in how they interact with their family, peers, society, and themselves (Choudhoury et al., 2006). They move from an idealistic opinion of parents during childhood, into increased conformity to peer group expectations and values, to the development of their own personal values and principles as they progress through early, middle, and late adolescence (B. Newman & P. Newman, 1999). This movement mirrors a shift in emotional support from family to peers and then to self and intimate partners. This is not to say there is or should be separation from the family, as healthy emotional development is highly dependent on continued positive interaction with parents throughout (Larson & Brown, 2007). However, there is gradual change until parents and the adolescent or young adult accept their individual roles and are able to share and challenge each others' personal views and beliefs in a healthy way.

As previously mentioned, emotional and cognitive development are inextricably linked as brain development progresses throughout adolescence into early adulthood. Cognition has a significant impact on expression of emotions, and conversely emotion and situational contexts have a significant impact on adolescents' behavioral choices (Steinberg, 2005). Emotional development during adolescence involves learning to recognize and master the control of emotions experienced so as to facilitate functioning within expected societal norms. Emotions serve many important functions including motivating positive behavior, achieving goals, providing information about self, and facilitating relationships, including intimacy (Larson & Brown, 2007). It involves self-discovery and self-characterization to acquire a specific role in society which is facilitated by the enhanced abstract thought acquired during adolescence. There is evidence to support an association between cognitive maturation and increased regulation of emotional behavior; however it has been proposed that these changes are non-linear unlike development during childhood and adulthood (Casey et al., 2010). The subcortical limbic system -including the amygdala is important in the processing of emotions and emotional responses to social stimuli, whereas the prefrontal cortex is responsible for the cognitive control or regulation of emotional behavior. An "Imbalance Model" has been put forward that proposes that an imbalance between the development of these two systems may be related to the development of psychopathology (Casey et al., 2010). Sensitivity to rewards seems to peak in adolescence and may have a positive impact, such as academic or athletic achievements or negative influence with thrill seeking through use of substances or other high-risk behaviors. This incentive response suggests behaviors may be defined from a motivational perspective, and the dorsal and ventral striata which receive input from the cerebral cortex have been found to be involved in these responses (Somerville & Casey, 2010). There is also a significant association between the pubertal stage of maturation and affective measures including sensation-seeking, sex and sexual arousal, emotional sensitivity, and sleep, with sensation-seeking peaking in middle adolescence (Steinberg, 2005).

High intensity emotions may also have a significant impact on adolescents' thought processes and by extension to their behavioral choices – these have been referred to as 'hot' and 'cold' cognitions (Dahl, 2004; Somerville & Casey, 2010). 'Hot cognitions' refer to thinking amidst high intensity emotions and often result in poor decision-making. 'Cold cognitions' refer to thoughts in a state of calm, more commonly resulting in appropriate decision-making. This may explain why the adolescent who is usually even-keeled may, under certain 'hot' circumstances, make an otherwise unexpected poor decision.

Healthy emotional development is a key developmental task for adolescents who are learning to negotiate increasingly complex and ambiguous social interactions and utilize lessons learned from previous experiences to assist in determining future choices. Discordance during this time of development may serve as the root of psychopathology. Adolescents who fail to learn how to modify their own emotions may become impulsive with progression to delinquent behavior or may become alienated both from peers and family, leading to parental conflict, relationship challenges, and an increased risk of depression, substance abuse, and suicide risk.

4. Interviewing the adolescent

Evaluation of an adolescent's psychosocial status is done through interview and may be an uncomfortable task for many healthcare providers. Because adolescents are generally the healthiest, contact with healthcare systems may be minimal; therefore, any contact should be considered an opportunity to obtain a psychosocial history and provide anticipatory guidance.

The literature available on the psychosocial interview of an adolescent is largely based on the North American experience. Even within North America, there are certain issues that need to be kept in mind based on the individual background of an adolescent, as will be discussed below. The psychosocial interview and history-taking in other parts of the world may vary from that conducted in North America depending on local norms, cultures, and existing or prevalent conditions. For this reason, three regions of the world, in addition to North America, will be presented below with particular focus given to one country per region. Unique issues and/or issues that are particularly relevant to that particular country/region will be emphasized in each section, in a manner that will be practical for a healthcare practitioner to utilize when providing care to an adolescent from the specified part of the world.

4.1 Interviewing the adolescent in North America

The HEADS acronym was introduced in North America (Goldenring & Rosen, 2004) to assist healthcare providers in obtaining a comprehensive adolescent psychosocial history in a sensitive manner and is seen by many to be universally applicable across the continent. It is important to remember that there is huge diversity in the adolescent population in North America, where right-wing fundamentalists, the descendants of African slaves, affluent youth, children of illegal migrant workers, rural youth, urban youth, and many others co-exist. Laws regarding consent and capacity vary, with many American jurisdictions allowing consent only to those over the age of 18 years, while many Canadian provinces have a functional definition that allows youth to give consent when they are capable of doing so.

Within all this diversity is a need to discuss basic psychosocial issues with children, adolescents, and youth. The original HEADS acronym now has many variations.

- *Home*: The vast majority of North American adolescents live with at least one parent. Careful questioning will elicit the family constellation, which may include grandparents, step-parents, siblings and step-siblings, and unrelated friends. Some young people may see a pet as being a member of the family. Questions must be asked in a way that allows for the teen to disclose that they are homeless, have difficult relationships, or have a non-traditional family, such as one with two fathers or two mothers.
- *Education*: Throughout North America, there is mandatory schooling, usually until age 16. Most young people continue through secondary education, which is usually grade 12 or age 18. Urban areas, particularly in the United States, have high rates of students who do not complete high school. If one asks a young person what their school performance is like, they all know that the correct answer is "fine" or "OK". Specific questions about marks, the level of the courses they are taking (with much variation in terms of level of schooling offered), how much school they miss, and career goals are all important.
- *Eating*: Eating disorders are prevalent in North America, resulting in young people being both underweight and overweight. The current focus in schools and health systems on obesity focuses on the importance of being thin, which may be a trigger for anorexia nervosa or bulimia. More and more, eating disorders are being diagnosed in pre-adolescents, often associated with significant anxiety or anxiety disorders. Poverty is strongly associated with childhood obesity, with less nutritious foods being available and limited opportunities for safe exercise for those living in inner cities.
- *Activities*: Some North American adolescents are extremely active as athletes, volunteers, or workers. Working more than 16 hours a week often interferes with scholastic achievement. Some places require volunteer work for students to graduate from high school. Direct questions about screen time are essential, with many young people spending 5 or more hours a day in front of a computer or TV screen. Many are unaware of the dangers of revealing personal information on the internet to a legion of "friends" they have never met. Peer relationships should also be addressed, including questions about how the young person spends their lunchtime, if they see their friends outside of school, whether their parents allow them to have friends outside their religious or cultural group, and if there are discrepancies in the rules about friendship for boys and girls within a family.
- *Adherence*: Chronic health conditions are not uncommon in North America, with adolescents surviving with conditions that were previously fatal. Adolescents have many reasons for not taking medications—their family might not be able to afford them, they may see them as a sign that they are different from their friends, a chaotic household does not lend itself to the organization needed to be adherent, and mental health issues can interfere with the ability to regularly take medication. Medications that affect physical appearance, such as steroids, can be quite problematic for young people. Questions need to be asked in a sensitive manner without making assumptions about adherence and the importance placed on medications within a family.
- *Drugs*: Most drugs are readily available to North American youth. Alcohol is the most common substance used by youth, followed by marijuana and tobacco. Young people may respond well to being asked about drugs in their environment first, such as asking, "At your school, do students tend to drink more or take drugs?" You can then go on to

ask about their friendship group and finally to their own personal use. Experimental use is common, but questions should be asked about the impact of use on their academics, family relationships, and friendships. Young people should also be asked about their parents' use of alcohol, tobacco, and other substances.

- *Safety*: Adolescence is a time of risk taking, and this can lead to personal growth and a feeling of satisfaction. It can also have severe and even fatal consequences. Safety is an issue in recreation, work, driving, and social relationships. Asking about physical safety such as drinking and driving or the use of bicycle helmets is important, but so is social safety, including questions about bullying and sexual assault.
- *Suicide*: An easy way to start a conversation about mental health is to enquire about mood, "On a scale of 1 to 10, with 1 being so sad you might kill yourself and 10 being the happiest you have ever felt, how would you rate yourself today and in the last week?" Questions about sleep, appetite, energy, and concentration are very useful. Young people usually don't want to admit to anything that might sound like a mental illness, but are often quick to endorse high levels of stress, so exploring the stress in their lives can be a good way to find out about these issues. If a young person admits that they have been thinking about suicide, it is important to find out if this is an active thought, if they have made a plan, written a suicide note, or done anything else to make this a reality. Suicide risk should be taken seriously, and parents need to be brought into the discussion to prevent this disaster from happening. In the United States and in rural Canada, many families own firearms. These should be removed from the home if there is any concern about suicidality.
- *Sex*: About 50% of North American youth have had heterosexual sexual intercourse by the time they finish high school. In the United States, teen pregnancy rates are high and abortions may be difficult to access. Young people need to be asked about their sexual activities in a non-judgmental way that does not assume that they have or do not have a particular sexual activity and that are non-gendered. A young person who is homosexual might not be sexually active, and they are as likely to have heterosexual sex as their heterosexual peers. Young people may have sex but not be in a relationship, so questions about sex must include both questions linked to a partner and ones that are separate. The question, "Have you ever had sex with anyone?" can lead to a fruitful discussion

The adolescent psychosocial history in three different regions will be discussed below: the Caribbean, the Middle East, and South East Asia, with Jamaica, Saudi Arabia, and Thailand being an example country from each region respectively. For consistency and practical purposes, the HEADS acronym will serve as a guide for the psychosocial interview in each region, with differences or variations in the acronym emphasized. The sequence of the topics addressed may vary depending on local sensitivities or significance. It is important to bear in mind that the reported experiences (unless otherwise referenced) are based on the authors' local experiences. Also keep in mind that some differences may apply to countries within the same region, and therefore it is important for one to familiarize himself with conditions or behaviors that may be particularly prevalent in a specific country.

4.2 Interviewing the adolescent in the Caribbean

Jamaica is the largest English-speaking Caribbean island, situated in the northern Caribbean Sea and is classified as a developing country with an upper-middle income economy by the

World Bank (The World bank, 2011). Adolescents aged 10-19 years account for almost 20% of the total population, with 10-24 year olds representing 27% of the population (Statistical Institute of Jamaica, 2011). Similarly, adolescents 10-19 years represent one-fifth of the total population in the Caribbean (Crawford et al., 2009). In Jamaica, pediatric services in the public health system stop at age 12 years; thereafter care is transferred to adult-centered services. In the past decade, the Ministry of Health has increased its focus on adolescent health care with the promotion of the adolescent friendly approach in health centers. There are currently no national guidelines for adolescent health care in Jamaica, and the practice of preventive health care for adolescents is at a less than optimal level (Harrison et al., 2011). A minority of physicians recommend regular health maintenance visits for adolescent patients, and so screening for potential health concerns should be performed at any visit, whether for acute or well care (Harrison et al., 2011).

Culturally, parents continue to assume primary responsibility for their adolescent's health care and usually accompany them for health visits or send an older family member. Some physicians report parents limiting access to teens for confidential discussion (Harrison et al., 2011), however with appropriate explanation of confidentiality policies to parents and adolescents together, confidential discussion with the adolescent is usually possible. It is most helpful to introduce the concept to parents as time alone with a health professional being an opportunity for adolescents to start accepting responsibility for their own health care. The provider's office should be promoted as a 'safe-place' for discussion of any concerns affecting an adolescent's health- physical, emotional, psychological, and not a place to "just talk about sex and drugs". Of course, it is appropriate that parents be kept 'in the loop' with regard to their adolescent's care, and once assured of this, most parents and adolescents seem to welcome confidential discussion with the health provider.

Many of the public healthcare facilities in Jamaica are understaffed, and this significantly impacts the time available for appropriate discussion with adolescents and parents. The well recognized psychosocial history acronym, HEADS, used widely internationally, was created to accommodate for this challenge. However in a recent survey, a minority of physicians in Jamaica reported being aware of HEADS, and as such, exposure to and training in the use of HEADS is being expanded for Jamaican physicians through continued medical education efforts.

As would be expected for any other cultural setting or geographic region, the tool has to be modified to be culturally sensitive for the specific population. Some of these modifications will be briefly discussed below.

- *Home:* Jamaica and many other Caribbean countries are matriarchal societies and have varied family units, including married, common-law, visiting, and single, with the most prevalent in Jamaica being the common-law marital relationship (UNICEF, n.d.). A positive male influence is therefore frequently absent, and the details as to how this affects the adolescent and the family in general, need to be explored. Many children and adolescents are also left in the care of extended family, as parents go overseas to seek employment, planning to support their family through remittances. Detailed information on household members and shared households must be taken including the level of supervision, age and gender of other household members or caregivers. The provider also needs to enquire about the frequency and quality of interaction with parents (verbal and/or physical), as there may often be concerns surrounding separation issues, family conflict, and safety within the home, with the resultant externalizing and internalizing behaviors in the adolescent.

- *Education/ Employment*: Similar to other countries, physicians need to enquire about the grade currently attained in school, whether the adolescent attends school, what grades they are getting, and whether they have been suspended or otherwise disciplined. In Jamaica, most adolescents attend public high/secondary schools (grade 7-11) with a student:teacher ratio of approximately 35:1. Adolescents with specific challenges or needs, such as those with Attention Deficit Hyperactivity Disorder (ADHD) or learning disorders, may go unnoticed in schools, and therefore physicians should enquire about these issues during health visits with adolescents. Another concern in Jamaican schools is bullying, which has recently started to receive more attention both from school administrations as well as in the public domain. Culturally, mild bullying has often been dispelled with the view that it is "just toughening you up", and "those little things should not bother you". More serious bullying is often settled on an individual basis with physical retaliation, as the culture is one that promotes the concept of "standing up for yourself". However some adolescents do not cope well with bullying, and physicians therefore need to ask questions about bullying, including physical, emotional, and relational bullying, in a sensitive manner. For example "Does anybody at school say things to you that bother you?", "Do you feel like you fit in or do people ignore you?", or "Does anybody force you to do things you don't want to... send you to buy lunch without giving you money?" A balanced approach is important when assessing for potential bullying as Jamaicans are a people who oftentimes speak bluntly, frequently not utilizing the Westernized social graces of saying things in a 'politically correct way'. Law mandates secondary level education in Jamaica; however, some adolescents may simply advance through the education system without actually acquiring the expected knowledge and skills. Ultimately, these adolescents leave school being unprepared for the adult work force with some becoming street youth with exposure to the attendant risks. Vocational/employment challenges are common as there are limited job opportunities for adolescents. As a result, some adolescents, particularly within 'inner city' societies, are wooed to establish an illegal lifestyle, joining 'gangs' and associating with 'area leaders or dons' in an attempt to make an easier living. These concerns have to be carefully asked about as many of these adolescents will not admit to being involved with illegal activity, however may respond in the positive if asked "Are any of your friends or other young people in your community linking up with gangs?"
- *Eating:* Anecdotally, there is limited awareness of disordered eating behaviors and attitudes in Jamaica both by lay persons as well as healthcare providers. Culturally, eating disorders have not been considered a problem in the society as a desire for the 'voluptuous', 'thick', 'full-bodied' woman has always been thought to be protective against body image concerns that focus on achieving low weight. However, national surveys have identified that Jamaican adolescents engage in disordered eating behaviors (DEB) (Fox & Gordon-Strachan, 2007), and a cross Caribbean survey found that although the prevalence of DEBs was less in the Caribbean than in North America, the use of extreme weight control measures was greater among Caribbean adolescents (McGuire et al., 2002). In clinical practice, the prevalence of DEBs anecdotally appears to

be increasing among Jamaican adolescents, perhaps due to increased globalization and internalization of the Westernized 'thin ideal'. Conversely, there is significant concern and more awareness about obesity in Jamaican adolescents (Wilks et al., 2007), secondary to increasingly inappropriate nutritional intake, fuelled by many popular fast-food restaurants. There is also limited emphasis being placed on physical exercise, including the removal of scheduled sessions for physical exercise in schools after grade 9. Additionally, there is limited access to safe outdoor spaces to facilitate exercise in some neighborhoods.

- *Activities:* Enquiring about activities engaged in, who time is shared with, and ensuring that adolescents have at least one trusted friend, referred to locally as a 'bredrin' or a 'bonafide' is important. Jamaican adolescents are technologically savvy, especially when Jamaica is still considered to be a developing country, with the vast majority of adolescents owning a mobile phone or having easy access to computers and the internet, often times with limited supervision. It is therefore important for providers to enquire about total media time to ensure this is not interfering significantly with schoolwork. It is also important to enquire about internet safety practices, for example "Do people you don't know try to 'friend' you… Do you accept people you don't know as friends?" Providers need to take the opportunity to reinforce positive practices and give appropriate advice, for example, "Be careful what pictures you send to your boy/girlfriend since you don't know what they'll do with them if you break up… Once the picture is out on the web, you can never get it back". Due to the small size and population of the Caribbean countries, it is particularly important to enquire about and advise against disclosing personal information online.
- *Drugs:* The local law states that substances such as cigarettes and alcohol are illegal for use in persons under 18 years. Monitoring and the consequences for sidestepping these are minimal and it is not difficult for 'under age' adolescents to access alcohol and cigarettes, with it being almost normative for many adolescents. However the level of binge-drinking among Jamaican adolescents is significantly less than that noted in North America. This more relaxed attitude towards use of these substances is pervasive and therefore health providers must ensure to enquire not only about use but also frequency and in particular, high risk behavior including driving under the influence. Initial questions should be more general, enquiring of friends and then becoming more specific: "Do you drink any alcohol, like beer or Smirnoff ice?", as many young people don't consider these 'real liquor'. There is generally little difficulty in acquiring marijuana although it is illegal in Jamaica. Many Jamaican adolescents do not think of marijuana as a "real" or "serious" drug. Additionally, many local musical artists identify with the Rastafarian faith which includes the use of marijuana as a part of their spiritual experience. A balanced harm-reduction approach with a gradual move towards abstinence is therefore most likely to be effective in cases of marijuana use by adolescents.
- *Sex and sexuality:* Jamaica, is a predominantly Christian country, and in many aspects a very religious society. This serves as a stabilizing and positive force in many adolescents' lives, and during the interview, enquiry into their level of involvement in church activities and how their religion informs their personal beliefs and practices is appropriate. However, religiosity can also have a negative impact, and Jamaican adolescents have reported the fear of contradicting church expectations as reasons for not seeking information from adult caregivers or accessing appropriate contraception

(Crawford et al., 2009). The age for consenting to sexual activity in Jamaica and the majority of the English-speaking Caribbean is 16 years, however the mean age for sexual debut is 13.5 years for males and 16.1 years for females (Jamaica Family Planning Board and Division of Reproductive Health, Centers for Disease Control and Prevention, 2008). The "Access to Reproductive Health Care Policy" guideline allows for the use of non-invasive contraceptives for adolescents who present for care and are unwilling to practice abstinence, however many health providers are still uncomfortable with this practice (Crawford et al., 2009). Many adolescents experience significant pressure to become sexually active from peers and the media, with a vibrant dancehall music culture that normalizes casual sex (Crawford et al., 2009). Discussion about adolescents and sexual activity is still considered taboo, and so health providers may have to first enquire about friends' sexual activity and then segue into the adolescent's personal activity, facilitating age-appropriate advice and care. Much of the local music and media promote men having relationships with multiple women, and many adolescent females feel that they cannot expect a monogamous relationship even though that is most times their preference. Healthcare providers therefore need to enquire of the power shift in relationships and if this is resulting in an unhealthy relationship. They may ask "Does your boyfriend refuse to wear a condom even if you ask?" or "Does your boyfriend get very jealous and check your phone calls or text messages?" It is not uncommon for young women to know that they are not the only sexual partner for someone but to still feel unsure of demanding condom use when the male partner argues against this. Female adolescents need to be empowered to make these demands by improving their concept of self-esteem and self-worth, if even to ensure they know how to put on the partner's condom. Jamaica is a very rigid society with regard to its approach towards homosexual orientation. Although often described internationally as a 'homophobic' society, Jamaicans in general have been found to be quite tolerant of homosexuality unless it 'directly' affects them. Though there is much homophobic rhetoric, many adolescents can identify at least one friend or schoolmate whom they think is homosexual and are not at odds unless specifically asked to say they are in agreement with homosexual relationships. This is felt to stem from a deep religious belief within the society that homosexuality is wrong. Although figures among adolescents are limited, and if available, likely to reflect underreporting (Crawford et al., 2009), anecdotally the prevalence of adolescent homosexual activity seems to be increasing. Healthcare providers must therefore care for their adolescents in a non-judgmental manner and enquire of adolescents' orientation and sexual history.

- *Safety:* In Jamaica, the prevalence of violent crimes is very high, and many of these are committed against and by adolescents including sexual offences, assault, and even homicides (Harriott, 2008). There are many neighborhoods that are unsafe with adolescents in these areas being under the added pressure of daily safety concerns. These concerns expand to some schools where students may carry concealed weapons as well. Questions such as "Do you feel safe in your home…school…community?" can be very revealing and the platform for further evaluation. Sexual safety may also be of concern as sexual offences are committed most frequently within the home or community. Questions such as "Has anyone ever touched you or done anything sexual to you that you did not want or like?" may be the only opportunity an adolescent has to discuss abuse.

- *Suicide:* Jamaican society is not one that generally embraces mental health treatment or mental health challenges as a viable diagnosis in many cases. This underscores the importance of screening for these concerns in teens who often have no one to freely discuss such things, for example mood disorders. However given the many challenges that adolescents face, it should be expected that at least a few are at high risk for significant psychopathology or the use of inappropriate coping strategies resulting in internalizing and externalizing behaviors. Many parents underestimate the effect of stressful changes on their adolescents, including separation from parents whether through death, even if by violent means, or migration and often do not seek professional help, albeit a somewhat scarce resource.

Jamaican adolescents face many challenges, a few unique to the local culture, but are also resilient, often going from a start with limited resources to becoming world renowned and respected figures.

4.3 Interviewing the adolescent in the Middle East

Population growth in the Middle East continues to be above the world's average. The most rapid growth of the overall population of young people in the region has been witnessed resulting in the "youth bulge" (Assaad & Roudi-Fahimi, 2007). Despite the significant numbers of adolescents, there continues to be lack of dedicated adolescent healthcare services in the Middle East. Similar to Jamaica and other parts of the Caribbean, in most parts of the Middle East, the age limit of Pediatrics is 12 years. Thereafter, individuals in their early adolescence are transferred to adult healthcare. This in part has to due with the cultural concept that once a young male or female has physical signs of puberty, he or she is assumed to be an adult. Years ago, the appearance of such signs signified that one was ready to enter a marital relationship and begin childbearing. In recent years, education has significantly improved, and secondary school enrollment rates have increased (Assaad & Roudi-Fahimi, 2007). This is especially true for females and has resulted in women pursuing higher education and delaying the onset of marriage and childbearing (Assaad & Roudi-Fahimi, 2007). Because of the changes seen in society, many in the Middle East have recently become aware of the changing needs of young individuals, and the term 'adolescent' or 'murahiq', in the Arabic language, has become more widely used. Murahiq used to previously have negative connotation to it, meaning that someone was still immature. In recent years, it has become a more socially acceptable term that correctly refers to the transitional period between childhood and adulthood.

Countries are recognizing the changing needs of adolescents and their impact on the economy and future of nations. In some Middle Eastern countries, investments in the education and health sectors, as well as providing more job opportunities for the young have been the focus in the new Millennium. When it comes to healthcare, most have not adopted any changes with regards to the age limits of Pediatrics practice, however, some institutions in the region have independently taken on the decision to increase the age limits to 14 years (Al Buhairan, 2010), and some are even discussing further increase.

Strong family ties generally exist in the Middle East, young individuals have close relationships with their family members, and respect of the elderly is a given. Young individuals are expected to continue to live at home with their families (sometimes extended family) until they get married; some even continue to live with their families after marriage depending on the family structure and possible financial matters.

When an adolescent male or female requires a health visit, it is the norm to be accompanied by a parent or older sibling. Health conditions are discussed in front of both adolescent patient and accompanying family member. This is not to say that adolescents do not keep certain information away from their parents or family members, but rather that it is culturally expected that parents have the right to know everything about their adolescent son or daughter. Interviewing an adolescent independently is foreign. However, when done, parents and adolescents have viewed it quite positively. When the healthcare provider explains to the family that he or she would like to talk to the adolescent patient independently because it is an opportunity for the young individual to begin to take on responsibility of his or her health, families are appreciative. Families also tend to appreciate the fact that an adult is willing to spend time and talk to the adolescent son or daughter, as some parents are sometimes unsure of how to address certain issues and know that the adolescent may not be sharing everything with them.

When it comes to consent taking, policies are institution based. Some policies state that the age for consent is 15 years, based on the fact that most males and females have developed pubertal signs by then and are therefore considered to be 'adults', while other institutions state that 18 years is the age for consent. This applies to consent for management or treatment of any sort of health condition. Confidentiality issues, therefore, lie within the constraints of consent policies.

As for the specific psychosocial history taking of a Middle Eastern adolescent, different points may need to be addressed and/or similar points may need to be addressed differently based on the specific country or even part of a country that the adolescent comes from. Though there are many cultural similarities between the different Middle Eastern countries, there are also some differences that exist. For the sake of the psychosocial interview, the information provided below is based on experience with adolescents from Saudi Arabia. The information may very well apply to adolescents from neighboring Arabian Gulf States, such as Bahrain, Kuwait, Oman, Qatar, and the United Arab Emirates, since culturally they are very similar. There may be certain conditions or practices that may be more prevalent in some of the other Middle Eastern countries, so it is recommended that each pediatrician familiarize himself with those matters based on the adolescent population he serves.

HEADS can be applied to Middle Eastern adolescents, with certain points to be kept in mind or specific modifications to be applied as outlined below:

- *Home*: It is necessary to be very specific in asking who lives at home with the adolescent, including extended family members and domestic helpers. When asking about one's relationship with family members, one should go beyond asking, "How would you describe your relationship with…." and ask "When something is bothering you, can you talk about it with your …" or "Who do you speak to when something is bothering you or you need to discuss a personal matter?" Polygamy is seen in some families, so asking if the father is married to more than one wife is important, as is asking about the presence of half-siblings. If the adolescent comes from a polygamous family, further questions regarding the living accommodations and paternal relationship with the adolescent and his/her full and half siblings should be pursued.

- *Education*: When asking about school performance, it is important to ask about changes in school/academic performance over the past year. Asking about one's relationship with peers at school is also important, including history of bullying (whether one is a victim or the offender), as this is often overlooked. Do not assume that all adolescents are enrolled in school. Even though some countries have laws for mandatory schooling for children and adolescents, these laws are not necessarily enforced. Adolescents with special needs are especially at risk of not being enrolled in school.
- *Eating*: Eating disorders, such as anorexia nervosa and bulimia nervosa, are not prevalent in the Middle East; however, this may be changing with the effects of globalization. There is also a lack of awareness of these conditions, so under-diagnosis may be another factor affecting the actual prevalence rates. Obesity, on the other hand, is a common condition with prevalence rates increasing over the years (El-Hazmi & Warsy, 2002). Fast food restaurants have infiltrated societies that were previously known to have healthy diets. Furthermore, the heat in many parts of the Middle East often precludes outdoor activities and exercise.
- *Activities*: Finding out who the adolescent spends time with during recreational or extracurricular activities is important; is it friends from school, the neighborhood, or extended family members? Some families may not allow their sons, but maybe more so their daughters, to spend time with their school friends outside of school hours; they may be expected to spend their time with their cousins or other family members. Technology has swept across the Middle East as it has globally. Time and activities spent on the Internet, including online chatting and cyber bullying should be asked about.
- *Drugs*: In some Middle Eastern countries, tobacco use is common among adults, and adolescents may be frequently exposed to family members who smoke. Tobacco use includes that found in cigarettes as well as sheesha (narghile or hookah). Sheesha use has gained increased popularity in the Arab world over the past two decades and has attracted adolescents and young adults to the extent that it has been declared a public health problem by the WHO (Martinasek et al., 2011). Other substance use, including alcohol, marijuana, and amphetamine use, attracts social stigma, and such a matter is not discussed openly. Directly asking about drug use may be considered offensive by some, as they may think that you assume that he or she is involved in substance use. This is considered to be a very sensitive topic, and so the pediatrician may decide to start off by asking about tobacco use among peers. Such a question may be posed: "Some individuals your age may be smoking; do you know if any of your peers are smoking?" This can then be followed by "Have you ever tried smoking?" and depending on the response you get, follow this by more questions related to smoking. Sheesha use should be asked about even if the young person denies cigarette smoking. After addressing tobacco, one should go on to address alcohol and other substances in a similar fashion. The substances that adolescents may be most exposed to in the Arabian Gulf States are cannabis (including hashish) and amphetamines. Captagon is a synthetic stimulant that is available and is abused and should be asked about. Certain areas have prevalent use of khat (or gat), an amphetamine-like stimulant that is usually chewed. Sniffing solvents and other materials should also be included in this section of the psychosocial history.
- *Safety*: Motor vehicle accidents are a significant cause of death among adolescents in this part of the world. Seat belt use has only been recently enforced in some countries, but nonetheless, lack of using them is not unusual. In countries with vast deserts and

sand dunes, recreational activities, such as sandboarding and others that involve motorbikes or four wheel drive vehicles, are often engaged in, and enquiring about safety measures pertaining to these should be included.

- *Suicide*: As in other parts of the world, adolescents in the Middle East are at risk of developing depression. Regularly asking about one's mood should be done during the psychosocial history taking. This can be done in a manner similar to that described previously with adolescents in North America. Many healthcare providers are uncomfortable asking about suicidal ideations or acts, and suicide is again another stigmatizing matter in the Middle East. However, when adolescents have been directly asked about this, they tend to respond honestly; for some, it has appeared that they were actually relieved that someone had finally opened this subject matter, as it is a very difficult matter to discuss.
- *Sex*: Sexuality and sexual activity are topics that are culturally inappropriate to address with most Middle Eastern adolescents. Young people have insufficient access to information on these matters, and in the few areas where educational curricula contain sexual and reproductive health, teachers often skip relevant sections because they are uncomfortable or embarrassed to teach them (DeJong et al., 2005). Sexual activity prior to the onset of marriage is unacceptable and regarded as shameful. Those adolescents that have engaged in some sort of sexual activity tend not to talk about it or discuss it freely, as it is considered taboo. The exceptions to bringing up sexuality issues more openly during a health care visit include the following: 1) an adolescent who has been exposed to any sort of abuse (asking specifically about sexual abuse is considered to be appropriate), 2) an adolescent who is involved in risky behaviors, and 3) a married adolescent.

4.4 Interviewing the adolescent in South East Asia

In Thailand, adolescent medicine is a relatively new field, and the psychosocial history and assessment is not consistently done during each adolescent visit. This may be due to lack of training and exposure to the field, the overwhelming ratio of physicians per capita, and also the healthcare provider's personal thoughts and attitudes towards conducting the psychosocial history itself. A survey conducted in a training institute in Thailand indicated that one third of the pediatric residents were not familiar with the HEADS acronym, one forth were not confident in conducting a psychosocial assessment, and 7% had never conducted the assessment prior to exposure to adolescent medicine (Areemit, In Press).

Thailand is a newly industrialized country, undergoing many changes. The number one cause of death for adolescents (age 13-18 years) is accidents, while child birth (23.7%) is the leading causes of hospital admissions (The Royal College of Pediatricians Thailand [RCOP], 2009). There are both nuclear and extended families; parents and relatives tend to be more involved in an adolescent's life and are commonly present at hospital visits. Depending on the institution, pediatricians see children until they are 15-18 years. Asking permission to interview the adolescent alone is not yet a part of regular practice. Without adequate approach, parents and adolescents may misinterpret this as an indication that the healthcare provider thinks there is something "wrong". Difficult encounters with the parents or the adolescent may be anticipated while asking for permission to conduct a psychosocial interview in private. However after establishing rapport and showing interest in the parents' and adolescent's issues, advocating that this is a part of a regular adolescent visit and that the adolescent can learn to discuss his or her own issues with the healthcare provider as an appropriate way of development and establishing confidentiality, interviewing adolescents independently has been found to be more welcome than anticipated. Providing confidential health care for adolescents themselves is more of an issue, especially as laws only provide confidential care for adults (18 years or older). In this situation, adolescents are given confidentiality with limits regarding issues that may harm their heath or somebody else's health. Healthcare providers then have to use their own judgment as to what can be kept confidential. Having said that, most issues that cannot be kept confidential will have to be discussed with the adolescent regarding appropriate care needed and how this will be addressed with the parents.

The sequence in conducting a HEADS assessment may differ slightly; when there is no urgent presenting issue around sexuality, this topic is preferably kept until the end of the interview. This is because sexuality is a very personal and private issue in Thailand, rarely discussed with adolescents, and may be considered impolite.

Discussed below are some pertinent issues for conducting a psychosocial interview for adolescents in Thailand.

- *Home:* It is not uncommon for parents to migrate from rural neighborhoods to big cities in order to earn more income. Twenty percent of children and adolescents live with their grandparents or relatives (National Statistical Office (NSO) Thailand, 2008), while the family may reunite only twice per year. This can have positive or negative effects, depending on the quality of care given. Positive effects include closer care by relatives when compared to the hard working parents who may have insufficient time. In an extended family, an adolescent may also have a wider range of adults who can be a source of support. However, this is not always the case for those who have low economic status, come from disrupted families, or are living with elderly or ill grandparents who do not have sufficient resources and energy that may be required for an adolescent. Co-sleeping or sharing the same bedroom with the care giver (parents or grandparents) is common practice. Though adolescents will eventually want privacy, many share their room with parents, grandparents, or siblings, especially when there is insufficient space within a house.
- *Education and Employment:* Usually, the parents and family financially support an adolescent/young adult until/if they complete education at the college/university level. Unless work is far from home, he or she is expected to live with the family until married and for some, even afterwards. If not working, the adolescent can help out in the house, thus moving out, getting a job, and living by themselves may not be a necessity. The secondary school attendance rate is 77.6%. The main reasons for not continuing secondary school are: achieving a certain degree of education already and economical issues. Most adolescents who do not continue secondary school will enter the workforce (49%), help with the family business (24%), look for a job (10%), or just stay at home (8%) (NSO, Thailand, 2008). Though there is a mandatory requirement to complete 9 years of school, there is insufficient data regarding the quality of education that adolescents receive. It is noted that some adolescents that have difficulties in school are allowed to pass through grades without sufficient evaluation and support for learning disabilities, attention deficit disorder, or other mental health issues. These

adolescents may have lower opportunities for employment (NSO, Thailand, 2008). When interviewing about education, in addition to the open ended non-judgmental approach, it is very reasonable to ask specifically about attending school, grades/changes in grades, and the school environment.

- *Eating, Body Image and Exercise:* Adolescents can be especially prone to hazardous eating behavior and unhealthy nutrition choices. Though a regular diet consists of 3 meals per day, meals and snacks tend not to be as structured as in Western countries. There is a wide variety of eating behaviors depending on lifestyle and the demand of one's everyday life. Skipping breakfast, having breakfast as the only meal of the day, having 4 meals including a late night meal, or snacking throughout the day may be normal for some. In addition, some individuals have religious and spiritual reasons to have only one meal per day. Eating disorders have been reported, but are uncommon in Thailand possibly due to a low prevalence or under detection (Limsuwan, 1983). On the other hand, the prevalence of obesity has increased from 6% in 1995 to 22% in 2008 (RCOP, 2009), and dieting is common among Thai adolescents (Aekplakorn & Mo-suwan 2010; Page & Suwanteerangkul, 2007). The media and peers play a major role in the formation of an ideal body image (Thianthai, 2006). Currently, K-pop (Korean pop) and J-pop (Japanese pop) are two popular trends (Winn, 2010). These trends portray adolescent girls, with small physique, white glowing skin, and big eyes. This has resulted in use of cosmetic contact lens to make the cornea look larger and/or change eye color, and complications found are associated with poor hygiene and below standard production of the contact lenses. Fake orthodontic braces worn to look young and wealthy has been associated with heavy metal intoxication. Skin whiteners, popular among adolescent girls and women, can pose toxic risks.
- *Activities:* Many adolescents in the school system in large cities use their spare time, up to 18 hours/week, to attend extracurricular academic school in order to achieve and get high scores on the national examination for university entrance. Others may participate in motorcycle gangs that race on public streets and highways in the night. These gangs may engage in other high risk behaviors such as alcohol use, other substance use, and unprotected sexual intercourse. Sixty nine percent of Thai children and adolescents use computers and have internet access. Of this group, 21% use it to play games including online games (RCOP, 2009). In areas where the internet is easily accessible, some internet cafés that are close to schools even provide clothes for students in school uniforms to change into.
- *Drugs:* Common drugs used are tobacco, alcohol, and amphetamine (NSO, Thailand, 2007; RCOP, 2009). Wood alcohol (methanol) can be found especially in areas near the northern, northeastern, and eastern borders of the country; teens should have information about this in order to avoid complications such as blindness. Other cosmetic medications that are used are macro-micro nutrient protein supplements for white glowing skin or for muscularity. There is usage of glutathione injection in order to have the glowing clear and fair looking skin. Herbal coffee is commonly used for dieting.
- *Suicide and mood:* Five to eight percent of Thai adolescents have been found to have depressive symptoms, and 1.1% have tried to commit suicide (RCOP, 2009). Due to culture, Thai adolescents may not be as verbal and may feel pressured to keep their feelings inside. Some may find it hard to verbalize their mood and emotions, especially negative ones; on the contrary, when asked in an appropriate manner, suicidal ideation can be discussed more openly.

- *Safety:* Though there are laws regarding helmet and seatbelt use, these are more strongly implemented in major cities, not in the rural areas. Thirty eight to eighty percent of Thai adolescents who drive motorcycles do not wear helmets, 14-45% do not wear seat belts, 18-32% were in a vehicle in which the driver had consumed alcohol, and 13-21% had consumed alcohol and driven a vehicle themselves (RCOP, 2009). There are drivers who drive without a driver's license. Helmets are mostly worn to avoid a penalty rather than for one's safety.
- *Sex: Sex* is a very personal and private issue; it is rarely discussed with adolescents, and can even be considered impolite. A study found that there are restrictions imposed by traditional culture and that sex education is not regarded as parental duty. The generation gap and 'better not bring it up' were the limitations in providing sex education by parents (Sridawruang et al., 2010). The majority of sexual education is taught in secondary school, most of it acknowledging the physical changes of puberty, sexually transmitted infections, and HIV. The psychosocial events that may occur during puberty are not yet widely addressed. Premarital sex is generally not accepted; there are double standard attitudes towards premarital sex, where it is acceptable for men but unacceptable for women. More adolescents (18%) are having sexual intercourse with only 14% using contraception. With lack of knowledge, misconceptions, and difficult access to low cost contraception, the teenage pregnancy rate has increased from 10% in 2001 to 15% of all pregnancies in 2004 and has become an issue for the country. It is considered very shameful for the unmarried adolescent girl and family, leading to late detection and complications. These pregnancies result in abortion (20-30%), continuation of the pregnancy and keeping the baby (60%), or continuation of the pregnancy but leaving the baby at the hospital for adoption (10%) (RCOP, 2009). Of those who continue the pregnancy, a majority will marry the baby's father, some will continue to be a single mother, and for others, the grandparents raise the baby as a child of their own. Thailand's HIV prevalence has been stable at 1.4 per 1000 since 2005; however 11% of the HIV positive cases are adolescents and youth aged below 24 years. This group is thought to be the majority of newly infected people each year (Joint United Nations Programme on HIV/AIDS [UNAIDS], 2009). When interviewing about this topic, the healthcare provider should ask for permission to ask some more personal questions. With a health promotion approach, questions about physical changes can be addressed first, followed by psychosocial changes including sexual identity. Sexual activity and high-risk behaviors should be addressed by asking about the adolescent's friends' experiences or common themes in the media first, then probing further as needed.

5. Conclusion

Adolescence is a dynamic stage of life, with so many changes occurring. Adolescents are a significant part of any country's population and much focus and attention on their needs is required, as they impact a country's health, social, economic, and political status. With the rapid global changes and advancement in technology, adolescents are often 'caught between tradition and progress' (United Nations, n.d.). However, among adolescents globally, there are more similarities than there are differences, and as healthcare providers, we can increase the number of adolescents that achieve health and success by optimizing their care, identifying their challenges, and finding resolutions, in addition to recognizing and promoting their positive attributes and intrinsic resilience.

6. References

Aekplakorn, W. & Mo-suwan, L. (2009). Prevalence of obesity in Thailand. *Obes Rev,* 10:589-92

Al Buhairan, F. (2010). Healthcare providers' opinions of adolescent healthcare in Saudi Arabia. Society for Adolescent Medicine Annual Meeting Program Issue, *J Adol Health,* 46(2):s11

American Academy of Pediatrics (1978). *Report by the task force on pediatric education. The future of pediatric education,* Evanston, USA

Areemit, R. (In press). Adolescent health care: attitudes and clinical practice of pediatric residents in a University Hospital in Northeast Thailand. *Proceedings of the 27th Faculty of Medicine annual conference: New trends in health care,* Khon Kaen, Thailand, October 2011

Assaad, R. & Roudi-Fahimi, F. (2007). Youth in the Middle East and North Africa: Demographic opportunity or challenge?, In: *Population Reference Bureau,* Accessed August 2011, Available from: http://www.prb.org/pdf07/YouthinMENA.pdf

Blakemore, S., Burnett, S., & Dahl, R. (2010). The role of puberty in the developing adolescent brain. *Hum Brain Mapp,* 31:926-33

Brown, B., Larson, R., & Saraswathi, T. (2002). *The world's youth,* Cambridge University Press, ISBN: 978-0-521-00605-7, New York, USA

Casey, B., Jones, R., Levita, L., Libby, V., Pattwell, S., & Ruberry, E. (2010). The storm and stress of adolescence: insights from human imaging and mouse genetics. *Dev Psychobiol,* 52(3):225-235

Choudhury, S., Blakemore, S., & Charman, T. Social cognitive development during adolescence. (2006). *Soc Cogn Affect Neurosci,* 1(3):165-174

Crawford, T., McGrowder, D., & Crawford, A. (2009). Access to contraception by minors in Jamaica: a public health concern. *North Am J Med Sci,* 1(5):247-255

Cromer, B. (2011). Adolescent Development, In: *Nelson Textbook of Pediatrics* (19th ed.), Kliegman, R., Stanton, B., St. Geme III, J., Schor, N., & Behrman, R. Saunders, Philadelphia, USA

Dahl, R. (2004). Adolescent brain development: a period of vulnerabilities and opportunities. Keynote address. *Ann N Y Acad Sci,* Jun;1021:1-22

DeJong, J., Jawad, R., Mortagy, I., & Shepard, B. (2005) The sexual and reproductive health of young people in the Arab countries and Iran. *Reprod Health Matters,*13(25):49-59

El-Hazmi, M. & Warsy, A. (2002). The prevalence of obesity and overweight in 1-18-year-old Saudi children. *Ann Saudi Med,* 22(5-6):303-7

Fox, K. & Gordon-Strachan, G. (2007). *Jamaican youth risk and resiliency behavior survey 2005: school-based survey on risk and resiliency behaviors of 10–15 year olds.* Accessed September 2011, Available from: http://www.cpc.unc.edu/measure/publications

Giedd, J., Blumenthal, J., Jeffries, N., Castellanos, F., Liu, H., Zijdenbos, A., Paus, T., Evans, A., & Rapoport, J. (1999). Brain development during childhood and adolescence: a longitudinal MRI study. *Nat Neurosci,* 2(10): 861-3

Gogtay, N., Giedd, J., Lusk, L., Hayashi, K., Greenstein, D., Vaituzis, A., Nugent III, T., Herman, D., Clasen, L., Toga, A., Rapoport, J., & Thompson, P. (2004). Dynamic mapping of human cortical development during childhood through early adulthood. *Proc Natl Acad Sci U S A* ;101(21):8174-9

Goldenring, J. & Rosen, D. (2004). Getting into adolescent heads: An essential update. *Contemp Pediatr,* January 2004;21:64

Harriott, A. (2008). *Bending the trend line: The challenge of controlling violence in Jamaica and the high violence societies of the Caribbean*, Arawak Publishers, Kingston, Jamaica

Harrison, A., Pierre, R., Gordon-Strachan, G., Campbell-Forrester, S., & Leslie, K. (2011). Adolescent health screening by physicians in Jamaica. *Pan Am J Public Health*, 29(4):252-58

Jamaica Family Planning Board and Division of Reproductive Health, Centers for Disease Control and Prevention (CDC). *Jamaica Reproductive Health Survey 2008*, Centers for Disease Control and Prevention (CDC), Atlanta, USA

Joint United Nations Programme on HIV/AIDS (UNAIDS). (2009). *Thailand HIV and AIDS estimates*, Accessed August 2011, Available from: http://www.unaids.org/en/regionscountries/countries/thailand/

Larson, R. & Brown, J. (2007). Emotional development in adolescence: what can be learned from a high school theater program? *Child Dev*, 78(4):1083-1099

Limsuwan, N. (1983). Anorexia nervosa: role of antipsychotic drugs in the treatment. *Ramathibodi Medical Journal*, 6:285-90

Luna, B., Padmanabhan, A., & O'Hearn, K. (2010). What has fMRI told us about the development of cognitive control through adolescence? *Brain Cogn*, 72:101-13

Martinasek, M., McDermott, R., & Martini, L. (2011). Waterpipe (hookah) tobacco smoking among youth. *Curr Probl Pediatr Adolesc Health Care*, 41:34-57

McGuire, M., Story, M., Neumark-Sztainer, D., Halcon, L., Campbell-Forrester, S., & Blum, R. (2002). Prevalence and correlates of weight-control behaviors among Caribbean adolescent students. *J Adolesc Health*, 31(2):208-211

Newman, B. & Newman, P. (1999). *Development through life. A psychosocial approach* (7th ed.), Wordsworth Publishing Co., Belmont, USA

Nugent, R. (2005). Youth in a global world, In: *Population Reference Bureau*, Accessed August 2011, Available from: http://www.prb.org/pdf06/YouthInAGlobalWorld.pdf

Page, R. & Suwanteerangkul, J. (2007). Dieting among Thai adolescents: having friends who diet and pressure to diet. *Eat Weight Disord*, 12:114

Paus, T. (2005). Mapping brain maturation and cognitive development during adolescence. *Trends Cogn Sci*,9:60-8

Radzik, M., Sherer, S., & Neinstein, L. (2007). Psychosocial Development in Normal Adolescents, In: *Adolescent Health Care: A Practical Guide* (5th ed.), Neinstein, L., Gordon, C., Katzman, D., Rosen, D., & Woods, E., pp 27-31, Lippincott Williams & Wilkins, Philadelphia, USA

Somerville, L. & Casey, B. (2010). Developmental neurobiology of cognitive control and motivational systems. *Curr Opin Neurobiol*, 20(2):236-241

Sridawruang, C., Pfeil, M. & Crozier, K. (2010). Why Thai parents do not discuss sex with their children: a qualitative study. *Nurs Health Sci*, 12:437-43

Statistical Forecasting Bureau, National Statistical Office (NSO) Thailand. (2007). *Alcohol and smoking report*, Accessed August 2011, Available from: http://service.nso.go.th/nso/nsopublish/themes/theme_2-4-7.html

Statistical Forecasting Bureau, National Statistical Office (NSO) Thailand. (2008). *Child and youth statistics report*, Accessed August 2011, Available from: http://service.nso.go.th/nso/nsopublish/themes/theme_2-1-11.html. Thai

Statistical Institute of Jamaica (2011). *Demographic statistics*. Accessed September 2011, Available from: <http://statinja.gov.jm>

Steinberg, L. (2005). Cognitive and affective development in adolescence. *Trends Cogn Sci,* 9(2):69-74

The Royal College of Pediatricians Thailand (RCOP). (2009). The Task force on Thailand's Child and Adolescent Health Situation, In: *Analysis of Child and Adolescent Health Situation,* pp. 161-188

The World Bank (2011). *Country classifications.* Accessed September 2011, Available from: http://data.worldbank.org/about/country-classifications

Thianthai, C. (2006). Influential sources affecting Bangkok adolescent body image perceptions. *Int J Adolesc Med Health,* 18:633-41

United Nations (n.d.). *United Nations report on global situation of youth shows changing trends,* Accessed August 2011, Available from: http://www.un.org/events/youth98/backinfo/yreport.htm

United Nations Children's Fund (UNICEF). (2011). *The State of the World's Children 2011: Adolescence an age of opportunity,* UNICEF, ISBN:978-92-806-4555-2, New York, USA

United Nations Childern's Fund (UNICEF). (n.d.). *Parenting in Jamaica,* Accessed September 2011, Available from: http://www.unicef.org/jamaica/parenting_corner.html

Wilks, R., Younger, N., McFarlane, S., & Van Den Broeck, J. (2007). *Jamaican youth risk and resiliency behaviour survey 2006: community-based survey on risk and resiliency behaviors of 15-19 year olds,* Accessed September 2011, Available from: http://www.cpc.unc.edu/measure/publications/tr-07-64

Winn, P. (2010). Warning: This fad may kill you, Korean trends tagged with deadly warnings in Thailand, In: *Global Post,* Accessed August 2011, Available from: <http://www.globalpost.com/dispatch/thailand/100823/korean-wave-fashion-thai-culture>

11

Comparisons of Bully and Unwanted Sexual Experiences Online and Offline Among a National Sample of Youth

Michele L. Ybarra, Kimberly J. Mitchell and Dorothy L. Espelage
Internet Solutions for Kids, Inc, University of Illinois, USA

1. Introduction

A dramatic increase in Internet use among young people in the past decade (Lenhart, 2009) has contributed to a heightened appreciation for the Internet's potential positive (Lenhart, 2009; Rideout, 2001; Ybarra & Suman, 2008) and negative impacts (Guan & Subrahmanyam, 2009; Juvonen & Gross, 2008; Katzer, Fetchenhauer, & Belschak, 2009; Li, 2006; Mitchell, Finkelhor, & Wolak, 2001, 2007; Raskauskas & Stoltz, 2007; Slonje & Smith, 2008; Smith et al., 2008; Wolak, Mitchell, & Finkelhor, 2006; Ybarra, Diener-West, & Leaf, 2007a; Ybarra, Leaf, & Diener-West, 2004) on the health and development of youth. Internet harassment and bullying victimization have received particular research attention, and are consistently found to be associated with psychosocial problems including depressive symptoms, poor caregiver-child relationships, social and behavior problems, and substance use (Guan & Subrahmanyam, 2009; Juvonen & Gross, 2008; Katzer et al., 2009; Li, 2006; Raskauskas & Stoltz, 2007; Slonje & Smith, 2008; Smith et al., 2008; Wolak et al., 2006; Ybarra et al., 2007a). Unwanted online sexual solicitation, defined as being asked to talk about sex, provide personal sexual information, or do something sexual when the youth does not want to when using the Internet, is another area of adolescent health concern. Online sexual solicitation has been associated with psychosocial challenges including depressive symptomatology (Mitchell et al., 2001, 2007; Ybarra et al., 2004).

Certainly, the Internet is but one environment in which youth must navigate. Victimization has been noted particularly at school, where youth spend a great deal of their time. Studies consistently report that victims of school bullying are significantly more likely to experience negative health and social consequences than non-bullied youth, including health problems, emotional and school adjustment problems, and poorer peer relationships (Due et al., 2005; Hawker & Boulton, 2000; Nansel et al., 2004; Sourander, Helstela, Helenius, & Piha, 2000). Unwanted sexual experiences in the schools is similarly associated with psychosocial problems, including alcohol use (Fineran & Bolen, 2006).

Many studies have reported relative rates of bullying online and offline (Juvonen & Gross, 2008; Katzer et al., 2009; Li, 2006; Raskauskas & Stoltz, 2007; Slonje & Smith, 2008; Smith et al., 2008; Wang, Iannotti, & Nansel, 2009); most report bullying more commonly occurring in the schools. These studies use varying definitions for online and offline bullying and/or focus on regional or convenience samples. Furthermore, rates in non-school environments are not reported. Little has been reported in terms of bullying perpetration across environments also. Of note, Wang and colleagues (Wang et al., 2009) report that among 6-10th graders nationally, 8% bully others online, 27% bully others socially, 37% bully verbally, and 13% bully others physically while at school. Online bullying is treated as a different *type* of bullying however; such that, for example, social bullying that occurs online is imperfectly measured. Importantly too, data are lacking about how the bullying *experience* may differ online versus offline. No data have been presented to compare relative rates of distress for bullying that occurs online versus offline. It also has been posited that a unique aspect of online bullying is the potential for anonymity; this assumes that all victims know their offline bullies. No research has examined however, whether this is a valid assumption.

Even less has been reported about unwanted sexual experiences online and offline. Ybarra and colleagues (Ybarra, Espelage, & Mitchell, 2007b) report overlaps in victimization for harassment and unwanted sexual experiences online; they do not report however, the relative rates of unwanted sexual experiences online and offline. To our knowledge, no other studies have reported relative rates of online and offline unwanted sexual solicitation in the general population of youth.

To address these gaps in the literature, we report data from the Growing up with Media study, a national survey of over 1,000 youth. Findings have implications for public policy initiatives as well as school and other community-based intervention efforts.

2. Methods

The Growing up with Media study is a longitudinal survey examining the associations between exposure to violent media - particularly new media (e.g., the Internet) - and violent behavior. Wave 1 data were collected August-September, 2006 with 1,588 youth-caregiver pairs; data were collected again November, 2007 - January 10, 2008 [Wave 2, (n=1,206)] and August - November, 2008 [Wave 3, (n=1,159)]. The survey protocol was reviewed and approved by the Centers for Disease Control and Prevention Institutional Review Board (IRB).

The sample was obtained from the Harris Poll Online (HPOL) opt-in panel (Harris Interactive, 2006), which is comparable to random telephone samples of adult populations once appropriate sample weights are applied (Berrens, Bohara, Jenkins-Smith, Silva, & Weimer, 2003; Berrens, Bohara, Jenkins-Smith, Silva, & Weimer, 2004; Schonlau et al., 2004; Taylor, Bremer, Overmeyer, Siegel, & Terhanian, 2001). Recruitment was balanced on youth age and sex. Participants were recruited through an email contact with randomly identified adult HPOL members who had previously indicated a child lived in the household. Adult respondents (one per household) were required to be equally or more knowledgeable than other adults in the home about the youth's media use, and to provide consent for their participation and permission for their child's participation. Youth participants were required to be 10-15 years old, read English, live in the household at least 50% of the time, have used the Internet in the last 6 months, and provide assent to participate in research.

On average, adult surveys lasted 5-minutes and youth surveys 21 minutes. Youth received a $20 gift certificate and caregivers a $15 check for their participation at Waves 1 and 2; and $25 and $20, respectively at Wave 3. The surveys were administered by Harris Interactive.

2.1 Sample

Although parallel questions of bullying online and offline were added at Wave 2, it was not until Wave 3 that measures of perpetration and distress were added. To fully answer the research questions posed, the current analyses are restricted to Wave 3. The baseline survey response rate, 26%, was within the expected range of similar online surveys (Cook, Heath, & Thompson, 2000; Kaplowitz, Hadlock, & Levine, 2004).

To maximize data, respondents were invited to take part in the Wave 2 and Wave 3 surveys irrespective of their participation at previous Waves. Response rates were 76% and 73% of baseline participants at Wave 2 and Wave 3, respectively. Survey participants in subsequent Waves were similar to participants in Wave 1 and also to the national population (See table 1 below). For example, using weighted data, 49% of the sample was male at Wave 3, and 49% was male at Wave 1. Seventy-three percent identified as White race at Wave 3 and 71% at Wave 1. Twenty-five percent lived in a household with an annual income of $35,000 or less at Wave 3 versus 26% at Wave 1.

Youth and Household Demographic Characteristics	Wave 1 (n=1,577) % (n)	Wave 2 (n=1,189) % (n)	Wave 3 (n=1,149) % (n)
Sex			
Female	51.0 (785)	50.3 (589)	50.8 (568)
Male	49.0 (792)	49.7 (600)	49.2 (581)
Age (mean)	12.6	13.7	14.5
Race			
White	71.3 (1155)	73.9 (900)	72.5 (855)
Black or African American	13.6 (213)	12.5 (140)	13.6 (145)
Mixed racial background	8.6 (113)	7.5 (80)	8.2 (84)
All other	6.5 (96)	6.1 (69)	5.7 (65)
Hispanic ethnicity	18.1 (206)	16.7 (144)	16.6 (137)
Annual household income			
<$35,000	25.7 (399)	24.3 (251)	24.8 (241)
$35,000 - $74,999	39.7 (685)	40.1 (525)	38.6 (490)
$75,000+	34.6 (493)	35.6 (413)	36.7 (418)

Table 1. A comparison of demographic charactaeristics of respondents across waves

2.2 Measures

Respondents were asked about bullying *victimization* as well as *perpetration* using Olweus' definition of bullying (Olweus, 1994): "We say a young person is being bullied or harassed when someone else or a group of people **repeatedly** hits, kicks, threatens, or says nasty or unpleasant things to them. Another example is when no one ever talks to them. These things can happen at school, online, or other places young people hang out. It is **not** bullying when two young people of about the **same strength** fight or tease each other. How often has this happened to you in the following environments?): 1) at school, 2) on the Internet, 3) on cell phones through text messaging, 4) on the way to and from school, and 5) somewhere else. For each environment, response options were: every day / almost every day; once or twice a week; once or twice a month; less often than once a month; never; and decline to answer.

Youth who reported bullying victimization in at least one environment were asked two follow up questions. First, these youth were asked to indicate how they felt when they were bullied in each environment, when thinking about the most serious incident. Responses were captured on a 5-point scale: not at all upset; somewhat upset; upset; very upset; extremely upset; and decline to answer. Second, youth were asked whether they knew their bully: "By "know" we mean you can recognize the person or you know who they are". Response options were: yes, no, not sure, and decline to answer.

Unwanted sexual experiences also were measured using parallel items for experiences when online, and experiences when at school. Note that other environments, including on the way to and from school, and 'somewhere else' were not queried. Text messaging-based experiences were queried, but using different measures and therefore are not included in the current analyses. Items were based upon those included in and referred to as "unwanted sexual solicitation" in the Youth Internet Safety Surveys (Finkelhor, Mitchell, & Wolak, 2000; Wolak et al., 2006). We choose to call these experiences "unwanted sexual experiences" to avoid connotation that these youth were necessarily solicited for sex. Youth endorsing at least one of the following questions were classified as having an unwanted sexual experience: 1) Someone tried to get me to talk about sex when I did not want to; 2) Someone asked me for sexual information about myself when I did not want to tell the person, e.g., really personal questions, like what my body looks like or sexual things I have done; 3) Someone asked me to do something sexual that I did not want to do. Response options were: everyday/almost every day; once or twice a week; once or twice a month; a few times a year; less than a few times a year; never; and decline to answer. Perpetration was asked solely for the online environment. Similarly, distress was only queried for youth reporting victimization online. Given that the focus of the current paper is comparisons across environments, these data are not reported.

2.3 Data cleaning and statistical analyses

Data cleaning indicated that 18 youth were likely 9 years of age, and 12 youth were 16 years of age at Wave 1. To maximize the amount of data; and because caregivers did not know the eligibility criteria (and, therefore, were unlikely to have misreported their child's age purposefully), these youth are included in the analyses.

Data were weighted statistically to reflect the population of adults with children aged 10-15 years old in the U.S. in 2006 (when the sample was first recruited) according to adult age, sex, race/ethnicity, region, education, household income, and child age and sex.(Bureau of Labor Statistics & Bureau of the Census, 2006) Adults were the weighting target as they were the ones first recruited into the survey. Survey sampling weights also adjust for adult respondents' self-selection into the HPOL (Berrens et al., 2003; Berrens et al., 2004; Schonlau et al., 2004; Taylor et al., 2001) as well as any differential follow-up of youth participants over time.

Missing data and "refused" responses were imputed using best-set regression (StataCorp, 2008). To reduce the likelihood of imputing truly non-responsive answers, participants were required to have valid data for at least 85% of the survey questions asked of all youth. Eleven respondents did not meet this criterion and were dropped from the Wave 1 sample; 17 were dropped from the Wave 2 and 10 from the Wave 3 samples.

Statistical comparisons across environments cannot be made because categories are not exclusive; youth can be represented in multiple categories.

3. Results

3.1 One-year prevalence rates across environments

3.1.1 Bully victimization

Frequency	Environment				
	School (n=1,149) % (n)	Internet (n=1,149) % (n)	Cell phone text messaging[a] (n=806) % (n)	To and From school (n=1,149) % (n)	Somewhere else (n=1,149) % (n)
Every day / almost every day	1.3 (15)	0.3 (4)	0.4 (1)	0.9 (3)	0.3 (3)
Once or twice a week	4.0 (43)	0.3 (5)	0.5 (6)	1.7 (16)	1.5 (13)
Once or twice a month	3.2 (46)	1.9 (22)	1.7 (13)	1.1 (15)	1.9 (22)
Less often	22.1 (254)	12.3 (150)	9.5 (73)	7.8 (88)	10.8 (114)
Never	69.4 (791)	85.3 (968)	88.2 (713)	89.2 (1027)	85.6 (997)

[a] Restricted to youth who sent and received text messages at least once in the past year (70%, n=806)

Table 2. A comparison of 1-year bullying victimization rates across environments

Overall, 40% of youth reported some bully victimization in the past year. Rates across environments are shown in Table 2. An examination of the school-online overlap suggests that most of these youth were bullied at school exclusively: 59% were bullied only at school; 13% were bullied only online; and 28% were bullied both at school and online

3.1.2 Bully perpetration

Frequency	Environment				
	School (n=1,149) % (n)	Internet (n=1,149) % (n)	Cell phone text messaging[a] (n=806) % (n)	To and From school (n=1,149) % (n)	Somewhere else (n=1,149) % (n)
Every day / almost every day	0.3 (5)	0.06 (2)	0.3 (2)	0.03 (1)	0.4 (3)
Once or twice a week	1.3 (13)	0.6 (7)	0.9 (6)	0.9 (8)	1.2 (11)
Once or twice a month	1.7 (22)	0.8 (15)	1.0 (11)	0.3 (8)	1.2 (15)
Less often	10.4 (107)	4.7 (47)	3.4 (25)	3.0 (34)	3.4 (44)
Never	86.4 (1002)	93.7 (1078)	94.3 (762)	95.8 (1098)	93.8 (1076)

[a] Restricted to youth who sent and received text messages at least once in the past year (70%, n=806)

Table 3. A comparison of 1-year bullying perpetration rates across environments

Eighteen percent of youth reported being bullies in the past year. Table 3 shows bullying rates by environment. The school-online overlap was similar to that noted for victims: among youth who bullied in either place, 59% bullied only at school, 10% bullied only online, and 31% bullied both online and at school.

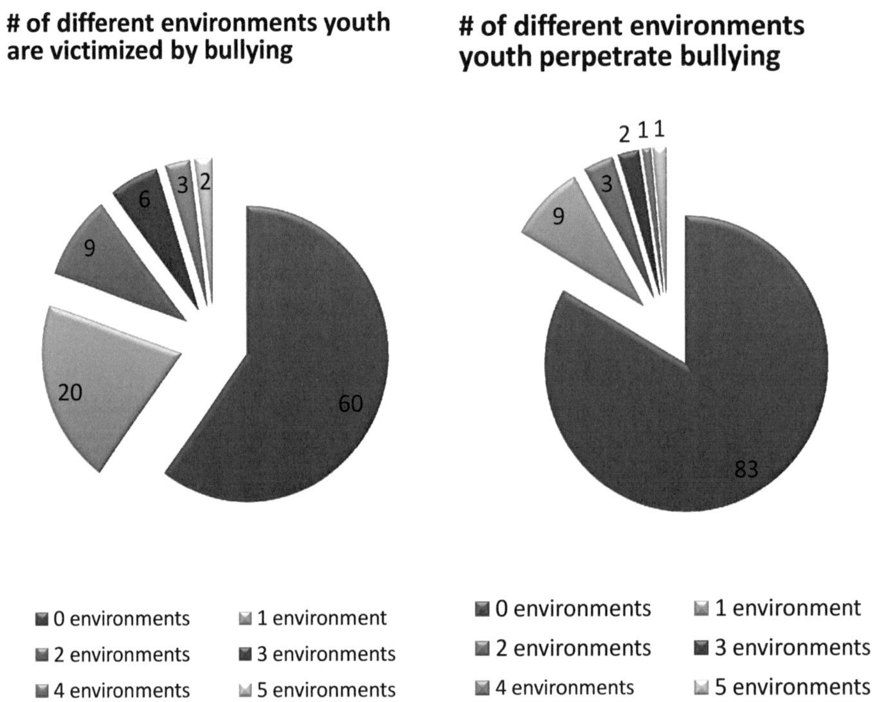

Fig. 1. Overlap of bullying experiences across environments

As shown in the Figure, the majority of youth were not victims (60%) or perpetrators (82%) of bullying in any environment. For those who were involved in bullying, the most common experience was victimization (20%) or perpetration (9%) in one environment. Fewer reported being victimized (9%) or perpetrating (4%) across two environments. Very few reported being bullied or bullying others in four or all five of the environments queried.

3.1.3 Unwanted sexual experiences

Frequency	Environment	
	School (n=1,149) % (n)	Internet (n=1,149) % (n)
Every day / almost every day	0.2 (5)	0.4 (7)
Once or twice a week	1.7 (14)	1.3 (9)
Once or twice a month	2.1 (17)	2.9 (29)
Less often	13.7 (169)	13.0 (154)
Never	82.3 (944)	82.4 (950)

Table 4. 1-year unwanted sexual experiences victimization rates across environments

Almost one in four youth (25%) reported being victims of unwanted sexual experiences in the past year. As show in Table 4, 18% of youth reported unwanted sexual experiences at school, and 18% online. Among victims, 29% reported being victimized at school only, 29% online only, and 42% both at school and online.

3.2 The bully victimization "experience" across environments

3.2.1 Distress

Youth who reported being bullied were asked to indicate how they felt about the most serious incident in each environment they were bullied. As shown in Table 5, more youth reported being upset by their most serious bullying incident at school (37.5%) than any other environment.

Environment	Very / extremely upset by the most serious incident % (n)	Not sure / Do not "know" the bully % (n)
School (n=358)	37.5 (128)	12.0 (44)
Internet (n=181)	15.4 (34)	45.8 (84)
Cell phone text messaging (n=95)	32.9 (28)	29.0 (23)
On the way to and from school (n=122)	38.8 (46)	22.4 (25)
Somewhere else (n=152)	36.7 (56)	27.2 (46)

Table 5. The bully victimization expereince: Victim distress and knowing one's perpetrator (n=1,149)

3.2.2 Knowing one's perpetrator

When asked to indicate if they "knew" the bully (i.e., the respondent could recognize the bully or knew who they were), almost half (46%) of youth bullied online said they were not sure or did not know who the bully was (see Table 5). About one in four youth said they were unsure or did not know their bully via text messaging (29%) and one in three said they were unsure or did not know their bully on the way to and from school (22%). Slightly more than one in ten youth bullied at school (12%) said they did not know or were unsure about the bully's identity.

4. Discussion

Based upon data from 12-17 year-olds surveyed nationally, involvement in bullying and unwanted sexual experiences appears common: 40% report being bullied, 18% report bullying, and 25% report being victims of unwanted sexual experiences in at least one environment that they navigate. Although it is difficult to compare these data with previous studies that have focused more specifically on experiences occurring either at school or online, it is fair to say that our findings provide further evidence that involvement in youth aggression, either as a perpetrator or as a victim, is widespread.

4.1 School bullying is more common than online bullying

Bullying is reported more frequently at school than online: 31% of youth report being bullied at school compared to 15% online; bully perpetration is reported by 14% of youth at school compared to 6% who bully others online. Moreover, an examination of the school-online overlap suggests that most youth are bullied or bully at school exclusively. Youth spend more hours in close immediate proximity with peers at school then they do at home or in their neighborhoods in the evening. Interactions in school are inherently social and the opportunities for conflict are plentiful (e.g., hallways, lunch, recess). It is not clear that online environments provide the same amount of time to bully others. Also too, school bullying is often perpetrated by individuals and groups of individuals with an audience present (O'Connell, Pepler, & Craig, 1999; Salmivalli, Lagerspetz, Björkqvist, Österman, & Kaukiainen, 1996) in order to promote the bully's popularity or maintain his or her high social status. The audience reinforces the behavior, thereby increasing the likelihood that it will continue. Although there is an audience online (e.g., Facebook), it is not clear what role this audience plays or how strongly their reinforcement is as it is being mediated through a computer screen. Perhaps part of the reason rates are higher at school is because the social reinforcement is stronger there.

4.2 School bullying is more distressing than online bullying

Online bullying may be different or more distressing than offline bullying because of the ability to hide one's identity, and the rapidity and breadth with which the information is disseminated. Our data do not support this hypothesis, however. Twice as many youth bullied at school (38%) indicate that they feel very or extremely upset by the most serious incident compared to youth bullied online (15%). Moreover, while many more youth (46%) report not knowing their bully online compared to school, 12% report they do not know their bully at school. It seems that the differential power inherent in keeping one's identity secret is more commonly utilized online, but it is possible offline as well (e.g., rumors spread around school).

4.3 Bullying happens other places as well

Importantly, 11% of youth report being bullied on the way to and from school, and 14% "somewhere else"; 4% and 6% report bullying perpetration in these respective environments. This serves as a useful reminder that the online/offline discussion does not implicitly mean online/school. Young people have to safely navigate a multitude of environments each day. Our challenge as researchers is to understand how the experiences of youth are similar and different by environment so that our public policy initiatives and interventions can be general when appropriate and environment-specific when need be.

4.4 Few youth have a never-ending bullying experience

Another concern some have is that technology has created a world in which victims cannot hide from bullies. This may be the case for some youth, but it does not appear to be the common experience. Most youth are not involved in bullying at all. Among victimized youth, the most common victimization experience is being victimized in one versus multiple environments, with school being the one environment most often reported. This suggests that for the majority of youth who are involved in bullying, it is not necessarily something that follows them from the time they wake to the tiime they go to sleep. Nonetheless, there is a very concerning 5% of youth who report being bullied and 2% who report bullying others in four or all five of the environments we queried. Certainly, for these youth, bullying is an experience that likely seems inescapable. Given that they are bullied in multiple environments, this may mean that there are more opportunities to reach them with support and other intervention efforts. It is essential to take steps to identify and target this group of kids.

4.5 Unwanted sexual experiences happen at school and online with equal frequency

Certainly, unwanted sexual encounters happening online have received the majority of academic research attention (Mitchell et al., 2001, 2007; Ybarra et al., 2004). A study conducted in 2000 among 2064 8-12th graders attending public school (American Association of University Women Educational Foundation, 2001) suggests that eight in ten students experience sexual harassment at school sometime in their lives. Rates of unwanted sexual experiences in the past year in the current study are the same at school (18%) and online (18%). Efforts to recognize and reduce unwanted sexual experiences in the schools need to receive just as much attention as those focused online.

While with good intention, recent public policy efforts to regulate social networking sites to reduce the risk of unwanted sexual encounters for adolescents (Berkman Center for Internet & Society at Harvard University, 2008) may not reach youth who are most vulnerable. Unlike bullying, youth who are victims of unwanted sexual experiences are more likely to report being targeted both online and at school (42%) compared to youth targeted at school only (29%) or online only (29%). Future research should focus on these dually-involved youth to better understand who they are and what researchers and other professionals working with adolescents might do to reduce their vulnerability online as well as offline.

4.6 Study limitations and strengths

This paper is the first to report rates of bullying involvement and unwanted sexual experiences online and offline, in school and out of school, using parallel measures among youth in a national US sample. It also is the first to report relative rates of distress and the frequency of "knowing" the perpetrator among bully victims. It is not however, without limitation. The measures for unwanted sexual experiences are less comprehensive than those for bullying. It is possible that the general prevalence rate for unwanted sexual experiences would be higher if other environments (e.g., cell phone text messaging) were queried. It also is possible that caregivers monitored their children while they were completing the survey. This may have led to under-reporting, although comparisons across environments should still hold as there is little reason to believe youth would be more willing to report bullying at school versus online, for example. The sample is based upon English-speaking households. Findings are not generalizable to households that do not read English.

4.7 Future research implications

Environments were queried with the assumption that they were distinct. With the convergence of technology, it is possible now for youth to be bullied on their Facebook profiles, which they could access on their web-capable cell phones during a break at school. In this scenario, youth could potentially click on all three 'environments'. Future research should focus on the conundrum of whether, and if so, how to disentangle these converging environments. This would improve our ability to compare prevalence rates of bullying across the environments in which young people live in order to better target scarce prevention dollars more effectively. It may be however that the "online" "offline" lines have so blurred that the question will quickly become 'have you been bullied', without respect to 'where'. The future challenge for researchers will be to determine when technology is an important characteristic to measure and when it is not.

4.8 'Real world' implications

With youth more likely to be involved in bullying as a victim or perpetrator at school versus online, programs need to continue to prevent and intervene on bullying behavior within schools. Certainly, schools are appropriately working to create protocols that address cyber-aggression and harassment. These prevention efforts should not replace programs that address face-to-face bullying, however; instead, they should be viewed as adjuncts to existing programming. Bullying experiences online could be incorporated into bully prevention programs by simply defining bullying online as bullying which is communicated through the online context.

The relative frequency of sexual harassment both at school and online speaks to the need for prevention programs at the school level. In contrast to the vigilance paid to bullying, sexual harassment is not a commonly discussed adolescent behavior. As noted above, this needs to change.

5. Conclusion

Data from 12-17 year olds nationally suggest that youth are more likely to be involved in bullying at school compared to online, on the way to and from school, and all other environments youth must navigate each day. They are as likely to be a victim of unwanted sexual experiences at school as online. Among bullied youth, 38% were very or extremely upset by their most serious bullying experience at school compared to 15% online. These data do not support a hypothesis that the Internet is introducing a more dangerous environment for youth, nor do they support the supposition that online victimization experiences are more distressing overall.

6. Acknowledgment

The Growing up with Media study was supported by Cooperative Agreement Number U49/CE000206 from the Centers for Disease Control and Prevention (CDC). The contents of this publication are solely the responsibility of the authors and do not necessarily represent the official views of the CDC. The funders were involved in the design and conduct of the study. They were not responsible for data collection, management, analysis, and interpretation of the data; nor were they involved in the preparation, review, or approval of the manuscript.

We would like to thank the entire Growing up with Media Study team from Internet Solutions for Kids, Harris Interactive, Johns Hopkins Bloomberg School of Public Health, and the Centers for Disease Control and Prevention, who contributed to the planning and implementation of the study. Finally, we thank the families for their time and willingness to participate in this study.

7. References

American Association of University Women Educational Foundation. (2001). *Hostile hallways: Bullying, teasing, and sexual harassment in school*. Washington, DC: AAUW Educational Foundation. Retrieved from http://www.aauw.org/learn/research/upload/hostilehallways.pdf

Berkman Center for Internet & Society at Harvard University. (2008). *Enhancing Child Safety & Online Technologies: Final Report of the Internet Safety Technical Taskforce to the Multi-State Working Group on Social Networking of State Attorneys General of the United States*. Cambridge, MA: The Berkman Center for Internet & Society, Harvard University. Retrieved from http://cyber.law.harvard.edu/pubrelease/isttf/

Berrens, R. P., Bohara, A. K., Jenkins-Smith, H., Silva, C., & Weimer, D. L. (2003). The advent of Internet surveys for political research: A comparison of telephone and Internet samples. *Political Analysis, 11*(1), 1-22. doi: 10.1093/pan/11.1.1

Berrens, R. P., Bohara, A. K., Jenkins-Smith, H. C., Silva, C. L., & Weimer, D. L. (2004). Information and effort in contingent valuation surveys: Application to global climate change using national internet samples. *Journal of Environmental Economics & Management, 47*(2), 331-363. doi: 10.1016/S0095-0696(03)00094-9

Bureau of Labor Statistics, & Bureau of the Census. (2006). Current Population Survey Retrieved July 5, 2006, from http://www.bls.census.gov/cps/cpsmain.htm

Cook, C., Heath, F., & Thompson, R. L. (2000). A meta-analysis of response rates in web- or Internet-based surveys. *Educational and Psychological Measurement, 60*(6), 821-836. doi: 10.1177/00131640021970934

Due, P., Holstein, B. E., Lynch, J., Diderichsen, F., Gabhain, S. N., Scheidt, P., ... Health Behaviour in School-Aged Children Bullying Working Group. (2005). Bullying and symptoms among school-aged children: International comparative cross sectional study in 28 countries. *European Journal of Public Health, 15*(2), 128-132. doi: 10.1093/eurpub/cki105

Fineran, S., & Bolen, R. M. (2006). Risk factors for peer sexual harassment in schools. *Journal of Interpersonal Violence, 21*(9), 1169-1190. doi: 10.1177/0886260506290422

Finkelhor, D., Mitchell, K. J., & Wolak, J. (2000). *Online victimization: A report on the nation's youth.* (6-00-020). Alexandria, VA: National Center for Missing & Exploited Children. Retrieved from http://www.unh.edu/ccrc/pdf/jvq/CV38.pdf

Guan, S. S., & Subrahmanyam, K. (2009). Youth Internet use: Risks and opportunities. *Current Opinions in Psychiatry, 22*(4), 351-356. doi: 10.1097/YCO.0b013e32832bd7e0

Harris Interactive. (2006). Online methodology Retrieved July 5, 2006, from http://www.harrisinteractive.com/partner/methodology.asp

Hawker, D. S. J., & Boulton, M. J. (2000). Twenty years' research on peer victimization and psychosocial maladjustment: A meta-analytic review of cross-sectional studies. *Journal of Child Psychology and Psychiatry, 41*(4), 441-455. doi: 10.1111/1469-7610.00629

Juvonen, J., & Gross, E. F. (2008). Extending the school grounds? - Bullying experiences in cyberspace. *Journal of School Health, 78*(9), 496-505. doi: 10.1111/j.1746-1561.2008.00335.x

Kaplowitz, M. D., Hadlock, T. D., & Levine, R. (2004). A comparison of web and mail survey response rates. *Public Opinion Quarterly, 68*(1), 94-101. doi: 10.1093/poq/nfh006

Katzer, C., Fetchenhauer, D., & Belschak, F. (2009). Cyberbullying: Who are the victims? A comparison of victimization in Internet chatrooms and victimization in school. *Journal of Media Psychology, 21*(1), 25-36. doi: 10.1027/1864-1105.21.1.25

Lenhart, A. (2009). *Teens and mobile phones over the past five years: Pew Internet looks back.* Washington, DC: Pew Internet & American Life Project. Retrieved from http://www.pewinternet.org/Reports/2009/14--Teens-and-Mobile-Phones-Data-Memo.aspx

Li, Q. (2006). Cyberbullying in schools: A research of gender differences. *School Psychology International, 27*(2), 157-170. doi: 10.1177/0143034306064547

Mitchell, K. J., Finkelhor, D., & Wolak, J. (2001). Risk factors for and impact of online sexual solicitation of youth. *Journal of the American Medical Association, 285*(23), 3011-3014. doi: 10.1001/jama.285.23.3011

Mitchell, K. J., Finkelhor, D., & Wolak, J. (2007). Youth internet users at risk for the most serious online sexual solicitations. *American Journal of Preventive Medicine, 32*(6), 532-537. doi: 10.1016/j.amepre.2007.02.001

Nansel, T., Craig, W., Overpeck, M., Saluja, G., Ruan, W. J., & Health Behavior in School-aged Children Bullying Working, G. (2004). Cross-national consistency in the relationship between bullying behaviors and psychosocial adjustment. *Archives of Pediatrics & Adolescent Medicine, 158*(8), 730-736. doi: 10.1001/archpedi.158.8.730

O'Connell, P., Pepler, D., & Craig, W. (1999). Peer involvement in bullying: insights and challenges for intervention. *Journal of Adolescence, 22*(4), 437-452. doi: 10.1006/jado.1999.0238

Olweus, D. (1994). Annotation: Bullying at School: Basic facts and effects of a school based intervention program. *Journal of Child Psychology and Psychiatry, 55*(7), 1171-1190. doi: 10.1111/j.1469-7610.1994.tb01229.x

Raskauskas, J., & Stoltz, A. D. (2007). Involvement in traditional and electronic bullying among adolescents. *Developmental Psychology, 43*(3), 564-575. doi: 10.1037/0012-1649.43.3.564

Rideout, V. J. (2001). *Generation Rx.com: How young people use the Internet for health information*. Washington, DC: The Henry J. Kaiser Family Foundation. Retrieved from http://www.kff.org/entmedia/20011211a-index.cfm

Salmivalli, C., Lagerspetz, K., Björkqvist, K., Österman, K., & Kaukiainen, A. (1996). Bullying as a group process: Participant roles and their relations to social status within the group. *Aggressive Behavior, 22*(1), 1-15. doi: 10.1002/(sici)1098-2337(1996)22:1<1::aid-ab1>3.0.co;2-t

Schonlau, M., Zapert, K., Simon, L. P., Sanstad, K. H., Marcus, S. M., Adams, J., Spranca, M., Berry, S. H. (2004). A comparison between response from a propensity-weighted Web survey and an identical RDD survey. *Social Science Computer Review, 22*(1), 128-138. doi: 10.1177/0894439303256551

Slonje, R., & Smith, P. K. (2008). Cyberbullying: Another main type of bullying? *Scandinavian Journal of Psychology, 49*(2), 147-154. doi: 10.1111/j.1467-9450.2007.00611.x

Smith, P. K., Mahdavi, J., Carvalho, M., Fisher, S., Russell, S., & Tippett, N. (2008). Cyberbullying: its nature and impact in secondary school pupils. *Journal of Child Psychology and Psychiatry, 49*(4), 376-385. doi: 10.1111/j.1469-7610.2007.01846.x

Sourander, A., Helstela, L., Helenius, H., & Piha, J. (2000). Persistence of bullying from childhood to adolescence--a longitudinal 8-year follow-up study. *Child Abuse & Neglect, 24*(7), 873-881. doi: 10.1016/S0145-2134(00)00146-0

StataCorp. (2008). Stata Statistical Software (Version 10.1). College Station, TX: Stata Corporation.

Taylor, H., Bremer, J., Overmeyer, C., Siegel, K. W., & Terhanian, G. (2001). The record of internet-based opinion polls in predicting the results of 72 races in the November 2000 US elections. *International Journal of Market Research, 43*, 1-8.

Wang, J., Iannotti, R. J., & Nansel, T. R. (2009). School bullying among adolescents in the United States: Physical, verbal, relational, and cyber. *Journal of Adolescent Health, 45*(4), 368-375. doi: 10.1016/j.jadohealth.2009.03.021

Wolak, J., Mitchell, K. J., & Finkelhor, D. (2006). *Online victimization of youth: 5 years later*. (07-06-025). Alexandria, VA: National Center for Missing & Exploited Children. Retrieved from
http://www.unh.edu/ccrc/pdf/CV138.pdf

Ybarra, M., Diener-West, M., & Leaf, P. (2007a). Examining the overlap in Internet harassment and school bullying: Implications for school intervention. *Journal of Adolescent Health, 41*(6 Suppl 1), S42-S52. doi: 10.1016/j.jadohealth.2007.09.004

Ybarra, M., Leaf, P., & Diener-West, M. (2004). Sex differences in youth-reported depressive symptomatology and unwanted internet sexual solicitation. *Journal of Medical Internet Research, 6*(1), e5. doi: 10.2196/jmir.6.1.e5

Ybarra, M., & Suman, M. (2008). Reasons, assessments, and actions taken: Sex and age differences in uses of Internet health information. *Health Education Research, 23*(3), 512-521. doi: 10.1093/her/cyl062

Ybarra, M. L., Espelage, D. L., & Mitchell, K. J. (2007b). The co-occurrence of Internet harassment and unwanted sexual solicitation victimization and perpetration: Associations with psychosocial indicators. *Journal of Adolescent Health, 41*(6 Suppl 1), S31-41. doi: 10.1016/j.jadohealth.2007.09.010

12

A New Approach in Adolescent Alcohol Intoxication – Clinical Pediatric Experience and Research Combined

E. Van Zanten[1], J.J. Van Hoof[2] and N. Van der Lely[1]
[1]*Department of Pediatrics, Reinier de Graaf Groep, Delft,*
[2]*Faculty of Behavioral Sciences, University of Twente, Enschede,*
The Netherlands

1. Introduction

Misuse of alcohol has become a pediatric health care issue during the last decade. In clinical practice, patients are first treated in an acute care setting. After sobering up, follow-up treatment starts in an outpatient department. To cope with the increasing numbers of underage patients with alcohol intoxication, special programs have been developed to improve follow-up treatment of these patients. The focus has shifted towards underlying neuropsychological and social problems. The main goals of the program are behavioral changes and prevention of new events.

The physiology of alcohol metabolism is clear, however in children and adolescents definitions of binge-drinking, problematic alcohol use and alcohol abuse are overlapping. Research is being done on epidemiology, risk factors and consequences that should be cleared up further. In particular, concerns about brain damage in young adolescents are a topic of interest.

Besides medical attention being paid to this new patient group, policymakers should increase awareness of the dangers of alcohol use. National and international policies differ substantially in legal drinking age and location of purchase. Media attention and marketing also have a huge influence on the drinking behavior of adolescents.

This chapter deals with the following subjects:

- Physiology
- Epidemiology
- Risk factors
- Consequences
- Acute care
- Hospital admittance
- Intervention / follow up
- Screening tools
- Prevention
- Protocol

2. Physiology

Ethanol is absorbed in the stomach or small bowel. Approximately 25% is absorbed directly from the stomach into the bloodstream; the remainder is absorbed by the small bowel. Ethanol cannot be stored; 90% up to 98% of it is broken down in the liver by oxidation. The other 2% to10% is removed directly via urine, breathed out through the lungs or excreted in sweat. Ethanol reaches its peak-blood-concentration within one hour, particularly when ingested on an empty stomach.

Oxidation of ethanol takes place in two ways. Most of it is done by enzymes known as alcohol dehydrogenase (ADH), which produces acetaldehyde, and aldehyde dehydrogenase (ALDH), which transforms acetaldehyde into acetate, a non-toxic metabolite. In this process, hydrogen is transferred from nicotinamide adenine dinucleotide (NAD+) to become NADH (figure 1). Acetate is further metabolized through the citric-acid cycle and leaves the body as carbon dioxide and water. A small amount is processed via an alternative pathway, known as the 'microsomal ethanol-oxidizing system', using cytochrome P-450. In young people, this system is hardly used, as it is mainly activated in regular drinkers or when the level of alcohol is very high (1).

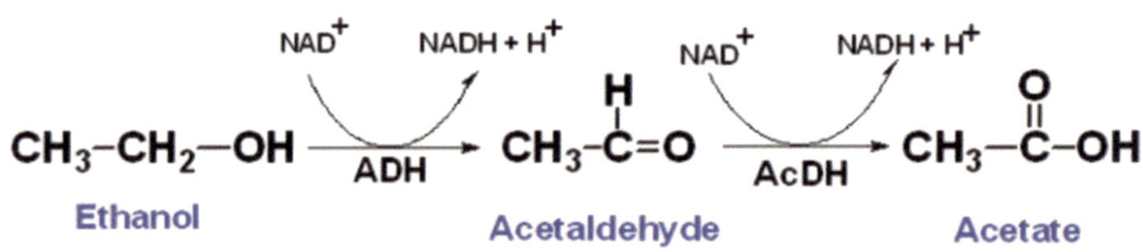

Fig. 1. Oxidation of Ethanol

Different subtypes of ALDH exist within the human body. Mitochondrial ALDH-2 has the biggest affinity with alcohol. About 50 per cent of East-Asian people have a genetic variation which causes their ALDH enzyme not to work very well, resulting in accumulation of toxic acetaldehyde.

The kinetics of alcohol has several metabolic consequences. Due to a changed NAD+/NADH ratio, which inhibits gluconeogenesis, the glucose metabolism can be affected. If existing glycogen deposits have been used, this might lead to hypoglycaemia. Young persons with low glycogen levels are particularly at risk. In other situations alcohol may favor, rather than inhibit, gluconeogenesis and may therefore cause hyperglycaemia (2).

In oxidation, several acid metabolites are being formed, such as lactate and hydroxyacid, which causes metabolic acidosis. In metabolic acidosis, renal potassium loss can cause hypokalaemia, which could be increased by vomiting. These metabolic alterations also favor liver damage. In practice, hypoglycaemia rarely occurs and acidosis is often mild (2) (see also Acute Care chapter).

Symptoms of alcohol intoxication usually appear at a blood alcohol concentration of 20-50 mg/dl (0.2-0.5%) (Table 3). However, interpersonal variability can be observed. Children have a smaller extracellular volume and could therefore experience symptoms at a lower blood concentration. Symptoms of alcohol use will be further discussed below.

3. Epidemiology

Of all the substances, alcohol is -by far- the most popular product. Almost all secondary school students try out alcoholic beverages at least once before they leave school between the age of 16 and 18. The percentage of students who abstain in their secondary school period is constant at around 10% (ref). Between 50% and 60% of all students consume alcohol every month.

Over the past years, this percentage has been rather stable. Since 2003, the youngest students (12 - 14 years) show an increase in lifetime prevalence of alcohol use and previous month alcohol use, especially among girls. Girls also seem to become an increasing cause of concern on other scales. Since 2003, young girls (<15 years) engage in binge drinking more often and have the same frequency of drunkenness as young boys (3;4).

Monitoring alcohol related hospital admissions in the Netherlands is part of the Dutch Pediatric Surveillance System (NSCK). This unique and effective signaling system collects information on several predetermined diseases, disorders or symptoms in Dutch general and academic hospitals. Nearly all the Dutch pediatricians participate (92%). Adolescent alcohol use was included in 2007, and ever since it has been one of the leading topics of the system.

When a patient under the age of 18 is admitted because of alcohol related problems, the pediatrician in charge reports the case. Questionnaires are distributed to the pediatricians by mail or they can download them from the website. The questionnaire consists of four parts, exploring (1) previous alcohol use circumstances and hospital treatment, (2) patient characteristics, (3) alcohol use patterns, and (4) control variables.

4. Questionnaire content

4.1 Intoxication and characteristics of hospital treatment

Time frame of intoxication (morning [6 a.m.–noon], afternoon [noon–6 p.m.], evening [6 p.m.–midnight], night [midnight–6 a.m.]), reason for hospitalization (traffic accident, other accident, aggression/violence, suicide attempt, reduced consciousness—if yes, period of unconsciousness in hours), blood alcohol concentration (BAC, grams of alcohol per liter blood), type of alcohol consumed (beer, wine, distilled spirits, premixed drinks, post mixed drinks [home-mixed or commercially mixed drinks], other), alcohol-obtaining practice (at home, from friends, supermarket, liquor store, hotel and catering industry, other), alcohol-consuming location (parents' home, adolescents' own home, friends' home, on the street, work place, at [a] school [party], public place [sports bar/canteen], commercial place [hotel and catering industry/bar/pub/discotheque], holiday, other), alcohol-consuming company (nobody, friends, parents, other relatives, strangers, other), and other (illicit) substances used (none, cannabis, cocaine, amphetamines / speed, magic mushrooms, Ecstasy, other). If respondents answered "yes" to the last question, method of confirmation was recorded (adolescents' own acknowledgment, other testimony, judgment of the pediatric doctor, laboratory values/urine, other), total time of hospitalization (days), hospital intensive care use (days), intravenous fluids (yes/no), and hospitalization aftercare (patient forwarded to any medical or aid agency).

4.2 General and demographic information about the adolescent

Patient code (control variable consisting of initials of the adolescent, confidential), date of birth (dd-mm-yy), gender, living area (first two numbers of postal code), daily occupation (educational level, work), school performance (normal, repeating of a class, dropout), family situation (traditional, foster parents, living alone), siblings (none, brother[s], sister[s], both), position to siblings (oldest, middle, youngest), cultural background (Dutch, Moroccan, Turkish, Surinamese, Antillean, other), religious background (none, Roman Catholic, Protestant Christian, Jewish, Muslim, Hindu, Buddhist, other), and adolescent registration to medical or aid agencies (none, pediatrician, psychologist, other professional, mental health care institution, The Netherlands Youth Institute, other).

4.3 Patterns of alcohol use and other substance use

Alcohol use in previous months (average number of units per week day [Monday–Thursday] and average number of units per weekend day [Friday–Sunday]), regular drinking places (parents' home, adolescents' own home, friends' home, on the street, work place, at [a] school [party], public place [sports bar/canteen], commercial place [hotel and catering industry/bar/pub/discotheque], holiday, other), regular (illicit) substance use (none, cannabis, cocaine, amphetamines/speed, magic mushrooms, Ecstasy [3,4-methylenedioxymethamphetamine, or MDMA], other), regular tobacco use (no, yes; if possible, estimated number of cigarettes per week), prescribed medication use (no, yes; if yes, what type of medication/name], and parental knowledge of alcohol use (parents know exactly, parents know approximately, parents believe their adolescent child consumes more or less), age of first alcoholic drink.

4.4 Control variables

Date of the intoxication, the date of filling in the questionnaire, pediatrician code number, and the hospital involved.

5. 2007 – 2010 Results

Over the years, the number of adolescents treated with alcohol intoxication increased, as also depicted in Table 1.

	2007	2008	2009	2010
Adolescents treated	297	337	500	684
Increase previous year		13%	48%	37%
Usable questionnaires (response)	231	288	440	566

Table 1. Number of hospitalized adolescents due to alcohol intoxication in Dutch hospitals

The actual number of adolescents suffering from alcohol intoxication must be higher due to the following considerations:

- not all hospitals participated in the data collection procedure;
- not all underage adolescents in hospitals see a pediatrician (instead, they are treated by an emergency doctor or other specialist)
- not all alcohol-related incidents might be diagnosed as alcohol related; and
- not all the adolescents with an alcohol-related injury or intoxication visit a hospital.

5.1 Demographic information

Boys and girls are admitted with alcohol intoxication in about the same percentages (52% male vs. 48% female). However, boys generally have a higher level of blood alcohol concentration (1.87 vs. 1.69 g/L). Intoxicated girls are younger (15.3 vs. 15.7 years) and are hospitalized for shorter periods than boys. Ages range from 11 years up to 17 years, with an average of 15.7 years.

The educational levels of youngsters with alcohol misuse seem to be similar to national statistics. Repeating a study year is not seen more frequently in adolescents with alcohol intoxication. In the Dutch multicultural society, the family structures and cultural and religious backgrounds in this group of patients also correspond with national statistics. The youngest child in the family is more frequently admitted with alcohol abuse (44% youngest child vs. 32% oldest child), children without siblings are relatively uncommon (7% of hospitalized patients have no siblings). These numbers show that adolescent alcohol intoxication occurs in all levels of society, making this pediatric health care issue a difficult but most important subject to deal with.

5.2 Intoxication characteristics and alcohol use patterns

On average, the adolescents admitted to hospital had a blood alcohol concentration of around 1.80 g/L. Depending on age, body weight, gender, tolerance and drug use, this represents an alcohol consumption of about 15 units.

	2007	2008	2009	2010
Average BAC*	1.8	1.9	1.8	1.8
Average reduced consciousness (hours)	2.2	2.9	3.1	3.1
Maximum reduced consciousness (hours)	16	24	22	48

* Blood Alcohol Concentration (grams of alcohol / liter blood)

Table 2. Intoxication characteristics

On average, reduced consciousness lasted for two to three hours (also known as alcohol coma). In 2010, one youngster stayed in a coma for 48 hours.

Questionnaires on the pattern of alcohol use demonstrate that more alcohol is consumed during weekends (0-15 units a day in the weekend, vs. 0-5 units on a week day). For 30% of the patients, the alcohol consumption is their first time; the other 70% do have experience in consuming alcoholic beverages. Most often they consumed beer (59%), followed by distilled spirits. Drinking locations mainly involve a friend's (54%) or parent's home (30%), but, strikingly, 35% of the adolescents treated with alcohol intoxication have been served alcohol in the catering industry (as well). Adolescents report that their parents 'know to some extent ' or even 'know exactly' how much alcohol they drink.

6. Risk factors

General risk factors for alcohol abuse are plenty. Individual, social, physiological and genetic factors influence alcohol use. Not all of these factors have the same level of importance, and some risk factors are still to be identified, as adolescents admitted with alcohol intoxication are a fairly new patient group. Also, risk seeking behavior overlaps with alcohol use. The different definitions of alcohol use, alcohol intoxication, problematic alcohol consumption etc., most likely lead to different outcomes in research and they should perhaps be looked at as different entities. However, known risk factors should be taken into account in individuals presenting with alcohol intoxication and are therefore discussed here.

A physiological process that could contribute to alcohol intoxication in adolescence is decreased sensitivity to most consequences of ethanol, which may lead to relatively high levels of alcohol consumption. For example, children do not have an explicitly stumbling walk when intoxicated. Possibly, sensitivity of cerebellar receptors is not yet fully developed. At the same time, adolescents seem to be more sensitive to other symptoms of alcohol use such as the social facilitation which occurs at low doses of alcohol (5;6).

Among adolescents admitted with alcohol intoxication, boys have a higher ethanol concentration than girls (7). Gender distribution is equal in the population, and duration of unconsciousness is equal between boys and girls. This shows that boys drink more, but it also suggests that girls become intoxicated at lower blood alcohol levels than boys (8). Girls probably are more sensitive to the toxic, suppressive effects of alcohol on the central nervous system.

The role of the socio-economic position in alcohol use is not completely clear. Negative health behavior is often confined to lower income families. More strikingly, it is one of the main factors by which socioeconomic health differences arise (9). Alcohol-related mortality is higher in lower socio-economic classes, mainly among middle-aged men (10). The educational level of the parent is associated with alcohol consumption. Highly educated mothers are correlated with less alcohol consumption (11). At the same time, unskilled occupational level of the father is positively correlated with the amount of alcohol consumed. Other reports conclude that children from families with higher incomes drink more frequently and they more often drink without supervision (12). Material factors such as financial worries and material scarcity can also reduce adolescent alcohol consumption (9). Lower intelligence scores, familial alcohol problems, peer influence and parental attachment can be possible confounders.

Students at pre-vocational secondary education or pre-university secondary education all drink from an early age. It appears that patients with alcohol intoxication on the pre-vocational level are younger and drink less. Higher educational level it is an independent risk factor for higher BAC at admittance.

Parental knowledge of alcohol use and parental rules influence alcohol use amongst adolescents (13). These aspects are striking in clinical practice, with examples of parents offering alcohol to their underage children. Parents who set strict alcohol-specific rules early on delay the age of onset and reduce the frequency and quantity of adolescent alcohol consumption (14) (Koning). A strict attitude of parents towards alcohol diminishes adolescents' involvement in alcohol use. To positively influence problematic alcohol use in their children, parental attitude should be addressed in the treatment of these patients.

Parental attachment can be another factor of interest in parental involvement. It has been described that poor parental attachment is related to an earlier onset of drinking. The inverse explanation can be that the younger the adolescent starts using alcohol, the less strong the attachment with the parents is (13). The influence of the relation between parent and adolescent needs to be clarified further.

A family history of alcohol use is associated with more alcohol consumption in adolescents; and with even higher transmission between parents and adolescents of the same gender (15). Alcoholism of the parents is associated with heavy drinking and binge drinking patterns during adolescence (16). The explanation of these tendencies can be found in the direct exposure to alcohol, as well as in assimilating certain standards and beliefs on alcohol use. Adolescents tend to imitate role models. On the other hand, a positive family history has been found to lead to a relatively lower sensitivity to alcohol.

Students living with peers during their college years drink more alcohol (17). Peer influence is a risk factor in many risk-seeking attitudes, such as smoking, substance abuse and sexual risk behavior. Children are particularly prone to the influence of peers during adolescence. Also, underage drinkers can gain access to alcohol through peers by having older friends who work in a store.

Alcohol use is related to substance use. Cannabis in particular is common, but amphetamines are used as well, as are ecstasy, happy mushrooms and cocaine. Co-occurrence is common and therefore patients admitted with alcohol intoxication should always be screened for substance abuse (18).

Cultural influences are connected to local politics, either nationally- or statewide. Determining legal drinking age has a strong influence on the availability of alcohol for adolescents (19;20). However, this seems to be just one of several factors to be considered. A prosperous society and a change in the available types of drinks are likely to have an effect on alcohol consumption. An increase in drinking among youngsters has been observed in the past decade (21). For Dutch adolescents purchasing alcohol is one of the leading expenses (22-24).

The relationship between alcohol or substance abuse and psychiatric disorders such as ADHD is described as a consequence as well as a cause (25;26). Symptoms like physical aggression, conduct disorders and violence as well as hyperactivity and oppositional behaviors at a young age appear to be risk factors for alcohol use in later life (27). In particular, higher quantities of alcohol consumption have been associated with a lack of restraint (disinhibition) (28;29). The interpretation of these associations can be causal and consequential and are interesting subjects of research still to be carried out. Depression and anxiety disorders in relation to alcohol use are mainly studies in adult populations (and not in adolescents or children). However, depression occurs more frequently in patients with alcohol abuse (30).

The clustering of social problems and alcohol intoxication was a particular observation of interest in a project carried out at the Reinier de Graaf Hospital in Delft, The Netherlands (see Protocol chapter). The rate of self-reported social problems was high among the adolescents admitted for alcohol intoxication. Among them were family histories of addiction (35.3%), divorce or a deceased parent (19.1% and 11,3% respectively); parent-child interaction was aberrant in many cases (44.6%), as were school problems (34.3%) and sexual abuse (4.4%) or life-events (e.g. severe illness, emotional problems (41.2%). Also common were underlying psychiatric disorders (40%) (autism, attention deficit hyperactivity disorder, depression or eating disorders).

These percentages show that the clustering of personal and social issues during puberty makes this group vulnerable.

7. Consequences

It is important to realize on the long term, that alcohol and substance abuse tend to track on into early adulthood and that alcohol use at a young age is a predictor for future alcohol use (31).

Adolescent drinkers are more likely than their non-drinking or experimenting peers to have school problems, drugs or engage in criminal activities such as stealing. In a follow up study carried out 10 years later, adolescents who had consumed alcohol were still more often involved in problem behaviors including unreliable work attendance, substance use problems, violent behavior and illegal activities during early adulthood. Early experimenters were also at higher risk than non-drinkers to have problems with substance use and criminal and violent behavior (32).

Heavy drinking has been shown to affect neuropsychological performance and could impair the growth and integrity of the brain structures. During adolescence, the part of the brain that is developing in particular is the frontal lobe. Here, the higher cognitive functions such as cognitive processing and executive functions are located (33;34).

Research with functional magnetic resonance imaging (fMRI) demonstrates that memory, attention and visuospatial abilities are negatively affected by alcohol. Alcohol and drug abusers perform worse than their peers (35). Increased vulnerability for these neurologic effects is seen in women, patients with a family history of alcohol use disorders, heavy episodic drinkers and alcohol use combined with drug use. The co-occurrence of psychiatric disorders is an important factor to consider in the evaluation of neurocognitive functioning in patients with alcohol abuse. As was mentioned before causality is not clear. The role of time of abstinence and age of first drink seem to be less related to neurologic damage (36).

Importantly, as young adulthood is a period when most people make important educational, occupational and social decisions, an impaired cognitive function could significantly affect their futures.

Alcohol use increases the risk of high-risk sexual intercourse. Young adolescents report that alcohol has caused them to engage in unplanned sex (27). Girls in particular are prone to participate in sexual relationships more readily, and even against their will, during intoxication. Afterwards, they often regret the incident and it is not uncommon that they are traumatized.

Alcohol consumption is one of the leading preventable causes of death in the United States (37). The WHO recently identified alcohol use amongst young people (10-24 years) as the most important factor contributing to disability adjustable life years (DALY's) (38). In particular, consumption of alcohol is associated with injuries and accidents, which are major contributors to mortality of adolescents.

Apart from the psychiatric disorders discussed before, alcohol use is also associated with medical conditions such as hepatitis and liver cirrhosis, hypertension, pancreatitis, cardiomyopathy, pneumonia and tuberculosis. Also cancers of the mouth, esophagus, pharynx, larynx and breast are more common in patients with excessive alcohol consumption. Neurologic disease is not uncommon, and alcohol use is associated with peripheral neuropathy and myopathy, as well as with central nervous diseases such as dementia and stroke.

8. Acute care

The acute care of an adolescent presenting with alcohol intoxication is being done conform the Advanced Pediatric Life Support protocol (APLS). Most hospitalizations occur during the evening or night (93%), (see Epidemiology section). The announcement of an adolescent having become unwell at a party or an unconscious youngster smelling of ethanol usually gives away the diagnosis. However, as the presentation is often severe, especially the level of consciousness, ABCD-assessment should always be done. Reports of reduced consciousness vary from a couple of minutes up to 48 hours (!), with an average of 2 hours and 11 minutes. According to Dutch research, average time of unconsciousness has risen during the past years from 2,2 hours in 2007 to 3,1 hours in 2010 (7). Other presentations include traffic accidents, aggression and violence and even suicide attempts (1%). These type of symptoms of alcohol intoxication (Table 3) usually appear at a blood alcohol concentration of 20-50 mg/dl (0.2-0.5%).

Blood Alcohol Concentration		Symptoms
Mg/dl	‰	
20-50	0,2-0,5	Gross motor impairment, difficulty concentrating
50-100	0,5-0,10	Decreased coordination and reactivity
100-150	1,0-1,5	Disturbed balance and gait
150-250	1,5-2,5	Stupor
300	3,0	Unconsciousness
400	4,0	Respiratory failure

Table 3. Symptoms of alcohol intoxication

At admission of a patient with alcohol intoxication, the following assessments should be done:

- Amount and type of alcoholic consumptions
- Other substances (e.g. marihuana, cocaine, amphetamines)
- Other medications (e.g. contraception, benzodiazepines)
- Blood (blood alcohol concentration, arterial blood gas, glucose, electrolytes, electrocardiogram, liver function)
- Urine toxicology screen.

The amount of alcohol consumed can be estimated by using the formula, based on the Widmark equation, in figure 2 (39). This can be of use in conversations with parents and patients about alcohol consumption.

$$\text{Cethanol} = \frac{A \times p \times 0{,}01 \times 0.8}{V \times Lg} \rightarrow A = \frac{\text{Cethanol} \times V \times Lg}{p \times 0{,}01 \times 0.8}$$

Cethanol	= Ethanol concentration (in g/L or o/oo)
A	= Amount of alcohol containing product consumed (in ml)
P	= Alcohol concentration in product (in %)
0,08	= Relative density of ethanol
V	= Volume of distribution (in L/kg) for a child: 0,7 L/kg
Lg	= Body weight (in kg)

Fig. 2. Formula to calculate amount of alcohol consumed

In general, acute medical complications are serious but mild. The complications seen most frequently are reduced consciousness (45%) and hypothermia (43.1%). Electrolyte disturbances are most often hypercloremia (31.1%) and low bicarbonate (22%), but hypokalemia (11.9%) and hypernatremia (7.7%) are also seen. Hypoglycaemia is not often reported, however hyperglycaemia can be seen in some patients (13.6%). Mild acidosis, more often metabolic but also respiratory, was observed in 28.8% of patients (2).

After admittance patients are directly monitored. Treatment mostly consists of administering intravenous fluids to rehydrate. Metabolic acidosis, hypoglycaemia and hypothermia are corrected. Gastric lavage and activated charcoal are not recommended since they are ineffective due to the rapid resorption of ethanol and because they possibly enhance the risk of aspiration.

9. Protocol

To standardize the care given to an intoxicated adolescent, a program was developed in the Reinier de Graaf Hospital, Delft, The Netherlands to follow up on patients with alcohol intoxication. The objective of the program is to structurally intervene in the growing problem of adolescents with alcohol intoxication. Four main goals were identified:

- To prevent repetition of intoxication
- To change the behavior of the adolescent towards alcohol
- To change the behavior and guidance of the parents
- To detect psychological co-morbidity

Consecutively, more insight is obtained into the epidemiology, social environment and psychological and cognitive functioning of these patients.

Based on the short-term and long-term complications mentioned above, the protocol is divided into different stages.

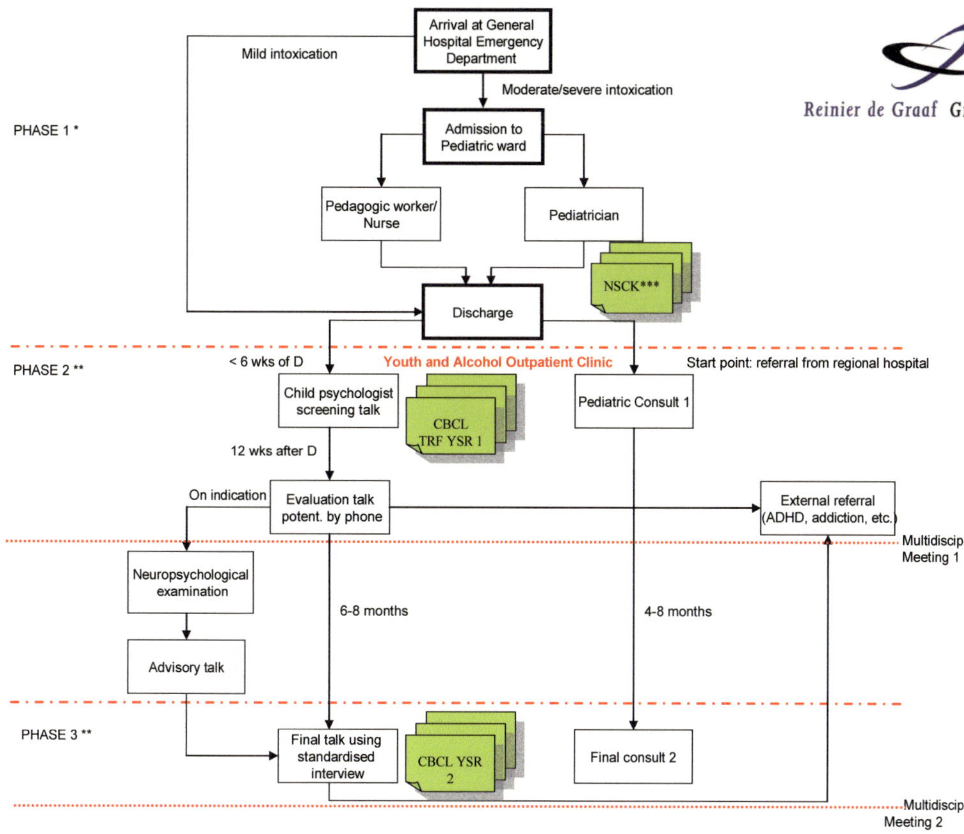

NSCK: Dutch Pediatric Surveillance System

CBCL: Child Behaviour Checklist

TRF: Teacher Report Form

YSR: Youth Self Report

Fig. 3. Flowchart alcohol treatment policlinic alcohol and youth

10. Hospital admittance

After acute care, the focus shifts towards treatment and education. By informing the patients and their parents about the dangers of alcohol consumption, the effect of hospitalization is broadened towards prevention and intervention. This will be of use during follow up at the outpatient department.

Most patients are admitted in the evening or at night (40). The next morning, they are woken on time to start a short program before being discharged from hospital. First, the pediatrician speaks both to the patient and the parents, explaining the reason for admittance and emphasizing the seriousness of the event. The patient's medical and social histories are checked and questions are asked about further alcohol use. The dangers of alcohol use are explained. This is seen as an important moment for intervention and education. Patient and parents pay more attention shortly after the incident occurred. Later on, a pedagogic employee or nurse will help the adolescent to answer questions on alcohol use on a government-funded website. Parents are also referred to websites for further information.

Most of the patients leave the hospital in good clinical health within a day after admittance. After discharge, a program starts at the outpatient department of pediatrics and child psychology.

11. Intervention & follow up

After treatment of the acute problems and sobering up, the multiple alcohol-use related problems mentioned above should be attended to in an evaluation.

Many treatments for alcohol use disorders can be applied to decrease alcohol use. Among them are family treatment, (short) motivational enhancement therapy and behavioral therapy, which all seem to have a significant positive effect on alcohol and substance use (41).

After receiving information in the hospital setting, the patients visit a pediatrician and a pediatric psychologist at the outpatient clinic. The program consists of several appointments.

At the appointment with the pediatrician, the patient's general alcohol and drug use, school problems and social issues are addressed. By means of a presentation several alcohol related problems are addressed, such as epidemiology, metabolism, neurological and physical consequences, case reports, peer pressure (for example at sport facilities), media attention and marketing strategies of alcohol industries. The role of the parents is emphasized as well; alcohol-specific rules are pointed out, such as; rules on vacation are the same as those at home, parents are not supposed to drink in front of their children, not to mention invite them to try. To optimize the effect of the intervention, these issues can be individualized depending on the patient's interest.

The child psychologist performs a psychological interview to screen for underlying problems. The patient is also evaluated based on behavioral questionnaires (Youth Self Report (YSR), Child Behavior Checklist (CBCL) and Teacher Report Form (TRF), to be filled in by patient as well as parents and teachers), and earlier and recent educational performance. The interaction between parents and adolescent is taken into account, and life events and psychosocial history also are important issues for discussion. Once again the dangers of alcohol use are explained.

When indicated, psychological, social, medical or addiction-related treatment is offered. Some services can be offered within the setting of the outpatient clinic, for others, the patient can be referred elsewhere. Although treatment is not always necessary, follow-up is done at all times. After the first appointments the patient will be contacted within 6 months after the event to discuss alcohol use and general well-being. However, often the pediatrician or child psychologist finds it necessary to see the patient in the mean time because of related issues.

In conclusion, underlying social and neuropsychological problems can come to light during psychological and pediatric screening and can be treated when indicated. The dangers of alcohol are being explained extensively to patients as well as parents. Help can consist of psychological treatment or referral to detox clinics or other youth care institutions.

Preliminary results of the project are promising. At follow-up, 84-88 % of the patients had stopped binge drinking and 61% had stopped the consumption of alcohol. Awareness of the parents was another factor of interest; at follow up 82,5 % of the parents applied specific alcohol rules, including prohibition of alcohol under 16 years of age. Behavioral questionnaires were filled in by 89% of the study population. Neuropsychological screening was done in 72% of the patients for whom it was indicated.

12. Tools for screening

Screening for problematic alcohol use can be useful during follow up of the patients. It can be expected that questions about lifestyle are delicate, particularly during adolescence and in the direct vicinity of parents or adults. At the same time, detection of problematic alcohol use at a young age can reveal alcohol dependency and ensure a more effective intervention. So far, no standard screening method has been identified.

Various self-report questionnaires are available for rapid assessment of drinking behavior, such as the Alcohol Use Disorders Identification Test (AUDIT), TWEAK (Tolerance, Worried, Eye-opener, Amnesia, Cut Down), the Michigan Alcohol Screening Test, CAGE (Cut Down, Annoyed, Guilty, Eye Opener) and the Alcohol Dependence Scale. The AUDIT was developed by the World Health Organization (WHO) as a measure for alcohol consumption, dependence and alcohol-related problems. The TWEAK focuses more on tolerance. It was specifically developed for women and aims to identify possible hazardous drinking patterns. The CAGE places emphasis on behaviors consistent with alcohol dependence.

These various screening methods are rapid, non-invasive and inexpensive, but they have different outcome parameters and were developed for adults. Applicability for adolescents has been investigated and seems to support the AUDIT as the better screening method (42), due to its focus on frequency of use, quantity and frequency of binge drinking. This can be an advantage in adolescents, because here the early detection of drinking problems is the main goal. However, reliability is low because of self-report.

Biological screening methods can offer more objectivity. Amongst them is the extensively used blood alcohol concentration, which is generally determined during the first care. However, this test only gives information during a short period after consumption of alcohol. It has no role in screening for alcohol use at the outpatient clinic.

Other traditional and new markers can add to the suspicion of problematic alcohol use. The more established markers of alcohol use are mean corpuscular volume (MCV), gamma-glutamyltransferase (GGT), aspartate aminotransferase (AST) and alanine aminotransferase (ALT). Increased values can lead to the differential diagnose of alcohol dependency. Direct markers, which are all products of ethanol metabolism, are acetyldehyde, acetic acid, fatty acid ethyl ester (FAEE) and ethyl glucuronide (EtG).

Newer biomarkers include carbohydrate-deficient transferrin (CDT), total serum sialic acid (TSA) and 5-hydroxytryptophol (5-HTOL). Transferrin is a plasma protein that carries iron through the bloodstream to the bone marrow. Transferrin is a polypeptide with two N-linked polysaccharide chains. The chains are branched with sialic acid residues. Consuming significant quantities of alcohol increases the proportion of transferrin with low saturation of sialic acid residues. They are referred to as carbohydrate-deficient transferrins (CDT). CDT testing is available in a regular hospital lab.

Sialic acid is a monosaccharide carbohydrate. As a consequence of excessive alcohol consumption, saturation of transferrin with sialic acid decreases and total serum sialic acid rises. Determination of TSA provides a means of detecting alcohol abuse. 5-hydroxytryptophol (5-HTOL) is a human metabolite of serotonin (5-hydroxytryptamine, 5-HT) and is excreted in the urine, where it mainly occurs conjugated with a glucuronic acid and, to a lesser extent, in free form or conjugated as a sulphate. After alcohol consumption, the 5-HTOL level in various body fluids will rise above normal values.

The value of these new biomarkers for screening purposes is still under discussion. Several factors are of importance; such as detection period after abstinence, patterns of alcohol use (episodic drinking, non-heavy chronic patterns, etc.), associated medical disorders, demographic differences and cost and availability. Sensitivity and specificity are of particular interest and are highly dependent on cut-off points, which have not yet been established (43;44)

The indirect marker CDT and direct marker EtG seem to have the most advantages for all-around utility. Combinations of different markers, especially CDT and GGT, have been studied, and application at multiple time points could significantly increase their usefulness.

Still, little research has been done among adolescents. Some studies among adults include a sub-analysis of patients under 20 years of age, and these show minimal association of alcohol consumption and markers (43;44).

In conclusion, biomarkers of alcohol use are of interest to pediatricians dealing with adolescents at the outpatient clinic for obtaining useful information on drinking patterns, which would otherwise be obtained by less reliable means like questionnaires. The exact role of biomarkers should be clarified further.

13. Prevention

Alcohol use in adolescents is influenced by internal and external factors. In the first place, health interventions such as government campaigns for mass media as well as smaller programs attempt to decrease youth alcohol use. Some studies show effects on knowledge, attitude and behavior. However, the effect is uncertain and these health effects can disappear over time (45).

Secondly, the alcohol industry has a major influence via alcohol commercials and brand visibility. Advertisements attempt to make the customer feel positive about a specific product or brand. Not only adults, but adolescents as well are persuaded to adopt a positive attitude towards alcohol and even drink more alcohol (46). Policies concerning alcohol advertisement focus on specific high-risk groups. Restricting outdoor alcohol advertisements near schools, banning alcohol commercials from television early in the evening or on youth-oriented channels and specific advertisement related rules are laid down in the law.

Another factor that influences alcohol use is media portrayals. The ambience that movies and television series create in relation to alcohol increases alcohol consumption, partly through the 'modeling theory' In particular, the so-called 'product placements' which are hidden in television shows and movies are often located tactically. Direct relations have been described between alcohol use in movies and early-onset teen drinking, drinking without parental awareness and acute alcohol consumption (47).

External risk factors that should be considered when carrying out prevention measures are matters of social, economic, physical and legal availability, which are the most important predictors of adolescent alcohol consumption, drinking patterns and alcohol-related harm (48).

Social availability refers to the social context into which drinking is incorporated. As was mentioned before, teens and adolescents drink alcohol in the company of their peers. Another social factor related to higher alcohol use is parental alcohol consumption. Economic availability relates to, prices of alcohol and especially to special promotions which increase alcohol consumption. The most frequently used governmental tool to prevent alcohol use is increasing taxes on alcoholic beverages. Higher prices lead to lower consumption (49). A third factor that can be used in prevention is physical availability, which focuses on outlet density and opening hours. Higher outlet density is related to higher availability. Especially outlet density and location should be considered, for example by decreasing availability near educational institutions.

A very important factor is legal availability. Alcohol policies for various age groups differ around the world, but the increasing number of patients admitted with alcohol intoxication demonstrates the infectivity of these laws. All legislation concerning the purchase, sale, consumption and possession of alcohol should be critically arranged for underage citizens. One of the prime governmental tools to influence alcohol consumption is setting age limits, because binge drinking, drinking at school and drinking and driving are related especially to the sale of alcohol to underage persons. Research has shown that higher legal age limits are related to a decrease of alcohol-related car crashes and other injuries. However, despite legal age limits it is still possible for many underage adolescents to obtain alcohol in commercial places. Strikingly, compliance with age legislation in commercial establishment is not guaranteed; and alcohol can easily be obtained and consumed (50). Falsification of identification cards is another way to obtain alcohol.

Prevention of alcohol use among adolescents should be aimed at patients, parents and politics. A conjunct of medical, political and sociological awareness of the dangers of alcohol use can decrease alcohol use within modern societies.

14. References

[1] Lieber CS. The discovery of the microsomal ethanol oxidizing system and its physiologic and pathologic role. Drug Metab Rev 2004; 36(3-4):511-529.
[2] Bouthoorn SH, van der Ploeg T, van Erkel NE, van der Lely N. Alcohol intoxication among Dutch adolescents: acute medical complications in the years 2000-2010. Clin Pediatr (Phila) 2011; 50(3):244-251.
[3] Monshouwer K, Verdurmen J, van Dorsselaer S, Smit, E, Gorter A, Vollebergh W. Jeugd en riskant gedrag 2007: kerngegevens uit het peilstationsonderzoek scholieren.

Roken, drinken, drugsgebruik en gokken onder scholieren vanaf tien jaar [Youth and risk behaviour monitor 2007]. Report from the Dutch Trimbos Institute 2008.
[4] Centraal Bureau voor de Statistiek Jeugdmonitor 2011 [Statistics Netherlands Youthmonitor 2011]
[5] Windle M, Brener N, Cuccaro P, Dittus P, Kanouse DE, Murray N et al. Parenting predictors of early-adolescents' health behaviors: simultaneous group comparisons across sex and ethnic groups. J Youth Adolesc 2010; 39(6):594-606.
[6] Spear LP, Varlinskaya EI. Sensitivity to ethanol and other hedonic stimuli in an animal model of adolescence: implications for prevention science? Dev Psychobiol 2010; 52(3):236-243.
[7] Bouthoorn SH, van Hoof JJ, van der Lely N. Adolescent alcohol intoxication in Dutch hospital centers of pediatrics: characteristics and gender differences. Eur J Pediatr 2011.
[8] Thomasson HR. Gender differences in alcohol metabolism. Physiological responses to ethanol. Recent Dev Alcohol 1995; 12:163-179.
[9] Droomers M, Schrijvers CT, Casswell S, Mackenbach JP. Occupational level of the father and alcohol consumption during adolescence; patterns and predictors. J Epidemiol Community Health 2003; 57(9):704-710.
[10] Siegler V, Al Hamad A, Johnson B, Wells C, Sheron N. Social inequalities in alcohol-related adult mortality by National Statistics Socio-economic Classification, England and Wales, 2001-03. Health Stat Q 2011;(50):4-39.
[11] Melotti R, Heron J, Hickman M, Macleod J, Araya R, Lewis G. Adolescent alcohol and tobacco use and early socioeconomic position: the ALSPAC birth cohort. Pediatrics 2011; 127(4):e948-e955.
[12] Bellis MA, Morleo M, Hughes K, Downing J, Wood S, Smallthwaite L et al. A cross-sectional survey of compliance with national guidance for alcohol consumption by children: measuring risk factors, protective factors and social norms for excessive and unsupervised drinking. BMC Public Health 2010; 10:547.
[13] van der Vorst H, Engels RC, Meeus W, Dekovic M. The impact of alcohol-specific rules, parental norms about early drinking and parental alcohol use on adolescents' drinking behavior. J Child Psychol Psychiatry 2006; 47(12):1299-1306.
[14] van der Vorst H, Engels RC, Meeus W, Dekovic M, Van Leeuwe J. The role of alcohol-specific socialization in adolescents' drinking behaviour. Addiction 2005; 100(10):1464-1476.
[15] van der Vorst H, Engels RC, Dekovic M, Meeus W, Vermulst AA. Alcohol-specific rules, personality and adolescents' alcohol use: a longitudinal person-environment study. Addiction 2007; 102(7):1064-1075.
[16] Chassin L, Pitts SC, Prost J. Binge drinking trajectories from adolescence to emerging adulthood in a high-risk sample: predictors and substance abuse outcomes. J Consult Clin Psychol 2002; 70(1):67-78.
[17] Boot CR, Rosiers JF, Meijman FJ, Van Hal GF. Consumption of tobacco, alcohol and recreational drugs in university students in Belgium and the Netherlands: the role of living situation. Int J Adolesc Med Health 2010; 22(4):527-534.
[18] Bava S, Tapert SF. Adolescent brain development and the risk for alcohol and other drug problems. Neuropsychol Rev 2010; 20(4):398-413.

[19] Nelson TF, Naimi TS, Brewer RD, Wechsler H. The state sets the rate: the relationship among state-specific college binge drinking, state binge drinking rates, and selected state alcohol control policies. Am J Public Health 2005; 95(3):441-446.
[20] Bieleman B, Kruize A, Nienhuis A. Monitor alcoholverstrekking jongeren 2005: naleving leeftijdsgrenzen 16 en 18 jaar. Drank- en horecawet: metingen 1999, 2001, 2003 en 2005. 2006. (Report)
[21] Laar MW, Cruts AAN, Verdurmen J, van Ooyen MMJ. Nationale Drug Monitor; jaarbericht 2004. 2004. (Report)
[22] Spijkerman R, van den Eijnden RJ, Huiberts A. Socioeconomic differences in alcohol-specific parenting practices and adolescents' drinking patterns. Eur Addict Res 2008; 14(1):26-37.
[23] Financieel gedrag van werkenden jongeren 2005. 2005. (Report)
[24] van den Eijnden RJ, Schutten M. Aankoop en gebruik van alcoholhoudende dranken door jongeren. 2005. (Report)
[25] Wilens TE, Biederman J. Alcohol, drugs, and attention-deficit/ hyperactivity disorder: a model for the study of addictions in youth. J Psychopharmacol 2006; 20(4):580-588.
[26] Tomlinson KL, Brown SA, Abrantes A. Psychiatric comorbidity and substance use treatment outcomes of adolescents. Psychol Addict Behav 2004; 18(2):160-169.
[27] Windle M, Spear LP, Fuligni AJ, Angold A, Brown JD, Pine D et al. Transitions into underage and problem drinking: developmental processes and mechanisms between 10 and 15 years of age. Pediatrics 2008; 121 Suppl 4:S273-S289.
[28] Earleywine M, Finn PR. Sensation seeking explains the relation between behavioral disinhibition and alcohol consumption. Addict Behav 1991; 16(3-4):123-128.
[29] Wiers RW, Bartholow BD, van den WE, Thush C, Engels RC, Sher KJ et al. Automatic and controlled processes and the development of addictive behaviors in adolescents: a review and a model. Pharmacol Biochem Behav 2007; 86(2):263-283.
[30] McKenzie M, Jorm AF, Romaniuk H, Olsson CA, Patton GC. Association of adolescent symptoms of depression and anxiety with alcohol use disorders in young adulthood: findings from the Victorian Adolescent Health Cohort Study. Med J Aust 2011; 195(3):S27-S30.
[31] Duncan SC, Alpert A, Duncan TE, Hops H. Adolescent alcohol use development and young adult outcomes. Drug Alcohol Depend, 1997;49: 1, 39-48.
[32] Ellickson PL, Tucker JS, Klein DJ. Ten-year prospective study of public health problems associated with early drinking. Pediatrics 2003; 111(5 Pt 1):949-955.
[33] Tapert SF, Schweinsburg AD, Barlett VC, Brown SA, Frank LR, Brown GG et al. Blood oxygen level dependent response and spatial working memory in adolescents with alcohol use disorders. Alcohol Clin Exp Res 2004; 28(10):1577-1586.
[34] Tapert SF, Pulido C, Paulus MP, Schuckit MA, Burke C. Level of response to alcohol and brain response during visual working memory. J Stud Alcohol 2004; 65(6):692-700.
[35] Schweinsburg AD, Schweinsburg BC, Cheung EH, Brown GG, Brown SA, Tapert SF. fMRI response to spatial working memory in adolescents with comorbid marijuana and alcohol use disorders. Drug Alcohol Depend 2005; 79(2):201-210.
[36] Tapert SF, Caldwell L., Burke C. Alcohol and the Adolescent Barin - Human studies. Alcohol Research and Health 2004; 28(4).

[37] Danaei G, Ding EL, Mozaffarian D, Taylor B, Rehm J, Murray CJ et al. The preventable causes of death in the United States: comparative risk assessment of dietary, lifestyle, and metabolic risk factors. PLoS Med 2009; 6(4):e1000058.
[38] Gore FM, Bloem PJ, Patton GC, Ferguson J, Joseph V, Coffey C et al. Global burden of disease in young people aged 10-24 years: a systematic analysis. Lancet 2011.
[39] Widmark EMP. Principles and Applications of Medicolegal Alcohol Determination. Biomedical Publications 1981;107-108.
[40] van Hoof JJ, van der Lely N, Bouthoorn SH, Van Dalen WE, Pereira RR. Adolescent alcohol intoxication in the Dutch hospital departments of pediatrics: a 2-year comparison study. J Adolesc Health 2011; 48(2):212-214.
[41] Deas D. Evidence-based treatments for alcohol use disorders in adolescents. Pediatrics 2008; 121 Suppl 4:S348-S354.
[42] Chung T, Colby SM, Barnett NP, Rohsenow DJ, Spirito A, Monti PM. Screening adolescents for problem drinking: performance of brief screens against DSM-IV alcohol diagnoses. J Stud Alcohol 2000; 61(4):579-587.
[43] Conigrave KM, Degenhardt LJ, Whitfield JB, Saunders JB, Helander A, Tabakoff B. CDT, GGT, and AST as markers of alcohol use: the WHO/ISBRA collaborative project. Alcohol Clin Exp Res 2002; 26(3):332-339.
[44] Kalapatapu RK, Chambers R. Novel Objective Biomarkers of Alcohol Use: Potential Diagnostic and Treatment Management Tools in Dual Diagnosis Care. J Dual Diagn 2009; 5(1):57-82.
[45] van Hoof JJ. Sweet Sixteen and Never Been Drunk? Adolescent Alcohol Use, Predictors and Consequences. 2010. (Report)
[46] Wyllie A, Zhang JF, Casswell S. Positive responses to televised beer advertisements associated with drinking and problems reported by 18 to 29-year-olds. Addiction 1998; 93(5):749-760.
[47] Dal Cin S, Worth KA, Dalton MA, Sargent JD. Exposure to Alcohol Use in Movies: Future Directions. Addiction 2008; 103(12):1937-1938.
[48] Paschall MJ, Grube JW, Kypri K. Alcohol control policies and alcohol consumption by youth: a multi-national study. Addiction 2009; 104(11):1849-1855.
[49] Purshouse RC, Meier PS, Brennan A, Taylor KB, Rafia R. Estimated effect of alcohol pricing policies on health and health economic outcomes in England: an epidemiological model. Lancet 2010; 375(9723):1355-1364.
[50] Gosselt JF, van Hoof JJ, de Jong MD, Prinsen S. Mystery shopping and alcohol sales: do supermarkets and liquor stores sell alcohol to underage customers? J Adolesc Health 2007; 41(3):302-308.

13

Infantile Hospitalisation and Chronic Disease

Camila Aloisio Alves[1] and Rosa Maria de Araújo Mitre[2]
[1]Gama Filho University and the Petropolis Faculty of Medicine,
[2]The Fernandes Figueira Institute / Fiocruz,
Brazil

1. Introduction

This chapter attempts to characterise the process of chronic disease and infant hospitalisation, the relationship between healthcare professionals, children and their families, in addition to considering the implications which chronic disease has throughout the life of the child and their family. The chapter also considers the changes in the field of pediatrics, its gaps and shortcomings and its position in the biomedical field, defining technical and scientific principles.

The chapter intends to contribute to the construction of knowledge within pediatrics in the face of contemporary concerns and reflections about chronic disease which can serve as a reference point for the promotion of healthcare strategies, principally specialised hospital care, for those children in hospital care.

With the evolution of diagnostic methods and new treatment methods there has been a great deal of discussion and research into chronic disease and its implications for the lives of child suffers. Chronic disease effects millions of people throughout the world, however, it is fundamental that we reflect upon the peculiarities involved when this experience occurs during childhood. To be able to speak of chronic illness and of infant hospitalisation, it is necessary to locate this stage of the child's development, which we refer to as childhood, whilst also considering the role which children occupy in contemporary society from the vantage point of healthcare.

Until the 18th Century children were the responsibility of the family which ensured the transmission of physical life, family possessions and names, but had no specific concern with educational. The State and charity were utilised only in cases of abandonment (Aries, 2009).

However, from the Renaissance to the Enlightenment the concern with children's health intensified, beginning from a sense of conservation and protection of childhood originating with mercantilism, and later, to capitalists with the intention of strengthening and expanding armies and a necessity for abundant labour power. Educational performance, which began to take centre stage in shaping children, was dominated by vigilance and discipline and was concerned with morality and a sense of responsibility. Likewise, the Family was elected as the principle cell in which to focus hygiene, nutrition and control (Aries, 2009).

Medicine fitted the function of guiding, controlling and instructing families and society with regard to treatments, clothing, toys, education and nutritional timetables, and was founded on the new knowledge of comprehensive childcare. A rational and scientific model emerged from within pediatric care providing the rules and norms for medical and educational practice towards children. (Rago, 1987; Zanoli & Merhy2001)

Childhood, as the object of study taken by medicine, focused its attention on the confluence of three privileged axes: high infant mortality rate, abandoned children and a repositioning of the doctor figure as central in the medicalisation of the family (Rago, 1987).

Raised to a privileged position of knowledge and understanding about the best ways to maintain a clean and healthy life, medicine now assumed the political role of recovering the trajectories of childhood, hitherto unproblematic, and began to the fulfil the task of intervening in private households.

In addition to education, impoverished and abandoned children were disciplined through professional institutions such as orphanages. They provided both discipline and new knowledge which was transmitted through the punitive and repressive model, restructuring both habits and customs (Rago, 1987).

The study of hygiene brought to social life new practices and norms of personal hygiene, familial hygiene and for the home, focusing principally on maintaining and sustaining healthy children and the formation of strong citizens, who would be able to work in the future. The relationship between childhood and adulthood was established and the way in which an individual had been treated during childhood came to be the main determinant for their future possibilities of a healthy adult life. Thus, hygiene became a central concern for governments and states in producing subjects and families and was directed towards protecting physical and emotional intimacy (Costa, 1983).

Later, children's health became harnessed to maternal health, originating in the binomial of mother-child. A proposal to protect the mother-child's health was developed, planned and implemented through specific programs and standards of healthcare. However, with this move towards preventative and communitarian medicine, a new proposal was presented focusing on comprehensive healthcare, both rationalising and hierarchical, establishing networks of hospital and outpatient services. There was a refocusing on the concepts of multiple causality and risk in the understanding of children's health. The fight against infant mortality was centred on discourses and practices directed towards understanding the social determinants of the health-disease process and of the necessity to expand assistance until adolescence. A shift occurred from focusing on childcare to focusing on disease, in which healthcare became organised and systematised into standards of care (Zanoli & Merhy, 2001).

An important characteristic of early pediatric hospitals is the absence of the mother or any other relative during the child's stay in hospital with the exception of official visiting hours. Contact, between healthcare teams and family members, was limited to passing on information during discharge, during visits and during more delicate procedures such as surgery.

During these moments of contact with the family, Winnicott (1982) highlights that whilst there were positives aspects for the child and their families they also generated mixed feelings amongst parents who assessed their children as being excessively sad. For professional healthcare workers it represented extra work re-stabilising and re-establishing the child after the conclusion of the visit.

With the subsequent inclusion of the family and/or the companion in the universe of hospitalisation, a change of focus was required from professional health workers, which had previously concentrated solely on the child and their pathology, in order to create a more comprehensive understanding of the condition of infant hospitalisation. Pediatric care once again came to have the family as its goal, which was considered as the primary unit of care, whilst not forgetting to take into account valued technological advances included within the healthcare perspective (Collet & Rocha, 2004).

Considering the course which infant care has taken since the 18th century it is possible to see that not only were concerns diversified, but that there were also changes in practices of care, control, education, training and protection.

Throughout the 20th Century, with the widening in scope of the role of medicine and increasing specialisation and technological development, infancy gained the same number of dedicated professionals as adults, composing a long list of healthcare professionals such as endocrinologists, neurologists, psychiatrists, infectologists and gastroenterologists amongst others.

Moreover, it is not possible to approach this subject matter without taking into consideration Human rights. If before the Enlightenment the child was just another familial entity, the 20th Century has repositioned the child at the centre of Human rights legislation with the stated objective of protecting them.

The United Nations (UN) adopted The Geneva Declaration of the Rights of the Child for the first time in 1924. However, with the changes to the political landscape during this period, the theme achieved a greater impact with the Universal Declaration of Human Rights (UN, 1948), through which it became universally recognised, for the first time, that the child should be subject to special care and attention, as stated in item 2, of article 25 (XXV) "motherhood and childhood are entitled to special care and assistance. All children, whether born in or out of wedlock, shall enjoy the same social protection".

Later, with the Declaration of the Rights of the Child (UN, 1959), ten basic principles were established - the right of the child to special protection; to be given the opportunities and facilities necessary for healthy and harmonious development; access to the benefits of social security, including adequate nutrition, housing, recreation and medical services; to receive education and protection against all forms of negligence, cruelty and exploitation - becoming a landmark and guide for the performance of both public and private institutions and professionals.

In Brazil, the federal constitution of 1988 establishes in article 227, the Rights of the child and the Statute of the Child and Adolescent (SCA, 1990) which regulated the article and was drafted based upon the International Instruments of Human Rights of the UN, and in particular, the Declaration of the Rights of the Child. Considered a landmark in Brazilian constitutional protection of children and adolescents, the SCA stipulates in article 4 that "It is the duty of the family, the community, society in general and public authorities to ensure, with absolute priority, the effective implementation of the right to life, health, nutrition, education, sport, leisure, professional training, culture, dignity, respect, freedom and family and community".

Five years later, Brazil promulgated resolution 41 on October 13th 1995 which was directed specifically towards the Rights of hospitalised children and adolescents. The resolution is composed of 20 rights including protection, care, use of procedures to minimise pain and the recognition of pediatric patients as subjects with rights within institutional healthcare.

However, it is not possible to discern the same concern and legal protections in relation to children and adolescents in different countries. The situations of war, famine, poverty and malnutrition produce refugees, orphans, and the displaced children of territorial and political conflicts on a daily basis.

The path to the concrete realisation of such rights is long and faced with many obstacles, which includes the way in which children are viewed and understood by adults - subjects who need to be represented by another voice in order to be heard.

The developmental approach to the child, of being in a process of formation which is incomplete and therefore requiring of norms and standards so that the social and cultural debt of becoming adult can be paid off through education and through the adult figure as a spokesperson for the child is criticised by Castro (2001), which brings to light a new concept of childhood.

In his theory, Castro (2001) emphasises the importance of legitimising children as being capable of exercising their rights through their capacity for action within and understanding of the world. Both adults and children become perceived and understood as belonging to different age-group categories with different roles and performances in society.

Qvortrup (2007) demonstrates in his study that the attitudes of society in relation to children are ambiguous because whilst at the same time as establishing rules and rights to protect children, society departs from these very same rules and rights in relation to adults. Without belittling the importance of ensuring these rights and protection to children, since childhood and politics are inextricably linked, present criticism and construction focuses on the movements of children only as edification materials for future generations and training as political subjects (Qvortrup, 2007).

However, this critical task becomes a great challenge when the conditions of chronically ill hospitalised pediatric patients, who find themselves with reduced levels of autonomy, are dependent upon technology, relatives, social support networks and the performance of professional health workers, are assumed.

2. Chronic disease in childhood

By chronic disease is understood those diseases that present prolonged periods of suffering, are incurable, and have profound effects on the everyday life of suffers, affecting social relations, the family and health institutions (Canesqui, 2007). Chronic diseases during infancy may be considered as events which have a biological, psychological and/or cognitive basis, with a prolonged periods of suffering which may produce limitations in functions or activities, a loss of social relationships, pharmaceutical dependency, special dietary requirements, medical technology, specialised equipment, personal assistance, comprehensive healthcare which not only includes medical attention but also other professional healthcare assistance such as psychologists, occupational therapists, nurses and physiotherapists amongst others, which need to be accommodated in different ways in the various spaces of sociability (Silva, 2001).

According to the World Health Organisation (WHO, 2003), a chronic condition constitutes a health problem which demands permanent health care and management over prolonged periods of time, even years or decades. Understanding chronic diseases involves addressing a vast array of diseases including both transferable diseases (HIV/AIDS) and non-transferable diseases (cardio-vascular, cancer and diabetes) and physical disabilities (amputations, blindness, and chronic joint diseases) which, although seemingly distinct from each other, all require permanent care.

Chronic diseases have assumed a new place in healthcare in light of the available technological support and scientific advances which have led to increased survival rates for this group of pathologies. There has been a demographic and epidemiological transition in pediatric care which can be characterised by the increase of chronic cases of overweight patients, infant obesity, reducing malnutrition and a reduction in infant mortality rates between the ages of two months and five years, actions aimed at increasing breast feeding, access to pre natal care, treating pneumonia, diarrhoea and the administration of vaccines (Moreira & Goldani, 2010).

This has had a profound impact on hospital care and point towards the construction of a new model of healthcare which should be expanded to included the prevention and treatment of infant diseases to guarantee the health of individuals so that they can grow and develop. The child is now dependent on technology - an increased population has grown quantitatively and now demands specialised treatments and services (Moreira & Goldani, 2010).

The wide variety of rare infant diseases which are genetic in origin and their subsequent survival is dependent upon both the type of healthcare offered and the available technology. The technologically dependent child, besides demanding new services, establishes a permanent relationship with the various stages of assistance. There are children who are born with chronic diseases, who are assisted by neonatology and in order to survive are transferred to pediatric wards. Institutional processes and transfers of responsibilities between professionals are developed as well appropriating hospital space for family members due to the changes involved in going from being part of life to being hospitalised.

Against this background of demographic and epidemiological changes, pediatric practices were being developed which included diagnostics and the administration of both human and financial resources in order to improve the assistance and healthcare given to patients (Moreira & Goldani, 2010).

However, the experience of chronic disease has at its core the uncertainty of future life and affects not only medical conduct, but above all, the course of the life of the patients who, in many cases, find themselves unable to plan long term for the future (Adam & Herzlich, 2001). Furthermore, chronic disease can alter our everyday routines and habits, which in the case of pediatric patients includes going to school, their circle of friends, visiting parks and practicing sports.

The diagnosis of chronic disease alters the everyday routine of the patient and their family, from initial investigation until confirmation of diagnosis, at which point patients begin to adapt to their new circumstances and learn to deal with the suffering, possible limitations and fear of dying (Pierre et. al., 1991).

Often, due to diagnostic examinations, this routine can even begin intrauterine with certain types of disability or disease being detected and corrective procedures initiated, for example in cases of spina bifida and heart disease. At other times, the baby can present signs or symptoms of chronic disease immediately from birth, thus initiating diagnostic procedures which can interfere with the construction of the mother-child bond and the establishment of the baby's routine.

Thus, the experience of living with chronic disease from birth implies a series of changes to the lives of the baby and family. Discipline is amongst the numerous challenges faced in everyday life, regardless of whether or not treatments require medication. This implies amongst other concerns, the frequency with which patients have to undergo examinations, consultations, medical procedures and hospitalisation (Vieira & Lima, 2002). Besides dealing with the behaviour and conduct of different healthcare professionals, chronic diseases can cause changes in routine which range from those effecting the family, such as those responsible becoming unemployed in order to care for the patient, having to move home in order to be closer to hospitals and health centres, structural changes to the house, to problems at school whether due to architectural barriers, adaptation or rejection of the pedagogical model or rejection by peers.

The constant concern with the care of the child from infancy becomes so great that it can interfere with the spontaneity of maternal care. Depending on the severity of the situation, accurate knowledge of the disease, the quality of interaction with healthcare staff and previous experience, the mother in question may think that she is incapable of providing the necessary care for her baby. The mother wrongly assumes that care is only a technical competence. Thus, it is fundamental that healthcare professionals are attentive to the need of encouraging and stimulating the participation of the mother, not only during the routine of medical treatments but also in nurturing the baby (Winnicott, 1988).

The chronic condition is presented as a delicate reality, becoming a private personal experience that the other does not access, dependent upon constant communication between the subjects. Because it is a private experience of the subject, it is not easily established making the job of deciphering chronic pain necessary amongst healthcare professionals (Baszanger, 1991).

The manner in which the child and the family face chronic disease is associated with the organisation and interaction of the family. The support of family and social ties, support networks for the family and protection of patients serve as a social fabric which permits a greater range for management of encounters and constructing ties which can ensure the well-being of patients (Adam & Herlizch, 2001; Viana et. al. 2007)

The physical pain, the psychic suffering and the deleterious effects of medical procedures are not always taken into consideration in healthcare practices. A narrow view of the experience of the chronic condition, which is defined as only discomfort and/or physical limitation, ignores or minimises the greater meaning and experience of the pediatric patient

(Charmaz, 1983). Considering that a child suffering from a chronic condition can become a chronic adult, it becomes essential that the individual stages of life and their respective experiences receive special attention in the context of hospitalisation and healthcare. For Moreira & Goldani, (2010: 324) *"health conditions in early life are strong determinants of adult health and this has not received sufficient attention"*.

For these authors the field needs more profound and systematic studies which are not limited to personal experiences, case studies, expert recommendations or small clinical trials which have made the child a *"therapeutic orphan"* (Moreira & Goldani, 2010: 325).

3. The hospitalisation process and the phases of infant and juvenile development

It is important to highlight that every child has a chronic disease, regardless of any diagnosis, first and foremost, that of being a child. This fundamental and obvious condition is unfortunately often forgotten by healthcare professionals, implying that the general level of maturity and response expected of these small patients is not consistent with the evolutionary period in which they find themselves. Thus, it is fundamental to consider the aspects of infant development and the principle characteristics of each phase when reflecting upon the attention paid to the health of chronically diseased children.

During the first two years of a baby's life the baby literally discovers the world through its relationship with the maternal figure and her corporal reactions and sensations. The child moves from a state in which everything resolves around them to the discovery of the outside world

The child's behaviour is based upon the perceptions constructed through the sensory exploration of the world and physical activities. Disease and medical procedures which cause pain and discomfort can seriously compromise the baby's relationship with their environment and themselves (Muriel et. al. 2011).

This is a period in which the child avoids the unknown, experiences distress and anguish at the mother's absence, what Bowlby (1984) describes as attachment. Because of this, situations of chronic disease and fear can trigger extreme reactions including crying, frightened expressions, inertia and greater dependency in their behaviour. Fear can be aroused by the presence of unknown persons, unknown places or situations, and the response will vary depending on a child's age, duration of separation and the degree of deprivation to which the child has been exposed (Bowlby, 1984). In spite of knowing the importance of early experiences in the baby's life, we still see, in practice, some healthcare professionals that believe that because of the fact that their client doesn't present a developed verbal language, chronic disease will somehow not have so many repercussions in their lives.

After this period, the child enters the Pre-operational phase (Piaget, 1976) where its first mental concepts are formed and the process of internalising reality commences. The imagination finds itself indulged in activity and mental reasoning but forms magical beliefs and inadequate concepts characterised by ego-centricism and animism. Accordingly, it is fundamental to take care with the information given to children because their thinking is egocentric and they are unable to articulate or relate to different points of view to their own.

Similarly, the notions of time and reversibility are still under construction. Because of this, children often find it difficult to understand why it is necessary for them to have to undergo certain treatment which they sometimes associate with discipline and punishment (Santa Roza, 1997).

Often, even simple activities like playing with other children or siblings can become compromised. This may occur because of limitations arising from the intense routine of treatment, the care taken when in contact with other people (avoidance of trauma or bacteria) or the parents fears in relation to any other eventuality that they think threatens the health (and consequentially the life) of their children.

At school age, between the ages of six to twelve, the child will gradually become increasingly mature for their physical, intellectual and social condition. It is a phase of investment in physical activities and of greater socialisation. However, sufferers of chronic conditions may find themselves unable to participate in conventional social interaction and banter, which gives rise to the possible loss of friendship ties and changes in familial relationships. Further, the comprehension of death which chronic disease brings with it becomes more accessible through language and abstract content (Muriel et. al., 2011).

Amongst adolescents, who experience a phase characterised by the involvement of formal identification, an appreciation of more abstract aspects through a greater intellectual and emotional contribution, the experience of chronic disease can place them in conflict with their desire to live a more autonomous life and the dependency imposed on them by their chronic condition (Muriel et. al., 2011).

In all of these phases, it is important to point out that school should be considered as a primary partner in this process, which implies the availability and time to receive children with special requirements, for example, those who have had tracheotomies, gastrostomies or colostomies, administered food absences due to prolonged periods of treatment, the possible structural and architectural barriers and the relationship with other children.

However, school may also represent a challenge for children with chronic diseases due to the fact that it may expose children to more vulnerable situations, to being stigmatised by their colleagues and even bullying. The corporal changes entailed as a result of chronic diseases may provoke changes in body-image, the generation of feelings of inferiority, depression and embarrassment from the perception that they are different from their peers (Castro & Moreno-Jiménez, 2007)

Because of this, it is important to point out that the monitoring of children with chronic diseases involves knowledge from various disciplines. The participation of different healthcare professionals aside from doctors, psychologists, social-workers, occupational therapists, physiotherapists, and speech-therapists is fundamental.

Another important aspect of treatment, frequent in the lives of chronically diseased children, is hospitalisation, whether due to the deterioration of the patient or as a strategy for administering specific medication and procedures. Regarding the hospitalisatision of a child or adolescent, in general, what is observed is conformation of this delicate moment for the family requiring a reconfiguration of the everyday life and the assimilation of the disease which may also induce subjective changes. At the moment of hospitalisation, the experience for the pediatric patient is marked by the rupture from the everyday routines of school, friends, family, peers and games. In general, "the activity and freedom characteristic of childhood are replaced by passivity, leaving few options for the child to make choices" (Mitre, 2006; 286).

This change produces an estrangement from the experience of being in hospital which will differ amongst patients and their relatives. The points of reference in a child's and adolescent's life are replaced by pale walls, invasive medical procedures, medication and machinery, new words and phrases and the sensation of pain and suffering changing the everyday routines of these patients (Mitre, 2006).

The hospitalisation of children may be considered as a potentially traumatic event when the full complexity of the human dimension is not fully considered (Santa Roza, 1997). Generally, models of care still favour the disease and view the child only as a sick body. We have to consider the diverse aspects involved in the process of hospital care when working with children, everything from the presentation of physical space to treatment routines, so as to avoid iatrogenesis (Santa Roza, 1997).

Bearing this in mind, we observe an increasing concern with the physical environment of hospitals and health centres, especially in pediatric wards. However, it is still common in hospitals and health centres to find the presence of unwelcoming and stressful stimuli. Unfamiliar and noisy equipment, a plethora of monitors with artificial lights, pipes and tubes and needles and tweezers comprise, in general, a threatening and unfamiliar setting.

With the evolution of technology, and this is not a criticism, merely an observation, some hospital wards nowadays resemble spaceships, both architecturally and in terms of the complexity of equipment. This is due to advancements in diagnostic and therapeutic procedures, modern criterias of optimising resources, and newly discovered diseases, micro-organisms and consequent treatments. However, this has led to an increased concern with creating healthcare spaces separate from society, isolating the infirm and setting the hospital in areas outside of cities apart from everyday life (Antunes, 1989).

In contrast, in economically disadvantaged areas, it is still common to find areas being used as pediatric wards which previously had been intended for use by another clientele, or still further, had been intended for completely different purposes. This may involve places with no windows or natural light, only cold light and few objects which remind you that this is a space for children.

The importance of windows to the outside world is discussed in the work of Antunes (1989), where he says, irrespective of what a patient sees, it can be a landscape, cars, people, they see what does not exist in the hospital, a life full of movement and they are reminded of the temporary suspension of their freedom and autonomy as a result of hospitalisation. In the case of infant hospitalisation it is not only the patient who is subject to the architecture of the hospital. The accompanying person, usually the mother, is also hospitalised together with the child and ends up feeling "trapped" in an environment which sometimes appears far removed from everyday life.

This can contribute to augmenting the feeling of anxiety caused by the concern for the sick child and as well as for other related situations, such as concern for another child who remained at home, the abandoned job, the lack of support from a partner or family. All of these questions will be reflected in the relationship established between the child and their carer, a relationship which, principally during hospitalisation, needs to be capable of providing the necessary support for the child experiencing this period (Mitre, 2000).

Compounding hospitalisation still further, the child is subjected to situations in which they do not have any choice. Despite the necessity and effectiveness of hospitalisations the child is extremely susceptible to experiences which can cause stress and suffering.

The feeling of discomfort and pain is one of the characteristics which may accompany the hospitalised child. This is both connected to the clinical condition of the patient, which is presented through painful symptoms causing discomfort, as well as certain medical procedures. The procedure may be a simple puncture, present in almost a hundred per cent of hospitalised children because of the need for effective and immediate medication, or other equally invasive procedures such as the insertion of different tubes to drain various bodily fluids and gasses, the use of catheters or other probes (Mitre, 2000). Depending on the child's age or clinical condition the child is unable to verbalise these feelings.

The simplest everyday routines are changed due to the fact of hospitalised. The hours of the day change, sometimes sleep is interrupted by the routines of the ward, having to constantly take temperatures, blood pressure, listening for respiratory and circulatory problems and the taking of medication.

Feeding habits and hygiene routines change as well. Sometimes food is restricted (or even temporarily suspended) depending on the clinical condition of the child or the particular procedure (examinations, intravenous procedures and punctures and surgery amongst others). Hygiene habits may change depending on the time and the place, some patients are required to make use of probes or even have to resort to using nappies. In certain cases patients have to be bathed in bed which can lead to discomfort and embarrassment especially with older children. Moreover, in some places, generally public hospital wards, many children and their families and friends have to share the same space without any privacy (Mitre, 2000).

Besides all this, during hospitalisation the child is kept away from their friends, family, toys and school; ultimately, their life. This period if often experienced by the child as a gap in their life and as if everything appears to be in parenthesis. Everyday life appears so distant that some patients lose their notions of time and space. Once, a child asked if the hospital had an exit door and elevator to descend to the street. For him, there only appeared to be an entrance (Mitre, 2000).

Santa Roza (1997) describes how in this environment the child experiences situations which, even when they don't constitute a new experience (as in the case of repeated hospital admissions), may still sometimes be perceived as frightening. During hospitalisation, the child begins to live intensely with the sliding fortunes of their body, experiencing their suffering, the suffering of their family and of other children. Sometimes they are present to witness death; other times, they fear their own. Fear, anxiety and anguish accompany the hospitalisation process. In general, the child is unable to comprehend why they have to pass through these unknown experiences which produce fear. This situation may stimulate fantasies and thoughts about guilt or punishment as well as the fear of abandonment and death.

For child sufferers of chronic disease and/or serious clinical conditions the situation is made worse because, in general, hospitalisations occur frequently and for certain children the hospital is the everyday routine. Some patients are hospitalised several times a year whilst others may stay in hospital for months on end. There are still those patients who come and go with such frequency that they begin to spend more time in the hospital than at home.

It is common to know the seriousness of the condition even if it has not already been clearly stated. The concern with death exists and manifests itself in different ways. Some children joke about this whilst others pass comments about other children who have died.

Kudo & Pierri (1993) point out that amongst the various factors which directly influence the way in which a child will react to the process of hospitalisation are; the type of and degree of the affective bond established between mother-child before being hospitalised, the child's personality, the length of stay and the attitude of hospital staff towards them and the child's age.

Gonzaga & Arruda (1998) highlight, based upon various interviews with hospitalised children, that care can be offered by various people during the administration of services but that the action of one doesn't minimise the effects of the others but instead the benefits are congregated. The different actors can become sources of care and of feeling cared for. However, examples of a lack of care were also mentioned including attitudes of disinterest shown by healthcare professionals (doctors and nurses), not executing procedures to alleviate pain or the execution of procedures in a cold and mechanical manner without due respect and understanding towards the condition and sensitivity of pain. All of these actions contribute to the increased anguish and stress that the hospitalised patient experiences.

It is important to note that the introduction of play and recreational activities presented positive results about the experience of infant hospitalisation. Considering that playing is a fundamental childhood activity it should also be present during the period of hospitalisation. Its absence can lead to the impairment of motor, cognitive, perceptive and emotional functions. (Mitre, 2006).

Play places the hospitalised child in a similar position to other children instead of the difference imposed on them by chronic disease (Mitre, 2004). It is an activity which furthers and supports the creation of alliances and interactions amongst children, carers and healthcare professionals allowing for the construction of a new social network whilst also helping to diminish the sensations of isolation and solitude that hospitalisation causes (Mitre, 2000). Also, in the child-carer relationship, play can help reconstruct ties which have become fragmented due to the familial breakdown caused by the illness (Mitre & Gomes, 2004).

Play and recreational activity also makes possible the expression of feelings, ideas, fears, affections and habits. Because play is something which belongs to an individual, social and cultural repertoire, it is conducive to the child identifying with familiar elements and situations whilst in the hospital environment (Mitre, 2006).

To value and stimulate play as a possible means of self-expression is to recognise that if you work with children it is necessary to respect the uniqueness and specific needs of each child. Thus, play in hospital can be considered as a democratic place where individual experiences are valued and the possibility of choice and the exercise of autonomy exist (Mitre, 2006).

4. Parental approach to chronic disease and the hospitalisation of the child

Chronic disease in children and adolescents, besides bringing new variables into the lives of the patients, imposes on the parents the need for developing new routines and acquiring new knowledge about the conduct and the care of children.

According to Alves (2009), mothers who live often with the hospitalisation process of children learn to provide care and are able to supervise the work of providing assistance, judging if they are "right or wrong" in accordance with what they have learnt.

By exercising their role of providing care to the child, mothers have a function which permeates meanings in the universe of nursing, whilst the nurse is, in these cases, in a place which does not have clearly demarcated boundaries in the delivery of healthcare. This confusing and ambiguous situation can create conflicts and disagreements with regards to knowledge and information. However, the disposition of mothers to provide care should not be taken as a rule in the same way that it is not specialised care (Alves, 2009).

The development of care by carers, in general, does not form part of the same option. The experience of chronic disease, gradually, inserts them into the hospital routine where they learn and act. The permanent presence of companions imprints another dynamic in the assistance process, because it provides the opportunity to learn some new technical abilities and to amplify other knowledge about the functioning of the hospital and of therapeutic techniques (Lima, Rocha e Scochi, 1999).

The presence of the family within the context of the hospitalisation of children and adolescents represented an advance in the relationship between the users and the hospital space, but as an isolated initiative it didn't recognise or take into account the need to understand the dynamics involved in the process of chronic disease in children and adolescents. The presence of the carer needs to be tracked by a therapeutic project which integrates patient care because the carer is attached to assistance and meaning is related to the patient's disease.

As a vehicle for providing access to the knowledge of patients and carers, dialogue and guidelines are indispensable resources. The construction of a therapeutic project, which integrates knowledge and establishes performance guidelines within each stage of patient care, can be a great resource for structuring and organising more harmonious and co-responsible relationships.

At this point the ability and capacity for communication, dialogue and a host of other demands and opportunities for the autonomous expressions of the family, comes into play. Sharing the provision of care with carers requires the exercise of co-participation. A space for dialogue is needed which enables the different actors to express their doubts and feelings. This space can not be attached to the duration of time in hospital, but rather instituted as a means for the management of daily services.

The investment in the relationships between healthcare professionals, patients, and their carers, founded and guided by such factors as the initial contact and dialogue between patients and doctors, may empower the role and autonomy of children and their carers.

The appreciation of knowledge of paediatric patients about the process of chronic disease and the relationships which they experience within the context of hospitalisation are as important as the experiences of carers. The right of children to express themselves can provide valuable information for healthcare practices which may be reconsidered in favour of a more comprehensive and friendly service.

Beginning with this understanding, it is possible to construct relationships within healthcare which will not be guided by the subjection and control of the patient, but where you can affirm the capacity of the paediatric patient to express, create and reinvent standards which make possible for autonomously administering the margin of risk to life, amplifying capacities for coping with the disease together with the most important relationships.

The recognition, on the part of healthcare teams, of the conditions in which the body is encountered, the subjectivity of the patient, is the first step towards incorporating a new understanding of the patient, taking into consideration the factors involved in the patient's life.

Taken as a proposal to consider care as a value (Pinheiro, 2007), understanding it as an integral action which has meanings related to the understanding of healthcare such as the right to medical and other specialised treatments, allows the patient to actively participate in the decisions taken in regard to the conduct of their own case.

Healthcare begins when a dialogical relationship between the patient and healthcare professionals is initiated, which transcends the simple game of the active questions of healthcare professionals and the passive responses of patients towards the construction of a space of exchanges, where the medical knowledge of the doctor incorporates itself into the lived experiences of the individual. With this, it is possible to establish relationships which are guided by partnership between people which have the objective of finding the shortest route to the restoration of health.

Caprara e Franco (1999) emphasise the need to overcome both the informative model that relays information and the paternalistic model which protects the patient from their own disease, towards a model of communication which includes other important actors in the life of the patient. It is an overcoming which requires a change in attitude and understanding about the healthcare process and the place of the other within this relationship.

For Deslandes (2004a), the possibilities of communication are related to the social position which individuals occupy. In the relationship between doctors and patients there exists, historically, a differentiation between the place and value of their speech.

However, the construction of an active communication begins by recognising the place of the patient as that of a subject in the relationship. According to Deslandes (2004b), the necessary movement in order to change this logic of attention within healthcare not only incorporates a new understanding of patients and their lived experiences, but also a change which observes the organisational culture in which are concentrated the relationships of knowledge-power, gender and social status. These are these factors present in the organisational culture which are able to feed certain types of relationships between the actors in institutions.

Healthcare taken as a value, (Pinheiro, 2007) proposes that we recognise the ethos of the cared for and of the provider of care, which requires including in the relationship the dimensions of individual life with its habits and customs and communitarian life, both being originating dimensions in the character and identity of the subjects. It is to be able to incorporate the ethos of the other in a process which extends itself making that therapeutic moment a unique moment of contact and dialogue.

5. Final considerations

It is important to highlight that working closer with chronically diseased children implies certain challenges can't be ignored by healthcare professionals. Firstly, every child, independent of their diagnosis, should be perceived as and treated as a child and not only as a clinical case or disease. It is not enough to have knowledge and mastery over techniques and procedures, it is also necessary to have knowledge of infant development and the perception that care is not limited to treating only symptoms. Part of the professional role should include helping children to deal with the barriers which originate with disease and expanding their limitations in favour of greater quality of life.

The various forms of healthcare need to be introduced to the child, not merely as the recipient of diagnostic and therapeutic techniques, but rather as a subject that possesses various ways to elaborate their experiences of living with chronic illness. The ways which children elaborate about the experience are different from adults, but this doesn't render them incapable of valuing the experience and extracting from it new meanings which healthcare staff can help to produce.

Hospitalisation contexts carry the potential to produce something new, transmuting into new pathways which allow for new perspectives as well as generating closure, diminishing the creative wagers of the subjects. The potential to change situations which cause fatigue, polarisations of care and dichotomies of knowledge is contained in the capacity to unite healthcare staff collectively towards an objective, the construction of which is shared between the patient, family and healthcare professionals (Alves, 2009).

In this sense, the meetings with each patient can promote changes in the perception of the subject because there are moments which are full of creative possibilities orientated towards solutions for coping with chronic infant disease, producing positive changes for the patients, families and healthcare professionals.

The participation of relatives in the hospitalised context and care of chronically diseased children also needs to be rethought so that the dichotomies and disputes of space and knowledge can be broken down. Learning about care inevitably occurs in families which accompany the daily care provided to the child making this experience a way to integrate different cultural knowledge and values.

Within the world of attention and assistance, acceptance and dialogue are wires, not only permeated by concepts and theoretical frameworks, but through the capacity to meet and produce subjectivity, revising values, perspectives and expectations.

To this end, necessary changes to the dynamics and processes of healthcare staff are needed, beginning with a management model which is shared and constructed in a collective fashion between healthcare professionals and the users of such services in order that it may become possible to break and minimise distance and to value the capacity for collective union.

Finally, to highlight the contribution of Ayres (2005), in relation to the concept which he calls Projects for human happiness. For the author, this concept refers to the idea of lived experiences, positively valued, which are not dependent on a state of complete well-being in the life of the subjects. In cases of disease, these projects can be constructed from the various values and guidelines which orientate healthcare. He makes the salient point that happiness materialises in the lives of individuals through the construction of everyday life projects, a concept which can't be defined universally or as an external entity. Projects for human happiness are associated with the capacity to overcome obstacles and move in the direction of values held by both the individual and collective.

The way to construct, in healthcare, Projects for human happiness involves the evaluation of values which orientate the processes of chronic disease and healthcare, as much as in regards to the integration of care by the different actors who participate, as well as the closer cultural, economic and social ties between healthcare professionals, patients and relatives. Above all, the view of the child should be complete, going beyond the supposed organic limitations and inability to express feelings and experiences.

There exist many different ways for the child to access the contents of pain and happiness. Nevertheless, a leading Projects for human happiness agent for carriers of chronic disease requires going beyond the implementation of technical methods and procedures or structural knowledge of disciplines, in order that new meanings and new ways of listening and new points of view can be expressed in spaces of care and attention.

6. References

Adam, P. & Herlizch, C. (2001). *Sociologia da doença e da medicina.* 1ª. Edição EDUCS: ISBN 85-7460-100-4, Bauru, São Paulo.

Alves, C. A. (2009). Desafios da humanização no contexto do cuidado da enfermagem pediátrica de média e alta complexidade. Dissertacão de Mestrado em Saúde da Criança e da Mulher. Instituto Fernandes Figueira. Rio de Janeiro.

Antunes, J. L.F. (1989). Por uma geografia hospitalar. *Tempo social, Revista Sociologia.* Vol. 1, No. 1: pp. 227-234. ISSN 0103 2070

Ariès, P. (2009) Por uma história da vida privada. In: *História da vida privada: da Renascença ao Século das Luzes.* Ariès, P. & Chartier, R. (orgs), pp. 7-19. 1ª. Edição, Companhia das Letras, ISBN 9788535914351, São Paulo.

Baszanger, I. (1991). Déchiffrer la douleur chronique: deux figures de la pratique médicale. *Sciences Sociales et Santé,* Vol. 9, No. 2, pp. 31-78. ISSN 10.3406/sosan.1991.1190

BRASIL. Constituição (1988). Constituição da República Federativa do Brasil: promulgada em 5 de outubro de 1988. Contém as emendas constitucionais posteriores. Brasília, DF: Senado.

BRASIL. (1990) Estatuto da Criança e do Adolescente. Lei nº 8.069 de 13 de julho de 1990. Dispõe sobre o Estatuto da Criança e do Adolescente e dá outras providências. Brasília, DF.

Bowlby, J. (1984) *Apego.* 1a. Edição, Martins Fontes, ISBN 0-465-00543-8, Rio de janeiro.

Canesqui AM. (2007). Estudos Socioantropológicos Sobre os Adoecidos Crônicos. In: *Olhares Socioantropológicos sobre os adoecidos crônicos*. Canesqui AM (org). pp. 9-49. HUCITEC/FAPESP, ISBN 8527107058, São Paulo.

Caprara A. & Franco A.L.Z. (199). A relação paciente-médico: para uma humanização da prática médica. *Cadernos de Saúde Pública*, Vol. 15, No. 3, pp. 647-654. ISSN 0102-311X

Castro LR. (2001) Da invisibilidade à ação: crianças e jovens na construção da cultura. In: *Crianças e Jovens na construção da cultura*. p.19-46. Nau Editora - FAPERJ, ISBN 9788585936471, Rio de Janeiro.

Castro E.K. & Moreno-Jiménez B. (2007) Resiliência em niños enfermos crónicos: aspectos teóricos. *Psicologia em estudo*. vol. 12, no. pp. 81-6. ISSN 1413-7372

Castro, E. K. & Piccinini, C. A. (2002). Implicações da doença orgânica crônica na infância para as relações familiares: algumas questões teóricas. *Psicologia: Reflexão e Crítica*, vol. 15, no. 3, pp. 625-635. ISSN 0102-7972

Charmaz, K. (1983). Loss of self: a fundamental form of suffering in the chronically ill. *Sociology of Health and Illness*, Vol, 5, No. 2, pp. 168-195. ISSN 10.1111/1467-9566.ep10491512

Collet, N. & Rocha, SMM. (2004) Criança hospitalizada: mãe e enfermagem compartilhando o cuidado. *Revista Latino-americana de Enfermagem* Vol. 12, No. 2, pp. 191-7. ISSN 0104-1169

Conselho Nacional de Defesa dos Direitos da Criança e Adolescente (Brasil). (1995) Resolução no. 41, 13 de outubro de 1995. Dispõe sobre os direitos da criança hospitalizada. Diário Oficial da República Federativa do Brasil (BR): Seção I, p.16319-20.

Costa, J .F. (2004). Ordem médica e norma familiar. 5ª. Edição Editora Paz e Terra, ISBN 8570380062, São Paulo.

Deslandes S.F. (2004a) A humanização e a construção política do lugar de sujeito no processo comunicacional. *Ciência e Saúde Coletiva*, Vol. 9, No. 1, pp. 15-29. ISSN 1413-8123

Deslandes SF. (2004b). A análise do discurso oficial sobre humanização da assistência hospitalar. *Ciência e Saúde Coletiva*, Vol. 9, No. 1, pp. 7-14. ISSN 1413-8123.

Gonzaga M.L.C. & Arruda E.M. (1998). Fontes e significados de cuidar e não cuidar em hospital pediátrico. *Revista Latino-americana de Enfermagem*, Vol. 6, No. 5, pp. 17-26. ISSN 0104-1169.

Lima R.A.G., Rocha S.M.M. & Scochi C.G.S. (1999) Assistência à criança hospitalizada: reflexões acerca da participação dos pais. *Revista Latino-americana de Enfermagem*, Vol. 7, No. 2, pp. 33-39.

Mitre R.M.A. (2006). O Brincar no Processo de Humanização da Produção de Cuidados Pediátricos. In: Humanização dos cuidados em saúde: conceitos, dilemas e práticas. Deslandes, S.F. (org). pp. 283-300. Ed. Fiocruz, ISBN 85-7541-079-2, Rio de Janeiro.

Mitre, R. & Gomes, R. A (2004). Promoção do Brincar no Contexto da Hospitalização Infantil enquanto Ação de Saúde. *Ciência e Saúde Coletiva*, Vol. 9, No. 1, pp. 147-154. ISSN 1413-8123

Mitre, R. (2000). Brincando para viver: Um estudo sobre a relação entre a criança gravemente adoecida e hospitalizada e o brincar,. Dissertação de mestrado, Rio de Janeiro: Instituto Fernandes Figueira, Fundação Oswaldo Cruz.

Moreira M.E.L. & Goldani M.Z. (2010). A criança é o pai do homem: novos desafios para a área de saúde da criança. *Ciência e Saúde Coletiva*, Vol. 15, No. 2, pp. 321-327. ISSN 1413-8123

Muriel, C. & Sourkes, B. (2011): Children´s voice: The experience of patients and their siblings. In: *Textbook of interdisciplinary pediatric palliative care*. Wolfe, J; Hinds, P & Sourkes, B (orgs). pp. 18-29. Elsevier - Saunders, ISBN 978-1-4377-0262-0, Philadelphia.

Organização das Nações Unidas. (1948) Declaração Universal dos Direitos do Homem. Proclamada pela resolução 217 A (III) da Assembléia Geral das Nações Unidas em 10 de dezembro de 1948.

Organização das Nações Unidas. (1959) Declaração Universal dos Direitos da Criança. Proclamada pela Resolução da Assembléia Geral 1386 (XIV), de 20 de Novembro de 1959.

Piaget, J. (2003) *Seis Estudos de Psicologia*. 24a. Edição Forense-Universitária ISBN 8521802463, Rio de Janeiro.

Pierre, A.; Faufmann, A. & Waissman, R. (1991) Vivre une maladie grave: analyse d'une situations de crise. *Revue Française de Sociologie*, Vol. 32, No. 4, pp. 652-655. http://www.persee.fr/web/revues/home/prescript/article/rfsoc_0035-2969_1991_num_32_4_4093

Pinheiro R. (2007). Cuidado como valor: um ensaio sobre o (re)pensar e a ação na construção de práticas eficazes de integralidade em saúde. In: *Razões públicas para a integralidade em saúde: o cuidado como valor*. Pinheiro R & Mattos RA (orgs.). pp. 15-28. IMS/UERJ: CEPESC: ABRASCO, ISBN: 978-85-89737-41-8., Rio de Janeiro

Qvortrup, J. (2007). Infância e política. *Conferencia Educação para a cidadania na sociedade: um desafio para os países nórdicos*. Escola de Educação de Professores da Universidade de Malmö, Suécia.

Rago, M. (1987). A preservação da infância. In: *Do cabaré ao lar – a utopia da cidade disciplinar*. pp. 117-135. Paz e Terra, ISBN 8521901860, São Paulo,

Silva, M. G. N. (2001). Doenças crônicas na infância: conceitos, prevalências e repercussões emocionais. *Revista de Pediatria do Ceará*, Vol. 2, No. 2, pp. 29-32. ISSN 1982-548X

Viana, V., Barbosa M.C. & Guimarães, J. (2007). Doença crônica na criança: fatores familiares e qualidade de vida. *Psicologia, Saúde e Doenças*, Vol. 8, No. 1, pp. 117-127. ISSN 1645-0086

Vieira M.A. & Lima R.A.G. (2002) Crianças e adolescentes com doença crônica: convivendo com mudanças. *Revista Latino-Americana de Enfermagem*. Vol. 10, No. 4, pp.552-60. ISSN 0104-1169

Winnicott, D. (1982) *A criança e o seu mundo*. 6ª. edição Guanabara Koogan, Rio de Janeiro. ISBN-13: 9788521611295

Winnicott, D. (1978). *Textos selecionados: da pediatria à psicanálise*. 1ª. Edição, Francisco Alves, ISBN 85-312-0739-8, Rio de Janeiro.

Zanolli M.L. & Merhy E.E. (2001) A pediatria social e as suas apostas reformistas. *Cadernos de Saúde Pública,* Vol. 17, No. 4, pp. 977-987. ISSN 0102-311X

14

How to Accompany Children and Parents During the Different Phases of a Severe Chronic Disease

Momcilo Jankovic and Giuseppe Masera
Pediatric Clinic, University of Milan - Bicocca, San Gerardo Hospital, Foundation MBBM, Monza, Italy

1. Introduction

Our experience is related to the treatment of a lifethreating disease (leukaemia) and from it should be applicable the same concepts or strategies to any other severe chronic disease.

Since the early 1970s, a cure for childhood cancer has become a reality: over 80% of cases are now cured. Yet, despite the relatively high cure rate, the diagnosis of leukemia continues to place a heavy burden on family functioning. The parents must walk the narrow line between focusing too much on the child's disease and treatment and maintaining a normal family life. Because cure is such a real possibility, the children must be prepared for a full and active participation in adult life, just like their peers. Proper discipline must be maintained within as normal a family life as possible. The child's continued attendance at school and participation in normal childhood activities is imperative in the child's preparation for adulthood.

For all these reasons, psychosocial intervention has become a necessity in the treatment of the child, even for those children who eventually will die from the disease.

Although there is little disagreement that the ultimate goal of treatment for childhood cancer is the total cure of the child-medical, educational, psychological, and social-the issue is how best to achieve this end. The literature is filled with research-based conclusions on which type of psychosocial intervention is best, including when and how one should communicate with the child about the diagnosis, how to help the parents maintain some sense of normality in their family life, how to help the child return to school, how to keep the siblings informed, how to start parent groups, how to involve parents in medical decision-making, how to prepare for the terminal phase when it occurs for some children, and how to continue to monitor long-term survivors. Problems occur whenever the approach must be modified to meet the needs and cultural preparation and expectations of the children and their families. This is especially true when one tries to apply conclusions that are appropriate in one culture to other centers and to other cultures.

What works in one cultural setting may not work as well in others. How might a center apply programs from one country or setting to another? Not all hospitals can afford a psychosocial team.

Not all cultures appreciate intervention by a psychologist or psychiatrist. What can pediatric hematologists do to modify their approach to the children and their families with maximal success, in a manner most appropriate to and respectful of the needs of the families within their own cultural setting? And above all, how can a center best monitor its intervention programs, to ensure that the needs of the children and their families are being met appropriately, in their best interests, and with greatest effectiveness and use of resources?

How do we help a family whose child has been diagnosed with a life-threatening illness? How do we help the children and their families cope with the illness and its treatment? As the medical treatment of childhood cancer has moved from an inevitable death sentence to an approximately 80% cure rate, the importance of including the psychosocial in the treatment of the children has now been so integrated that the majority of the pediatric cancer centers throughout the world now view treatment as a biopsychosocial process.

From the very beginning, with the shock of the diagnosis itself, the children and their families undergo a critical change in their lives. The illness has a high social and economic cost, even if the treatment itself is done free of charge to the families. Whether the child is treated in countries with limited resources or in the wealthier countries, personal, family, and cultural circumstances can block access to a full cure, a cure that treats the child at all levels: medical, psychological and social. As the families face the task of adjustment to this new reality, with the support of the hospital health care team the families can find a source of renewed energy and the inner strength to cope with the disease and the treatment process.

Each phase of treatment has its own characteristic that contribute to the reaction of parents and children. The phases are the following: acute phase, during treatment, after treatment, long-term follow-up, end-of-life.

2. A Multidisciplinary effort: Type of strategy in all the phases of the disease

From the earliest years, the effort to care for the child with cancer has been multidisciplinary, multi-institutional, and international, involving a highly cooperative and collaborative effort of physicians, nurses, psychologists, social workers, and allied health care professionals all working together across national borders. When, thirty years ago, physicians treating the children found themselves struggling with the psychological and social repercussions of the cancer on their young dying patients and their families issues that ranged far beyond their medical expertise and training, psychosocial practitioners helped in dealing with these broader human concerns. The pediatric oncologists and hematologists from countries throughout the world began working cooperatively with psychiatrists, social workers, nursing care specialists, and psychologists. To the credit of all involved, this cooperative multidisciplinary, multi-institutional and international effort has been from the very earliest years and continues to be the hallmark of the treatment of childhood cancer. It is important that all members of the health care team engage in psychosocial support, and not just the psychosocial personnel.

3. Research: Psychosocial research is essential to build up different clinical approaches

The primary psychosocial concern in child cancer care is to help the children and their families cope with the diagnosis of cancer and its aftermath. The children and their families, the great majority of whom are struggling with the new diagnosis but who do not show signs of falling apart, need our support. How can we most effectively help mentally healthy children whose lives have been suddenly turned upside down with the diagnosis of a life-threatening illness? We can't expect the families to wait for intervention until we can fully determine which intervention works most effectively and validly. We must try to help the child and family who have an immediate here-and-now need for support, while pursuing scientifically valid controlled research designed to sort out effective from ineffective interventions. The optimal clinical service is the application of the best available evidence-based findings applied locally in cultural context. Well done research is costly and difficult to accomplish in centers with limited resources. However, the health care team even a center with limited resources can listen carefully to the children and their families to find out how they are functioning and how they are responding to the service that is offered. It is recommended that parents be asked formally how well they view the center's functioning and this satisfaction within a simple nonrandomized like study. Modifying one's approach based on a reflection on the families' level of satisfaction with the service can help make the service better. Even in countries with limited resources, it is possible and critically essential to give full attention to the psychosocial needs of the children and their families.

4. Alliance between parents and physicians: The basis in all the phases of the disease

It is clear that a hospital health care team can not do it all. Parents should be invited increasingly to participate actively in their child's medical, psychological and social care, brought in as part of the decision-making process and support system. There should be a healthy, cooperative, and open alliance between the parents and the members of the health care team, including the establishment of parent groups for self-help and for raising supplementary and critical funding.

Wasteful expenditure of negative energy by anyone involved might be more profitably used, and in turn mobilize new and even more powerful positive energies, by cooperating toward fighting the disease in a therapeutic alliance. This alliance may take one or both of two forms: (a) an alliance between individual family members parents and children and individual medical staff members; and (b) an alliance between families as a group and health care team members as a group. These therapeutic alliances are formed when both parties work together with a common purpose pooling resources toward a common goal: curing the cancer and minimizing its medical and psychosocial side-effects, and mobilizing the energies of all members of society to this end.

The role of physicians and health care team members working together in cooperation with parents as equal partners is to:

1. Dedicate time, energy and creativity to collaborate with parent associations by suggesting and arranging joint meetings and acting in advisory capacities.

2. Encourage all parents, especially shy or cautious parents, to join a parent association and help activate parents to organize such associations where they do not already exist.
3. Have parent association members, together with members of the health care team, cooperate in deciding upon a global medical, psychosocial and social-cultural intervention program, toward which they all can converge their united energies.
4. Do all in their power to ensure that cured children and young adults are successfully reintegrated into society, without being penalized in school, work, social relations or insurability for having had cancer as a child.

5. Open communication: At diagnosis, during treatment, at the end of life

Communicating the diagnosis and how best to do is the first step in a communicative process and relationship that involves the medical team and the family, and that allows for growth and change over time. As the evidence mounts that the children, siblings, and parents would be best served by being encouraged to bring into the open their anxieties about the illness and its possible consequences, studies have been paying more attention to how parents and medical personnel communicate with the child. The initial diagnosis is a model for all future interchanges of information between the medical professionals and families and between the family members themselves, especially between parent and child. As the families of the children diagnosed with cancer struggle to face the new emotional crisis which is challenging the relationships among the family members and the very balance of family life, we need to help the families strengthen their coping skills, alleviate their anxiety and offer the type of support the children and families are seeking, in specific ways that are most important to the children and families at a given moment. Basic to effective family coping is the belief that communication of both happy and painful thoughts and feelings, by the parents and by the children, is a healthier state of mental well being than retaining those thoughts in silence. This belief is a prerequisite to mutual support among family members. The families which allow open discussion of the illness and its prognosis are able to cope more effectively with the illness within their own family, and are also able to give and receive the support of other parents in the clinic.

Management of this communicative process has an important influence on how all involved child, parents, other family members, and medical staff work and care for the child together.

At diagnosis the child and family's level of anxiety is very high, and their level of prior information and understanding varies greatly. Most parents want to know as much as possible about the disease, treatment procedures, prognosis, practical coping details, and emotional impacts. The staff's communication of the diagnosis and treatment plan should be done in a way that is responsive to these needs, and that develops confidence and trust among the pediatric cancer staff, patient and family.

Our general view is that full and open communication between the medical care team and the family (including the child), and within the entire family, is the ideal situation. However, this is not always possible or preferable. It also must be done in a way that is sensitive to different cultural styles and preferences.

The communicative session should be conducted in a private space, with comfortable seating and an environment conducive to discussion of painful issues, as a conversation between equals. Both parents and the chairman or a senior medical staff member should be present, as well as the head nurse or another staff member. The attendance of the family's local physician should be encouraged unless parents do not agree. If requested the child with cancer (according to age), other family members (e.g. grandparents: they are significant sufferers that often receive little attention!) or close friends also may attend this session.

When communicating with the child, the physician should explain the disease at the level of development of the child, using pictures and analogies such as the flower garden to help the child's understanding. The physician should make sure that the dialogue is truly a two-way interaction, with the child invited to ask questions and having the answers explained as clearly as possible. Depending on age and level of development, the physician should talk to the siblings as well, explaining to them the basic elements of the disease and its treatment, and having them as well communicate back to the parents what they understand about the illness. In this way, an open system of communication is set up within the family.

6. The siblings: At diagnosis, during treatment, over the time

From the earliest intervention periods, the health care team members have all they can do, first to focus on the needs of the children with cancer, and then on the needs of the parents. The parents are overwhelmed by their concerns for the sick child, giving their immediate and full attention to the medical treatment of their sick child. Without any ill intention on the part of already overburdened parents, siblings are often inadvertently ignored. We should try to give attention to the needs of the siblings as well, and not let them be forgotten. During this time of crisis, when the parents are already giving their almost undivided attention to the sick child, how does one bring the needs of the siblings to parents' attention? How does one encourage and help the family to return to as normal a family life as possible as soon as possible? There are general principles for helping take care of the needs of siblings that apply throughout the treatment process, and there are principles specific to each phase of treatment: what to expect both for themselves and for their brother or sister now versus after physical changes occur, or changes in their relationships with their brother, sister, and parents, and what they can do to help during these transitions; and what adverse effects the siblings might have on the patient (for example, "spreading germs," e.g., a cold, or picking fights). Members of the health care team can speak with parents about the need to support the siblings, despite all of the other burdens that go into caring for the ill child. They can encourage the parents to share and generate suggestions regarding how to involve the siblings from the very beginning. Parents need to communicate with and listen to siblings. As an instinctively human reaction, in the absence of factual information, siblings tend to fear the worst, even for their own health. When parents and members of the health care team attempt in good faith to shield the siblings from knowledge about the illness, such well-intentioned hiding of the truth often drives the siblings to fear even worse possibilities, and can lead to feelings of isolation, guilt, and resentment.

At the time of diagnosis, health care team members and other parents when feasible should share with the parents of a newly diagnosed child the need to keep siblings informed from the very beginning, demystifying the illness and the treatments; parents should be encouraged to bring the siblings to the hospital if the siblings wish to go, let them visit with their brother or sister, and let them see how the hospital looks; parents should be encouraged to explore the benefits of immediately telling the siblings, and should help choose which person will be the one to inform the siblings, using simple and age-appropriate language and phrasing when delivering the news of the diagnosis; and siblings should have explained to them that they were in no way responsible for causing the cancer.

7. Living a normal life/back to school: During treatment

Improvements in the ability of medical care made it possible for children diagnosed with cancer to live longer and, in increasing frequency, to be cured. The children are able, while in remission, to live a relatively normal life, somewhat free of their concerns about their illness. We need to help the children to engage in the educational and social activities that accompany normal growth and development . It is not enough for young people simply to survive what was once a life-threatening illness. Survival means that the children have to continue to be educated toward one day becoming fully functioning adult members of society. Thus, parents and professionals have the increasing responsibility of promoting sound academic and social development as the children go through the treatment process.

Going back to school has a very normalizing influence on the child. Integration into school is a critical and essential part of the normal psychological and social development of any child. Children with cancer are not only entitled to attend school, but they must be stimulated to do so. Even while in the hospital, children should continue their schooling, as an indication to them of hope for cure, that their life will continue as normal, despite the illness. Programs should be developed to help the children continue their schooling while in the hospital, and to help them return to their normal life as school children as soon as possible, and their teachers trained to treat the children as normally as possible. We should pay special early attention to patterns and difficulties of socially adaptive behavior in the children and most importantly be aware of the strong link between the use of cranial radiation and subsequent learning deficits. As a group, children with cancer function at less socially adapted levels in school than peers, have a tendency not to reach out to others, not to initiate activities, not to try new things, and not to express feelings freely. The children retain a self-protective attitude. And so, in addition to already being devastated by the emotional stresses associated with a child having cancer and undergoing what to them were extraordinary medical treatments, we know that the cognitive side effects of the therapy place a group of the children at a higher risk not only for learning difficulties, but also for subsequent adaptive behavioral problems.

We cannot freeze children for years during treatment while their peers continue to grow and develop, leaving the children with cancer developmentally far behind and in a catch-up mode. We must prepare children for their future. Not only should we give priority to the children continuing to live a normal life during the course of treatment, we have in fact come to view childhood cancer as a golden opportunity for the children to learn skills in coping that can give them a running start on their preparation for engaging in a fully functioning adulthood.

8. Long-Term survivors or better "cured" subjects: After treatment, long-term follow-up

How well are the children responding to the increasingly successful treatments? Programs oriented to the needs of the long-term survivor should begin when the child goes off therapy, with centers focusing on the sequelae specific to each form of illness, treatment, toxicity, and future problems specific to each child's needs. Centers should offer counseling programs for the more serious medical and psychosocial problems, adapted to the need of each individual and local culture. Centers should develop specialty clinics, managed by the pediatric oncologist who treated the children, and having available a full range of adult and young adult specialists as consulting physicians. Each long-term survivor should be monitored for special conditions related to their unique history as well as their age-specific developmental concerns. Programs should include psychological counseling for the survivors experiencing adjustment difficulties and significant side effects.

As medicine continues to achieve an increasingly higher success rate in long-term survival, we should follow survivors to determine further potential long-term sequelae. The long-term role of each pediatric hematology/oncology center is to follow the survivors until there is assurance that the child will have no further long-term sequelae. It is important and critically necessary to follow the child until the disease is considered "cured" (at about five years). After that time, one should not over-medicalize the survivor, but help the child to make the transition to normal health-care status. When specific sequelae (such as heart problems) are known for a particular child, that child should be followed for the issue of concern specific to that child.

The clinic should keep a careful computerized record of essential data particular to each survivor so that in the future, when the now-adult survivor is seen by an adult physician, the data on the survivor's previous cancer experience will be available upon request.

Psychological research studies that have followed the survivors of childhood cancer for many years after successful treatment have found, not only that the now-adult-survivors are doing well, but that in many way having learned from the challenges of their childhood cancer experience they are better prepared for the more pressing challenges of adulthood than are their peers. The so-defined resilience is not an utopia but a always more visible reality.

9. Impending death: At the end of life

Despite the remarkable growth in the percentage of cures and the increasing sense of hope being given to newly diagnosed children and their families, many of the children are not able to be cured. Death for some remains a reality. There are three periods of time surrounding this final phase of life that have become the subjects of research. The first is the period when treatment is judged to be no longer effective and the difficult decision is made to move from curative intent to the palliative phase of care. The second is the period from the beginning of palliative care to the death of the child. The third is after the child dies, with the staff counseling the parents in their grief following the death of their child.

A child with cancer is considered by his/her physician to be moving from curative to palliative care when the child cannot be successfully treated by presently available therapies, and the child needs specific treatments, identified to be palliative and not curative, for physical or mental distress. There can be a long delay between the moment when the physician determines that the child will not be cured and the moment when everyone involved agrees that the child has entered the last or final phase of life.

In managing this transition from the curative to the palliative phase of the child's treatment, it is critical to protect the child. The expectations of the family must be considered to help them avoid feelings of guilt for not having done everything possible. However, a real dilemma is created for everyone if aggressive therapy is continued when the possibilities of cure are virtually not existent.

The decision to move from the intent to cure to palliative care should be made with the parents and the full health-care team, certainly including the nurses. Depending on age and level of development, the child should also be involved in the decision, with older children especially participating more actively. The child should know as much as possible and developmentally appropriate about the seriousness of his/her situation. However, if the child wishes to remain less informed, this wish should be respected, and whatever information is given should allow the child to retain a margin of hope.

The continuation of curative treatment beyond the point when cure is no longer possible should be avoided (the so-called "ruthless obstinacy" treatment).

After a child dies, that individual child's medical history should be evaluated. This evaluation should be made by the health-care team as a group. It is very important to reflect on all events, even minor ones, that occurred during the course of the child's treatment. It is critical to reflect on the choices that were made and why, in order to help the staff come to terms with their own grieving and to learn from the experience in order to help future families.

The center's health-care team should be prepared to modify its overall philosophical goals and reset directions and guidelines when appropriate, based on such review of individual cases and parental comments.

After the child dies, hospitals should offer bereavement counseling on the part of physicians and nurses to help clarify past care and guide future grieving. Parents and siblings, when appropriate, can be invited to discuss with the physician both the level of care and the surviving family members' current needs. A first-step aid to bereavement is for the physician, about three to four months after the child dies, to call back the parents (and siblings, when age-appropriate) and to discuss with them the details of the terminal phase, to help them work through their understanding of what happened. If at this point, some families need further help in grieving, they can be referred to parent-self-help grieving groups or to one-on-one therapy. For the majority of the families, the one follow-up interview appears to be a sufficient step in helping them to move forward through the grieving process.

10. Final recommendations for application: Since diagnosis on

Psychosocial interventions have become so fully incorporated into the care of children with cancer that they are now considered, not just an appendage, but a critical component in the care of the child with cancer. Where do we go from here?

1. As we health care professionals become more experienced in dealing with the children with cancer and their families, we cannot forget that for each newly diagnosed family, it is truly all brand new. Each case is individual. We should continue to bring to the newly diagnosed children and their family a fresh sensitivity that acknowledges the newness of their experience.
2. Children, even the youngest, sense the seriousness of their illness. They pick up the fears and anxieties of the adults around them. They do their best to communicate with us, at all ages. Even the youngest try to talk to us, often without words, often just by their body language. How well do we listen? Do we truly listen? We need to develop more effective ways of attending to what the children are experiencing and their mode of communicating that awareness.
3. Many of our interventions have proceeded far ahead of our success in measuring their effectiveness. While many new instruments have been developed and older instruments have been creatively applied specific to the study of the children and their families, we need to continue this creative effort and plunge more deeply into the study of the effectiveness of our interventions.
4. Parent groups are critical to the continued success of each clinic's efforts, not only by forming support services for one another on mutual psychosocial needs, but as importantly in teaming with physicians in raising funds to keep the clinic up-to-date and growing both in research and in intervention. Health care professionals and parents should strengthen their alliance, making it a priority to continue sharing decision-making, not only in individual cases, but in parental support of the clinic's growth.
5. Among the newly diagnosed families, there will be a small percentage 15% or so who bring with them pre-diagnosis problems that can seriously interfere with the child's treatment. We should continue to develop ways to help identify these families at the very beginning, so that we can refer them for the extra psychosocial help that they will need in order to cope with the treatment. With our remaining resources, we will then be better able to help the families who bring with them a stronger history of coping abilities and who are less encumbered by long-standing behavioral, social, financial, or legal problems.
6. Burnout is a very serious possibility for those working with children with cancer and their families. Acknowledging this very real fact and talking about it openly within the health care team can help prevent serious burnout and alleviate the milder and more subtle forms of burnout.
7. While there is an ongoing need for professionals to publish their findings in refereed journals, it is equally important to translate these findings into readable, clear, and simple booklets or pamphlets for the children, for their parents, and for their teachers. We owe it to the children and their families to continue developing clear and simply written booklets that can help explain some of the complexities of the treatment in ways that they can understand.
8. Much of our psychosocial long-term follow-up study during these past years has focused on potential negative sequelae of the illness and how best to prevent and/or ameliorate them. The next step in helping the children as they grow into adulthood should be to focus on the potential for growth associated with their illness. The children-becoming-young-adults, by overcoming their illness, have a golden opportunity to develop their skills in coping and learning to deal with future life's problems as they enter adulthood.

9. Medicine advances most effectively by narrowing its scope. Psychology advances by broadening its scope and generalizing to theory. Both together are necessary in the treatment of the child with cancer. As we continue to develop the research and intervention efforts with the children with oncological and hematological illnesses, we have seen our biopsychosocial efforts become a model for the increasing integration of the psychosocial in the treatment of children with a variety of chronic illnesses (Roberts, 2003). We should continue to disseminate our research and intervention findings among pediatric practitioners who are dealing with similar issues in different settings and with different chronic childhood illnesses.

11. References

[1] Van Eys, J. (Ed.) (1977) The truly cured child. Baltimore, MD: University Park Press.
[2] International Society of Pediatric Oncology (SIOP). (2004). Online Access: www.siop.nl.
[3] Roberts, M. C. (Ed.). (2003). Handbook of Pediatric Psychology. (3rd edit.) New York: The Guilford Press.
[4] Global Alliance for the Cure of Children with Cancer (GACCC). (2004). Online Access: www.inctr.org/projects/other.shtml.
[5] Masera, G. & Biondi, A. (1999). Research in low-income countries. Annals of Oncology, 10, 137-138.
[6] Masera, G., Baez, F., Biondi, A., Cavalli, F., Conter, V., Flores, A., et al (1998). North-south twinning in paediatric haematology-oncology The La Mascota programme, Nicaragua. Lancet, 351, 1923-1926.
[7] Naafs-Wilstra, M., Barr, R., Greenberg, C., Magrath, I., Cardenas, F., Chesler, M. et al (2001) Pediatric oncology in developing countries: Development of an alliance of stakeholders. Medical and Pediatric Oncology, 36, 305-309.
[8] Candlelighters Childhood Cancer Foundation. (2004). Online Access: www.candlelighters.org
[9] International Confederation of Childhood Cancer Parent Organisations (ICCCPO). (2004). Online Access: www.icccpo.org
[10] Spinetta, J. J., Rigler, D., & Karon, M. (1973). Anxiety in the dying child. Pediatrics, 52, 841-845.
[11] Spinetta, J. J., Rigler, D., & Karon, M. (1974). Personal space as a measure of the dying child's sense of isolation. Journal of Consulting and Clinical Psychology, 42, 751-756.
[12] Spinetta, J. J., & Maloney, L. J. (1975). Death anxiety in the out-patient leukemic child. Pediatrics, 56, 1034-1037.
[13] Bluebond-Langner, M. (1977). Meanings of death to children. In H. Feifel (Ed.), New meanings of death. New York: McGraw-Hill.
[14] Bluebond-Langner, M. (1978). The private worlds of dying children. Princeton, NJ: Princeton University Press.
[15] Jankovic, M., Loiacono, N. B., Spinetta, J. J., Riva, L., Conter, V., & Masera, G. (1994). Telling young children with leukemia their diagnosis: The flower garden as analogy. Pediatric Hematology and Oncology, 11: 75-81.
[16] Koocher, G. P., & O'Malley, J. E. (Eds.) (1981). The Damocles syndrome: Psychological consequences of surviving childhood cancer. New York: McGraw-Hill.

[17] Eden, O. B., Black, I., & Emery, A. E. (1993). The use of taped parental interviews to improve communication with childhood cancer families. Pediatric Hematology and Oncology, 10, 157-162.

[18] Masera, G., Beltrame, F., Corbetta, A., Fraschini, D., Adamoli, L., Jankovic, M., et al (2003). Audiotaping communication of the diagnosis of childhood leukemia: Parents' evaluation. Journal of Pediatric Hematology Oncology, 25(5), 368-371.

[19] Chesler, M. A. & Barbarin, O. A. (1987). Childhood cancer and the family. New York Brunner/Mazel.

[20] Deasy-Spinetta, P., & Spinetta, J. J. (1980). The child with cancer in school: Teachers' appraisal. American Journal of Pediatric Hematology/Oncology, 2, 89-94.

[21] Deasy-Spinetta, P., & Spinetta, J. J. (1989). Educational issues in the rehabilitation of long-term survivors. In P. A. Pizzo & D. G. Poplack (Eds.), Principles and practice of pediatric oncology. Philadelphia, PA: J. B. Lippincott.

[22] Adamoli, L., Deasy-Spinetta, P., Corbetta, A., Jankovic, M., Lia, R., Locati, A., et al (1997). School functioning for the child with leukemia in continuous first remission: Screening high risk children. Pediatric Hematology and Oncology, 14:121-131.

[23] Spinetta, J. J., & Deasy-Spinetta, P. (Eds.). (1981). Living with childhood cancer. St. Louis, MO: C. V. Mosby.

[24] Spinetta, J. J. & Deasy-Spinetta, P. (1986). The patient's socialization in the community and school during therapy. Cancer, 58, 512-516.

[25] Kupst, M. J., & Schulman, J. L. (1988). Long-term coping with pediatric leukemia: A six-year follow-up study. Journal of Pediatric Psychology, 13, 7-22.

[26] Van Dongen-Melman, J. E., Pruyn, J. F., De Groot, A., Koot, H. M., Hahlen, K., & Verhulst, F. C. (1995). Late psychosocial consequences for parents of children who survived cancer. Journal of Pediatric Psychology, 20, 567-586.

[27] Spinetta, J. J. (2005). Survivors of teenage cancer: Family dynamics and long-term effects. In O. B. Eden (Ed.), Proceedings of the Third International Conference on Cancer and the Adolescent. British Medical Journal.

[28] Parry, C. (2002). The psychosocial experiences of long-term survivors of childhood cancer across the life span. Ann Arbor, MI. University of Michigan PhD Dissertation in Sociology & Social Work.

[29] Jay, S. M., & Elliott, C. H. (1990). A stress inoculation program for parent whose children are undergoing painful medical procedures. Journal of Consulting and Clinical Psychology, 58, 799-804.

[30] Walco, G. (2005) Pain and procedure management. In R. T. Brown (Ed.), Pediatric hematology/oncology: A biopsychosocial approach. Oxford, England: Oxford University Press.

[31] Walker, C. (1989). Use of art and play therapy in pediatric oncology. Journal of Pediatric Oncology Nursing, 6, 121-126.

[32] Hilgard, J. R. & LeBaron, S. (1984) Hypnotherapy of pain in children with cancer. Los Altos, CA: William Kaufman.

[33] Jacobsen, P. B., Manne, S. L., Gorfinke, K., Schorr, O., Rapkin, R., & Redd, W. H. (1990). Analysis of child and parent behavior during painful medical procedures. Health Psychology, 9, 559-576.

[34] Boman, K., & Bodegard, G. (2000). Long-term coping in childhood cancer survivors: Influence of illness, treatment, and demographic background factors. Acta Paediatrica, 89, 105-111.

[35] Eden, O. B., Harrison, G., Richards, S., Lilleyman, J. S., Bailey, C. C., Chessells, J. M. et al (2000). Long-term follow-up of the United Kingdom Medical Research Council protocols for childhood acute lymphoblastic leukaemia, 1980-1997. Leukemia, 14, 2307-2320.

[36] Deasy-Spinetta, P., Spinetta, J. J., & Oxman, J. B. (1989). The relationship between learning deficits and social adaptation in children with leukemia. Journal of Psychosocial Oncology, 6 (3/4), 109-121.

[37] Hewitt, M., Weiner, S. L.. & Simone, J. V. (Eds.) (2003) Childhood cancer survivorship: Improving care and quality of life. Washington, DC: The National Academies Press.

[38] Jankovic, M., Brouwers, P., Valsecchi, M.G., Van Veldhuizen, A., Huisman, J., Kamphuis, R., et al (1994). Association of 1800 cGy cranial irradiation with intellectual function in children with acute lymphoblastic leukaemia.The Lancet, 344: 224-227.

[39] Spinetta, J. J., Murphy, J. L, Vik, P. J., Day, J., & Mott, M. A. (1989). Long-term adjustment in families of children with cancer. Journal of Psychosocial Oncology, 6 (3/4), 179-191.

[40] Stuber, M. L. (1996). Psychiatric sequelae in seriously ill children and their families. Psychiatric Clinics of North America, 19, 481-493.

[41] Zebrack, B. J., Zeltzer, L. K., Whitton, J., Mertens, A. C., Odom, L., Berkow. R. et al (2002). Psychological outcomes in long-term survivors of childhood leukemia, Hodgkin's disease, and non-Hodgkins's lymphoma: A report from the Childhood Cancer Survivor Study. Pediatrics, 110, 42-52.

[42] Jankovic, M., Masera, G., Uderzo, C., Conter, V., Adamoli, L., & Spinetta, J. J. (1989). Meetings with parents after the death of their child from leukemia. Pediatric Hematology and Oncology, 6, 155-160.

[43] Martinson, I. M. (1993). Hospice care for children: Past, present, and future. Journal of Pediatric Oncology Nursing, 10, 93-398.

[44] Sourkes, B. (1996). The broken heart: Anticipatory grief in the child facing death. Journal of Palliative Care, 12, 56-59.

[45] Spinetta, J. J., Swarner, J. A., & Sheposh, J. P. (1981). Effective parental coping following the death of a child from cancer. Journal of Pediatric Psychology, 6, 251-263.

[46] Stuber, M. L., & Mesrkhani, V. H. (2001). "What do we tell the children?": Understanding childhood grief. Western Journal of Medicine, 174, 187-191.

[47] Masera, G., Jankovic, M., Adamoli, L., Corbetta, A., Fraschini, D., Lia, R., et al (1997). The pychosocial program for childhood leukemia in Monza, Italy. Annals of the New York Academy of Sciences, 824: 210-220.

[48] Pizzo, P. A. & Poplack, D. G. (Eds.) (2001). Principles and practice of pediatric oncology. 4th edit. Philadelphia, PA: Lippincott Williams & Wilkins.

[49] Kazak, A. E. (1993). Psychological research in pediatric oncology. Journal of Pediatric Psychology, 18, 313-318.

[50] Spinetta, J. J. (1984). Development of psychometric assessment methods by life cycle stages. Cancer, 53 (10, Suppl.), 2222-2226.

[51] Van Dongen-Melman, J. E., DeGroot, A., Hahlen, K., & Verhulst, F. C. (1996). Commentary: Potential pitfalls of using illness-specific measures. Journal of Pediatric Psychology, 21, 103-106

[52] Masera, G., Spinetta, J. J., D'Angio, G. J., Green, D. M., Marky, I., Jankovic, M. et al. (1993). SIOP Working Committee on Psychosocial Issues in Pediatric Oncology: Critical Commentary. Medical and Pediatric Oncology, 21, 627-628.

[53] Masera, G., Jankovic, M., Deasy-Spinetta, P., Adamoli, L., Ben Arush, M. W., Challinor, J., et al (1995). SIOP Working Committee on Psychosocial Issues in Pediatric Oncology: Guidelines for School/Education. Medical and Pediatric Oncology, 25: 321-322).

[54] Masera, G., Chesler, M., Jankovic, M., Eden, T., Nesbit, M. E., Van Dongen-Melman, J., et al (1996). SIOP Working Committee on Psychosocial Issues in Pediatric Oncology: Guidelines for Care of Long-Term Survivors. Medical and Pediatric Oncology, 27: 1-2.

[55] Masera, G., Chesler, M. A., Jankovic, M., Ablin, A.R., Ben Arush, M. W., Breatnach, F., et al (1997). SIOP Working Committee on Psychosocial Issues in Pediatric Oncology: Guidelines for communication of the diagnosis. Medical and Pediatric Oncology, 28, 382-385.

[56] Masera, G., Spinetta, J. J., Jankovic, M., Ablin, A., Buchwall, I, Van Dongen-Melman, J., et al (1998). SIOP Working Committee on Psychosocial Issues in Pediatric Oncology: Guidelines for a therapeutic alliance between families and staff. Medical and Pediatric Oncology, 30, 183-186.

[57] Masera, G., Spinetta, J. J., Jankovic, M., Ablin, A. R., D'Angio, G. J., Van Dongen-Melman, J., et al (1999). Guidelines for assistance to terminally ill children with cancer: A report of the SIOP Working Committee on Psychosocial Issues in Pediatric Oncology. Medical and Pediatric Oncology, 32(1): 44-48.

[58] Spinetta, J. J., Jankovic, M., Eden. T., Green, D., Martins, A. G., Wandzura, C., et al., (1999). SIOP Working Committee on Psychosocial Issues in Pediatric Oncology: Guidelines for assistance to siblings of children with cancer. Medical and Pediatric Oncology, 33, 395-398.

[59] Spinetta, J. J., Jankovic, M., Ben Arush, M. W., Eden, T., Epelman, C., Greenberg, M. L., et al (2000). SIOP Working Committee on Psychosocial Issues in Pediatric Oncology: Guidelines for the Recognition, Prevention, and Remediation of Burnout in Health Care Professionals Participating in the Care of Children with Cancer. Medical and Pediatric Oncology, 35, 122-125.

[60] Spinetta, J. J., Masera, G., Eden, T., Oppenheim, D., Martins, A. G., van Dongen-Melman, J., et al (2002). SIOP Working Committee on Psychosocial Issues in Pediatric Oncology: Refusal, non-compliance, and abandonment of treatment in children and adolescents with cancer. Medical and Pediatric Oncology 38(2), 114-117.

[61] Spinetta, J. J., Masera, G., Jankovic, M., Oppenheim, D., Martins, A. G., Ben Arush, M. W., et al (2003). SIOP Working Committee on Psychosocial Issues in Pediatric Oncology: Valid informed consent and participative decision-making in children with cancer and their parents. Medical andPediatric Oncology, 40(4), 244-246.

[62] Jankovic, M., Spinetta, J., Martins, A. G, Pession, A., Sullivan, M., D'Angio, G. J., et al (2004). Nonconventional therapies in childhood cancer: Guidelines for

distinguishing non-harmful from harmful therapies. Pediatric Blood and Cancer 42, 106-108.
[63] Jankovic M., Spinetta J.J., Masera G., Barr R.D., D'Angio G.J., Epelman C., Evans A., Kosmidis H.V., Eden T. (2008); Communicating with the dying child: An invitation to listening--a report of the SIOP working committee on psychosocial issues in pediatric oncology. Pediatr Blood Cancer. May;50(5):1087-8.
[64] Spinetta J.J., Jankovic M., Masera G., Ablin A.R., Barr R.D., Ben Arush M.W., D'Angio G.J., Van Dongen-Melman J., Eden T., Epelman C., Martins A.G., Greenberg M.L., Kosmidis H.V., Oppenheim D., Zeltzer P.M. (2009); Optimal care for the child with cancer: A summary statement from the SIOP Working Committee on Psychosocial Issues in Pediatric Oncology. Pediatr Blood Cancer. Jul;52(7):904-7.
[65] Edelstein K., D'agostino N., Bernstein L.J., Nathan P.C., Greenberg M.L., Hodgson D.C., Millar B.A., Laperriere N., Spiegler B.J. (2011); Long-term neurocognitive outcomes in young adult survivors of childhood acute lymphoblastic leukemia. J Pediatr Hematol Oncol. Aug;33(6):450-8.
[66] Reulen R.C., Frobisher C., Winter D.L., Kelly J., Lancashire E.R., Stiller C.A., Pritchard-Jones K., Jenkinson H.C., Hawkins M.M. (2011); British Childhood Cancer Survivor Study Steering Group. Long-term risks of subsequent primary neoplasms among survivors of childhood cancer. JAMA. Jun 8;305(22):2311-9.
[67] Oeffinger KC, Tonorezos ES. (2011). The cancer is over, now what?: Understanding risk, changing outcomes. Cancer. May 15;117(10 Suppl):2250-7.
[68] Pivetta E., Maule M.M., Pisani P., Zugna D., Haupt R., Jankovic M., Aricò M., Casale F., Clerico A., Cordero di Montezemolo L., Kiren V., Locatelli F., Palumbo G., Pession A., Pillon M., Santoro N., Terenziani M., Valsecchi M.G., Dama E., Magnani C., Merletti F., Pastore G. (2011); Italian Association of Pediatric Hematology and Oncology (AIEOP) Group. Marriage and parenthood among childhood cancer survivors: a report from the Italian AIEOP Off-Therapy Registry. Haematologica. May;96(5):744-51.

Part 5

Professional Liability

15

Risk Management in Obstetrics and Neonatal-Perinatal Medicine

Jonathan Muraskas, Lindsay Ellsworth,
Eric Culp, Gretchen Garbe and John Morrison
Loyola University Medical Center,
University of Mississippi Medical Center,
USA

1. Introduction

The professional liability crisis remains a common problem for obstetricians. Approximately 90% of American College of Obstetricians and Gynecologists fellows have been sued at least once and 25% have been sued four or more times. Approximately 15% of obstetricians have ceased obstetric practice because of exorbitant premiums and the prevalence of nonmeritorious claims in this field of practice. The average age at which an obstetrician/gynecologist stops providing obstetrical care is currently 48 years of age; the age at which most physicians approach the peak of judgment and experience.

This current liability crisis is very relevant to all practitioners who care for newborns. Neonatologists, pediatricians, hospitalists, and nurse practitioners all provide critical care to sick newborns in different venues. These newborns are younger, more fragile, often extremely small and the risk of life long chronic disease, pain and disability are significant for these patients. Parents often experience emotional and economic distress when their newborn is in the NICU. These factors have contributed to an increased number of allegations against practitioners of neonatal/perinatal medicine.

Juries tend to have a natural sympathy for disabled children even when allegations are nonmeritorious. In addition, many states exempt minors from the statute of limitations for medical liability which can lead to a physician defending claims 10-20 years after the alleged incident. Capping noneconomic damages in children is difficult. The increase in litigation cases is mirrored by an increase in the awards received by the plaintiff. Today the average jury award for poor obstetric and neonatal outcome exceeds $3,000,000. Obstetricians pay some of the highest insurance premiums, up to $300,000 per year in some states. Efforts at tort reform, award caps and the policing of junk science have not been uniformly successful.

The purpose of this Chapter is to identify the etiology, pathology and prevention of common allegations of professional liability for the obstetrician and practitioner of neonatal-perinatal medicine. The author has reviewed 100 closed cases of alleged professional liability against obstetricians for causation of poor neonatal outcome and 100 closed cases of alleged professional liability involving practitioners of neonatal perinatal medicine as an expert. These cases were reviewed over a 25 year period (1985-2010). Approximately 75% of the cases were reviewed for the defense and 25% for the plaintiff. Of these, 75% of the cases were settled, 19% were dismissed and 6% went to trial with a favorable jury verdict for the defense in 75% of the trial cases. Based on our experience, we developed an evidence-based work-up that can confirm or refute allegations of acute intrapartum asphyxia sufficient to cause cerebral palsy.

2. Common allegations of obstetrical professional liability

Table 1 lists the eight major categories that resulted in allegations of obstetric professional liability. The most common obstetrical allegation was failure to perform a timely C-section. The inability to recognize and react to nonreassuring fetal heart tones was the dominant allegation. Poor communication between the nurse, obstetrician and anesthesiologist in making the decision and provisions to perform an emergency C-section was common. The ability to perform an emergency C-section as a rescue procedure for the patient and/or fetus is a necessary part of the practice of moderate obstetrics. Although only accounting for 3% of all cesarean sections, the timeliness of cesarean sections is a frequent source of litigation. Even today it is unclear if this 30 minute rule from decision to incision is valid and more studies need to be performed. In fact, a recent study showed that approximately one-third of primary C-section deliveries were performed for emergency indications and were commenced more than 30 minutes after the decision to operate, mainly for nonreassuring fetal heart rate tracings. In this study, adverse neonatal outcomes were not increased. Unfortunately despite limited data, the 30 minute response time has become a medical/legal benchmark for adequacy of obstetrical care when a cesarean section is indicated.

Failure to triage a mother appropriately was the next most common allegation of professional liability against practitioners of obstetrical care. It is essential that all emergency rooms have specific protocols in the evaluation and management of the pregnant patient even when the primary complaint may not be obstetrically related. Misdiagnosis of preeclampsia/HELLP syndrome can be fatal to the mother and newborn. More common in group practices, the problems that result from a failure to follow-up on specific tests ordered in the prenatal period. The failure to follow-up on fetal ultrasounds that demonstrated twin to twin transfusion is a specific example. "If you do not document it, you did not do it" is a common cause of speculation

Complicated deliveries can result in catastrophic neonatal outcomes. Many high-risk situations, such as delivering a poorly controlled diabetic, VBAC, forceps, and vacuum require that the obstetrician initiate pediatric/neonatal presence in the delivery room. Infants born under these situations can appear stable and decompensate 12-48 hours after the initial event. The pediatrician needs to be alert for signs and symptoms of anemia, seizures and any altered neurologic status. A twin pregnancy is high risk and should command the presence of appropriate personnel for the delivery.

Regionalization continues to have a role and is in the best interest of the mother and newborn. The state and perinatal centers oversee the rules and regulations that dictate the level of care of the high risk mother and newborn provided at specific hospitals. Triplets and higher order pregnancies, newborns with known congenital anomalies and extremely low birthweight newborns are best delivered and cared for in a tertiary center. The best ambulance is the uterus. Ego can cloud good judgment and compromise the care and outcomes of the mother and fetus.

Cause for Obstetric Allegations	Case Examples		N = 100
1. Failure to perform a timely C-section	Non-reassuring fetal heart tones Poor communication between OB's and Anesthesiologists Obstetrical nurse failure to interpret ominous fetal strip Nurse spent too long trying to obtain FHT when none were present Inadequate fetal monitoring for prolonged periods of time	Postponing aggressive treatment for the next shift Inadequate physician sign out at change of shifts Failure of midwife to recognize ominous fetal heart tracings Failure of midwife to have appropriate resuscitation equipment and personnel for home delivery	40%
2. Failure to triage mother appropriately	Failure to follow-up test results Failure to give antenatal steroids Emergency room triage errors (misdiagnosis of Mirror Syndrome) Misdiagnose pre-eclampsia as gallbladder disease in ER Mother sent home at 39 weeks in active labor Failure to detect rupture of membranes	Failure to rule out abruption Failure to diagnose HELLP syndrome Diagnostic difficulties due to maternal obesity Failure of triage nurse and/or house staff to present an accurate picture of the case to the attending	21%
3. Complicated delivery	Shoulder dystocia Uterine rupture with VBAC Double footling breech delivered vaginally	Neonate born with fractured ribs, skull fracture, fractured clavicle Twin pregnancy in which in utero demise of viable twin was due to nonviable twin death	17%
4. Failure to transport mother to tertiary case center in appropriate timing	Expected difficult delivery with complicated neonate was not preemptively transferred to a tertiary care center Delivery of triplet or higher order pregnancy in a level 2 center	Congenital anomalies Complicated twin pregnancies, triplets, quadruplets (twin to twin transfusion, significant discordancy) 24 weeker	11%
5. Pharmacologic error	Dosing errors with Pitocin Using Pitocin instead of Magnesium Failure to follow Pitocin protocol	Failure to discontinue Pitocin with non-reassuring fetal heart tones and/or hyperstimulation	5%
6. Failure to diagnose maternal infection	Failure to diagnose chorioamnionitis Failure to obtain and document GBS status Failure to recognize fetal tachycardia as a sign of chorioamnionitis		3%
7. Inappropriate use of labor induction	Maternal request Physician convenience	Late preterm newborns	2%
8. Failure to educate patient	Patient not instructed exactly when she should go to the hospital for labor		1%

Table 1. Common Allegations of Obstetrical Professional Liability

Another common allegation of professional liability with poor neonatal outcome involves the use of Pitocin. In our experience, many obstetricians and obstetrical nursing personnel were not familiar with their hospital specific protocol for the use of Pitocin. Failure to discontinue Pitocin with nonreassuring fetal heart tones and the inability to recognize hyperstimulation generates arguments for poor neonatal outcome. Since 1994 the use of antenatal steroids to enhance fetal pulmonary and brain maturation has become the standard of care. Failure to give antenatal steroids between 24 and 34 weeks gestation with evidence of imminent delivery can result in poor newborn outcomes.

Neonatal sepsis can have significant morbidity and mortality. Failure to obtain and document Group B Streptococcus (GBS) status was common. Failure to recognize fetal tachycardia as a fetal response to chorioamnionitis was noted. Chorioamnionitis is one of the most common causes for newborn depression often requiring significant resuscitation in the delivery room. The presence of maternal chorioamnionitis which can include a fever, elevated white count, left shift, fetal tachycardia and foul-smelling amniotic fluid should mandate the presence of pediatrics/neonatology for the delivery.

In the last decade a significant awareness on the dangers of induction for convenience and/or maternal request has evolved. Numerous studies have shown that the late preterm newborn has significant morbidity and mortality compared to their term counterparts. One should never assume that a late preterm newborn at 34-36 weeks will have an uneventful nursery course. In our experience and supported by numerous studies, the male infant is at least one week behind in maturation compared to their female counterparts. Some of the most severe cases of hypoxic respiratory failure can occur in these late preterm newborns.

A common pathway leading to litigation from the previous eight categories of the obstetrical allegations discussed is whether with a reasonable degree of medical certainty a deviation in the standard of care caused morbidity and/or mortality in the newborn. The proportion of cerebral palsy associated with intrapartum hypoxia-ischemia is 8-14.5%. Despite this fact, the use of junk science, unethical expert witness testimony, and speculation in childbirth litigation persist.

3. Proposed work-up to confirm or refute allegations of acute intrapartum asphyxia

The next section summarizes our work in developing a workup for the newborn to confirm or refute the 4 essential and 5 suggestive criteria proposed in defining an acute intrapartum event sufficient to cause cerebral palsy as defined in the 2003 ACOG and AAP Task Force publication on Neonatal Encephalopathy and Cerebral Palsy. (Table 2)

Each case of alleged intrapartum asphyxia is unique and no single test can time an alleged event. The College criteria have been criticized for being too restrictive and potentially not being able to identify many cases of intrapartum asphyxia. Many consider a sentinel event to be a critical and essential first step in linking intrapartum asphyxia to neonatal encephalopathy. Aside from a sentinel event during labor, the College criteria are postdelivery assessments. Despite this controversy, we feel this proposed workup will provide significantly more objective evidence-based data in the medical record to support or refute allegations of intrapartum asphyxia. Table 3 outlines an evidence-based work-up to be considered in term and near term newborns with unexplained depression at birth with evidence of encephalopathy including seizures.

ESSENTIAL CRITERIA (Must meet all four)	Clinical work-up
Evidence of a metabolic acidosis in fetal umbilical cord arterial blood obtained at delivery (pH < 7.0 and base deficit ≥ 12 mmol/L)	Arterial Cord Gas
Early onset of severe or moderate neonatal encephalopathy in infants born at 34 or more weeks of gestation	EEG
Cerebral palsy of the spastic quadriplegic or dyskinetic type	MRI Head
Exclusion of other identifiable etiologies such as trauma, coagulation disorders, infectious conditions, or genetic disorders	Newborn Weight, Length and Head Circumference Placental Pathology CBC with Differential, blood cultures U/S Head MRI Head
Criteria that suggest an intrapartum timing	**Clinical Work-Up**
A sentinel (signal) hypoxic event occurring immediately before or during labor	Electronic Fetal Heart Rate Interpretation CBC with Differential, Platelets, NRBCs
A sudden and sustained fetal bradycardia or the absence of fetal heart rate variability in the presence of persistent, late, or variable decelerations, usually after a hypoxic sentinel event when the pattern was previously normal	Electronic Fetal Heart Rate Interpretation CBC with Differential, Platelets, NRBCs
Apgar scores of 0-3 beyond 5 minutes	Apgar Score 10 and 15 min
Onset of multisystem involvement within 72 hours of birth	PT, PTT, Fibrinogen, LFTs, Creatinine, Electrolytes, Glucose, Calcium, ECHO
Early imaging study showing evidence of acute nonfocal cerebral abnormality	Ultrasonography of the head MRI of the head

EEG: electroencephalogram; MRI: magnetic resonance imaging; NRBC: nucleated red blood cell; PT: prothrombin time; PTT: partial thromboplastin time; LFT: liver function tests; ECHO: echocardiogram

Table 2. Criteria to define an acute intrapartum event sufficient to cause cerebral palsy

Umbilical cord blood gas assessments are the most objective determinants of the fetal metabolic condition at the moment of birth. Umbilical arterial blood reflects fetal status more directly and umbilical venous blood more closely reflects whether the oxygen exchange of the uteroplacental unit is optimal. Westgate et al recommend obtaining cord blood from the artery and vein. However, in clinical practice this is not practical and an umbilical cord arterial gas is most often obtained. Fetal scalp blood sampling has been virtually eliminated in clinical practice without an increase in adverse newborn outcomes. An ongoing dilemma with the College criteria is the requirement of metabolic acidemia to determine whether an insult occurred intrapartum. Many term newborns who are delivered in the presence of fetal acidemia are not recognized by intrapartum events and are triaged to the regular nursery with an uneventful hospital course. Studies have demonstrated when the umbilical artery pH was less than 7.0 at birth, 67% had a metabolic component in their acidemia compared with 14% for those with pH of 7.0 to 7.2. One study showed with an umbilical arterial pH less than 7.0 at birth, neurologic damage was found in 23%, with the remaining 77% being neurologically normal at the time of neonatal discharge. The pH is a direct measurement, whereas the base deficit is a calculated value obtained by the Siggard-Andersen alignment nomogram. This nomogram can confirm the biochemical authenticity of arterial cord blood gases. Umbilical arterial pH decreases and the base deficit increases during the course of normal labor, because a buffer base is depleted before the pH declines. The pH decreases approximately 0.07 units for every 10-mm Hg increment increase in PCO2. The respiratory component of acidosis cannot damage the newborn, and when present, the onset of hypoxia can be established because this component cannot last more than 20 to 30 minutes. In our experience, the absence of a cord arterial blood gas leads to more speculation between the plaintiff and defense experts than any other laboratory value and should be drawn in all deliveries and sent for analysis when clinically indicated.

Clinical Work-Up		Days of Life			
		1	2	3	7
1	Arterial Cord Gas	X			
2	Apgar Scores at 10′ and 15′ (if 5 minutes ≤ 6)	X			
3	Physical Exam: Newborn weight, length and head circumference	X			
4	Placental Pathology	X			
5	CBC with differential, Platelets, blood cultures	X			
6	U/S Head	X	X		
7	NRBCs	X	X	X	
8	PT, PTT, Fibrinogen, LFTs, Creatinine, Electrolytes, Glucose, Calcium, ECHO		X		
9	EEG		X		
10	MRI Head				X

Table 3. Proposed Clinical Work-Up of Newborns > 34 weeks GA with Alleged Perinatal Asphyxia in the First Week of Life

Neonatal encephalopathy is a clinically defined syndrome of disturbed neurological function in the earliest days of life, manifested by depression of tone and reflexes, subnormal levels of consciousness, and often times, seizures. After intrapartum asphyxia, hypotonia is the norm and, in general, early hypertonia or absence of hypotonia (normal tone) point to other neurological abnormalities. The grading of neonatal encephalopathy as mild, moderate, or severe was originally described by Sarnat and Sarnat. The presence of seizures is required to meet the Sarnat criteria for moderate to severe encephalopathy. Neonatal seizures can be subtle, often presenting with oxygen desaturations and focal motor abnormalities such as eye deviation, smacking of lips, and staring. Also, the presence of atypical apnea with desaturations frequently was not identified as seizures and delayed appropriate therapy. An electroencephalogram can be used to confirm the presence of seizures. Seizures soon after birth (1–6 hours or more than 24 hours of life are not consistent with acute intrapartum asphyxia). When seizures occurred within 24 hours, 48% of newborns were significantly negatively affected compared with when the seizures occurred after 24 hours.

Cerebral palsy (CP) is most often not diagnosed until well after the first year of life. White matter lesions such as cystic periventricular leukomalacia is a common lesion of prematurity (less than 34 weeks of gestation), often results in spastic diplegia, and is usually not associated with intrapartum asphyxia in the term infant. However, focal noncystic white matter injury is increasingly recognized in term newborns with neonatal encephalopathy. In term newborns, the gray matter is the most metabolically active and therefore most vulnerable to an acute intrapartum event. Although spastic quadriplegia with a dyskinetic, chorioathetoid component is the most common subtype of CP associated with an acute profound hypoxic intrapartum event, it is not specific to intrapartum hypoxia.

The majority of cases involving neonatal encephalopathy and CP are associated with maternal and antenatal factors such as intrauterine infection, maternal/fetal coagulation problems, antenatal hemorrhage, abnormal presentation, preterm birth, and developmental/chromosomal abnormalities. Plotting out weight, length, and head circumference is a vital component of the initial newborn assessment. The presence of microcephaly at birth can be consistent with an earlier pregnancy insult and usually results in a poor neurological outcome. The presence of intrauterine growth restriction and status of small for gestational age at birth can be associated with poor neurodevelopmental outcomes.

The placenta can be an excellent source of information to confirm alternate etiologies such as metabolic disorders, adverse growth events, and infections. Intraamniotic infection is the most common antecedent to birth depression, low Apgar scores, and neonatal encephalopathy in term newborns. The presence of chorioamnionitis and funisitis are significant risk factors for CP in term/near-term newborns. Fetal inflammatory response syndrome caused by cytokine expression in the fetus after exposure to maternal infection can also result in neonatal encephalopathy, often with negative cultures, cord arterial pH more than 7.0, and Apgar scores more than 3 to 5 at 5 minutes. Infection, inflammation, thrombosis, and coagulopathy are recognized as being associated with white matter-mediated damage caused by the elevated fetal cytokines and are ultimately associated with periventricular leukomalacia and encephalopathy. A newborn with neutropenia (absolute neutrophil count less than 2,000) and a band-to-segmented neutrophils ratio of more than 0.2 on a complete blood count more probably than not has clinical sepsis despite negative cultures. Newborn blood cultures should be obtained any time sepsis is suspected. A genetic work-up may be helpful to direct postnatal testing. Newborn thrombophilias also can be a congenital cause of abnormal neonatal outcome and may present as a hemorrhagic or thrombotic lesion. Many known thrombophilias, such as antithrombin III deficiency, protein C or S deficiency, prothrombin genetic deficiencies, hyperhomocystinemia, and factor V Leiden mutation, can all lead to strokes in the newborn, which can cause neonatal encephalopathy with CP and mental retardation and/or fetal/neonatal death. Meconium stained amniotic fluid is often erroneously associated with intrapartum fetal distress. In reality, 15% of the 4,000,000 annual births in the United States have meconium-stained amniotic fluid.

Vaginal bleeding during labor can signal trauma, such as a ruptured uterus, abruptio placenta/placenta previa, or fetal bleeding from a vasoprevia. When bleeding leads to fetal damage, it is usually associated with a significantly abnormal electronic fetal heart rate tracing such as bradycardia (usually less than100 beats per minute for more than 10 minutes) and/or repetitive late decelerations with absent fetal heart rate variability. Bleeding can also be concealed and such fetal heart rate tracings may be the only suggestion of fetal compromise.

The presence of anemia in the newborn at birth also can point to nonpreventable etiologies such as maternal-fetal transfusion as well as chronic abruption. Unexplained anemia in the newborn should prompt the pediatrician/neonatologist to request a maternal Kleihauer-Betke test. In the newborn, a complete blood count with differential and a platelet count at birth as well as nucleated red blood cell often can be helpful in differentiating the patient with intrapartum asphyxia from other causes of encephalopathy.

The presence of thrombocytopenia (less than 150,000) as well as an elevated hemoglobin (greater than 18 g/dL) and hematocrit (greater than 55%) in the newborn can be consistent with chronic hypoxia in utero. Serial nucleated red blood cell counts in the first 3 days of life can provide helpful information because an elevated nucleated red blood cell count at birth with delayed clearance (greater than 72 hours) does not support a diagnosis of acute intrapartum asphyxia. The proportion of CP associated with intrapartum hypoxia-ischemia is 8% to 14.5%.Certain preexisting conditions such as perinatal ischemic stroke, neuromuscular disorders, and certain in-born errors of metabolism can present at birth with a clinical picture not unlike intrapartum asphyxia. Likewise, elevated lymphocyte counts in the fetus may be predictive of earlier hypoxia that antedates labor. Finally, a detailed note by the obstetrician after delivery that summarizes the intrapartum course may be helpful in ruling out asphyxia in labor as the cause of newborn depression.

Nonspecific criteria collectively suggestive of intrapartum timing include sentinel hypoxic intrapartum event. Cord prolapse, ruptured uterus, maternal shock amniotic fluid embolus, and acute bleeding can result in catastrophic intrapartum asphyxia.

The National Institute of Child Health in Human Development's Research Planning Workshop on electronic fetal heart rate monitoring offers standardized definitions for such tracings. The participants agreed that tracings with a normal fetal heart rate pattern including baseline heart rate within the normal range and normal fetal heart rate variability with the presence of accelerations and absent of decelerations (type I) confers an extremely high likelihood of a normally oxygenated fetus. At the other end of the spectrum, when there is bradycardia or repetitive (greater than 50% of contractions) late or significant variable decelerations, each with absent fetal heart rate variability (type III), there is a substantial risk of impending damaging asphyxia. However, the false positive rates of these patterns (type III) are very high, and the majority of nonreassuring fetal tracings during labor are associated with normal outcomes. Thus, none of these patterns can be used to predict CP and mental retardation as an outcome ascribed to intrapartum asphyxia. However, if accelerations occur above a normal baseline and variability of any degree is present, then it frequently rules out intrapartum acidosis or asphyxia as a cause of neonatal encephalopathy and CP. An in-depth review of the fetal heart rate tracing is helpful in confirming or refuting asphyxia as the cause of newborn depression.

Apgar scores can be subjective. Numerous factors can affect the Apgar scores, including intrapartum maternal sedation or anesthesia, congenital malformations, the individual assigning the score, resuscitative efforts, and the presence of an infection. This can result in speculation on the quality and response to resuscitation. Although low Apgars are poor predictors of long-term neurologic outcome, there is a good correlation with extremely low Apgars (0, 1, and 2) at 15 to 20 minutes and subsequent neurologic dysfunction. For example, Apgar score of less than 3 at 15 minutes was associated with a 53% neonatal mortality rate and a 36% CP incidence. Conversely, it is also true that 75% of children with CP have normal Apgar scores. The fine details of resuscitation require documentation or they could be used erroneously to support intrapartum asphyxia. Inability to achieve an adequate airway in a depressed newborn or failure of a previously damaged fetus to transition to extrauterine life are common etiologies of low Apgar scores and can erroneously lead to the assumption that this depression is attributable to the obstetric care. This is also important because the 30-minute decision–incision guideline may impact Apgar scores, as well as umbilical and neonatal blood gas sampling. It is paradoxical to note, however, that in 50% to 65% of cases, the decision–incision interval exceeds 30 minutes, but the lower Apgar scores and blood gases are usually found in those who have an interval of less than 30 minutes and often less than 15 minutes.

Multisystem organ dysfunction is physiologically related to the diving reflex. In the majority of cases, intrapartum asphyxia deprives all other organs of oxygenated blood before the flow of oxygen to the brain is diminished. Studies have demonstrated that a cord pH 6.92 or less is the threshold linked with neonatal organ dysfunction at 72 hours of birth. Many expert witnesses erroneously consider a transient decrease in urine output (less than 2 $mL/kg^{-1}/h^{-1}$) or a slight elevation in liver enzymes to be signs of

multiorgan failure. The presence of pulmonary hypertension, tricuspid insufficiency, hypocalcemia, hypoglycemia, abnormal cardiac enzymes, and coagulopathy may be more supportive of multiorgan failure after a significant intrapartum event if other causes cannot be ruled out.

Several patterns of brain injury may result from hypoxic-ischemic episodes in the fetus and depend on the severity of cerebral hypotension, the maturity of the brain at the time of injury, and the duration or recurrence of the event. Cerebral edema usually appears approximately 24 hours after a significant asphyxial episode and resolves in 3 to 5 days. The presence of cerebral edema on an ultrasonogram on the first day of life would not be consistent with an acute intrapartum asphyxial event. The evolution of cystic periventricular leukomalacia in preterm newborns takes 2 to 3 weeks after an insult to be visualized using conventional imaging studies such as computed tomography and ultrasonography scans. Magnetic resonance imaging has emerged as a valuable tool for determining the timing and etiology of neonatal brain injury. Hypoxia-ischemia in term newborns typically results in one of two characteristic patterns of brain injury: 1) a basal ganglia distribution pattern involving deep gray nuclei, hippocampus, and perirolandic cortex with additional cortical involvement when severe, and 2) a watershed distribution pattern involving intervascular boundary-zone white matter plus cortical gray matter when severe. Acute total asphyxia mainly involves the brain stem nuclei, thalami, and basal ganglia and is associated with dystonic CP and brain stem deficits. Prolonged partial asphyxia involves mainly the cerebral cortex, especially parasagittal regions, and is associated with spastic quadriplegia and microcephaly. In term newborns, basal ganglia and thalamic lesions evolve through a neurotoxic cascade during the first week after the insult. Imaging studies obtained too early after birth may appear normal even when there has been severe injury to the brain. It is important to consider not only which imaging studies to obtain but also when to schedule them to optimize the results in attempting to determine the timing of the alleged insult. Neuroimaging can be helpful in approximating a window of time when the injury might have occurred.

4. Allegations of professional liability in neonatal-perinatal medicine

We next identified the most common events in the care of sick newborns leading to litigation against practitioners. Multiple allegations were common due to the prolonged care of the newborn. Table 4 lists the top ten allegations of professional liability against practitioners of neonatal perinatal medicine. The ten most frequent allegations brought against practitioners who care for newborns included: inadequate airway/intubation (21%), failure to recognize air leak (18%), delayed transfer to Level III facility (14%), inadequate treatment of seizures (11%), delayed attendance at delivery (10%), cardiac tamponade (malpositioned central line) (6%), failure to perform eye exam (6%), medication error (6%), midgut volvulus (5%), and hyperbilirubinemia (kernicterus) (3%). Meritorious allegations against practitioners in newborn care are frequently preventable events. Substandard neonatal resuscitation in the delivery room can also propagate non-meritorious allegations against obstetricians.

Allegation	**N = 100**
Inadequate airway/intubation	21%
Failure to recognize air leak (pneumothorax)	18%
Delayed transfer to Level III facility	14%
Inadequate treatment of seizures	11%
Delayed attendance in the NICU/delivery room	10%
Cardiac tamponade (central line)	6%
Failure to do eye exam (blindness)	6%
Medication error (overdose)	6%
Midgut volvulus	5%
Hyperbilirubinemia (kernicterus)	3%

Table 4. Top ten allegations against practitioners of newborn medicine

We found that the most common allegations were a result of difficulties in the management of airways and air leaks in newborns. The procedural skills, including proficiency in intubation and thoracentesis, require a significant amount of clinical experience. Evolving technology over the last two decades with steroids, surfactants and ventilation have reduced the acuity of neonatal lung disease with concomitant reduction in intubations and chest tube placement. The recent restrictions on the time that pediatric residents are allowed to spend in intensive care units, set by the Accreditation Council for Graduate Medical Education, has contributed even more to their reduced experience with these procedures. More than half of all intubation attempts by pediatric residents are unsuccessful leading to multiple attempts by caregivers to properly place the endotracheal tube. Also, general pediatricians are often the primary caregiver when resuscitation of newborns in the delivery room is required. Their residency programs must ensure they become proficient in the resuscitation and care of the newborn.

Procedural skills teaching based on observing the skill, performing the skill, then teaching the skill is not adequate for proper training. Improving opportunities for clinical experience with intubation and thoracentesis may reduce legal actions against practitioners. Simulation-based training can have a role to provide a realistic medical situation in which learners can gain exposure to clinical tasks and anatomical regions. Approximately 10% of newborns require some form of resuscitation at birth, and a skilled resuscitator is necessary for all deliveries even when they are considered low risk. In our clinical experience, the most common etiology of decompensation in a newborn is airway related, with chest compressions rarely indicated when an adequate airway is effectively established. When an adequate airway is achieved, but newborns do not respond to resuscitation, one needs to expediently consider a pneumothorax in the differential diagnosis. Failure to recognize an air leak was the second most common allegation found in this study. An unrecognized air leak is the most common etiology for sudden unexplained death in unsuccessful newborn resuscitation. A tension pneumothorax is an acute life threatening event that may not allow the time for x-ray confirmation. Prompt recognition and needle aspiration of the pleural space should result in rapid clinical improvement for these newborns. It has been our experience that poor newborn outcomes as a result of improper delivery room resuscitation often are erroneously attributed to the delivering obstetrician. A depressed newborn requiring vigorous resuscitation with poor Apgars more often than not creates the mindset that it must be the obstetrician's fault.

Due to the critical state of newborns in the NICU, numerous protocols have been instituted to reduce iatrogenic events. When set protocols were not followed rigorously, we found that cardiac tamponade and blindness resulted in allegations of malpractice. Central lines are frequently used in the treatment of newborns for both medication and nutrition infusion, but their use carries significant risks. The possible malposition and migration of a central catheter can result in perforation of the myocardium or pericardial effusion which can be fatal. It is recommended that the central line be optimally placed outside of the right atrium to reduce these risks. Newborns with central lines must be carefully monitored with serial radiographs to confirm the position of the central line throughout the course of their treatment. Another protocol set forth in the care of newborns is an eye exam for all preterm newborns less than 33 weeks gestational age at 4 to 6 weeks chronological age. A newborn is almost never too sick for an eye exam, although nurses may feel that their patient is too unstable to be dilated and examined.

The potential for rapid decline in an unstable newborn requires that their caregivers not delay in proper treatment measures. A prolonged response time for physicians during an emergency situation, as well as delayed transfer of newborns to a proper level NICU were common allegations found in this study. All hospitals have contracts that require trained personnel to be at a high-risk scenario within a certain time frame. A delayed response to a page, and the lack of an alternative plan to notify a skilled resuscitator can result in catastrophic consequences for a compromised newborn. In addition, critical care of a newborn often requires advanced services that are not available in all NICUs. Level I, II, II+, and community Level III centers have set policies and regulations overseen by their regional perinatal center. The lack of experience of nursing and respiratory personnel in a low volume NICU can contribute to deviations in the standard of care. Regionalization continues to have a role, and is in the best interest of mothers and their newborns.

Common allegations in this study also resulted from a failure to recognize life-threatening conditions including seizures and intestinal mid-gut volvulus. Newborn seizures can be difficult to clinically diagnose due to subtle abnormal ocular and focal movements. Subtle motor abnormalities with concomitant desaturation and/or apnea often represent seizure activity. The first line of medication in the treatment of seizures in newborns is phenobarbital at a loading dose of 20 mg/kg to achieve therapeutic levels of 20-40 μg/mL. An adequate airway is essential if one desires to increase phenobarbital dosing. Persistent seizures may require the addition of phenytoin or ativan. Inadequately treated seizures can result in permanent neuronal cell damage due to enhanced metabolic activity. Malrotation of the intestine is usually observed in the neonatal period and presents with signs of acute intestinal obstruction and often bilious emesis. Mid-gut volvulus is a true surgical emergency, where delay can result in ischemic necrosis of the entire gut which is most often lethal. The upper GI series is the method of choice for diagnosing malrotation. Importantly, an acutely ill newborn with a history of bilious emesis needs immediate surgical consultation. Early diagnosis and treatment of these two conditions is essential in facilitating good outcomes.

Medication errors are preventable events that frequently occur in the NICU and are a common source of allegations. It has been previously reported that out of every five adverse drug events in pediatric patients, three of those events occurred in an NICU. Errors are particularly dangerous in the NICU due to the fragile state of newborns. The rapidly changing body weight, different rates of organ development affecting drug pharmacokinetics, and need for dilutions of medications contribute to the common occurrence of medication errors in the NICU. In this study, medication errors occurred as a result of incorrect dosing, documentation, or processing. Morphine, sodium supplementation, and aminoglycosides were the most frequent pharmacological agents administered inappropriately. With the advent of computerized order entry, a reduction in ordering errors is expected due to standardized templates for physicians and nurses. The computerized system also provides an additional way to intercept errors before they affect the newborn. Documentation, communication, and attention to detail can help to reduce preventable medication errors.

In the 21st century, kernicterus still occurs throughout the United States. The most common allegations in our experience were delayed contact and response of the blood bank as well as the inability to perform a timely exchange transfusion. An umbilical venous line is relatively easy to place, even in a newborn up to a week old. However, withdrawing blood is often problematic when using a 3.5 or 5.0 umbilical venous catheter due to the thin walled umbilical vein that collapses with minimal negative pressure. An exchange catheter in the exchange transfusion tray should be utilized whenever possible to expedite the procedure. Too often, subspecialty services are called to gain vascular access, which can greatly delay initiation of the exchange transfusion. A thorough physical exam documenting any signs or symptoms of kernicterus should be charted prior to, during, and after the exchange transfusion.

Although tort reform in some states has reduced non-meritorious legal suits, professional liability involving caregivers of mothers and newborns is significant. We have identified common areas in obstetrics and newborn medicine that resulted in malpractice claims. All practitioners in our field need to examine these areas within their practice and address any deficiencies, implement new protocols, and improve communication and documentation in the medical record. Addressing the issues described can potentially have a favorable impact on the medical malpractice crisis, and more importantly avoid potentially preventable devastating outcomes. We cannot overemphasize the importance of honesty, humility, compassion and competency in all our interactions with our patients.

5. References

ACOG Committee on Obstetric Practice. Umbilical cord blood gas and acid-base analysis. *Obstet Gynecol* 2006; 108: 1319-22.

American Academy of Pediatrics, John Kattwinkel ed, Neonatal Resuscitation Textbook, 5th ed, 2006:16-17.

American College of Obstetricians and Gynecologists, American Academy of Pediatricians. Chapter 5: Neonatal assessment. In: Van Eerden P, Bernstein PS (eds). *Neonatal encephalopathy and cerebral palsy.* ACOG: Washington, DC, 2003, pp 53-62.

Arnon S, Litmonovitz I, Regev RH, Bauer S, Shainkin-Kestenbau R, Dolfin T. Serum amyloid A: An early and accurate marker of neonatal early-onset sepsis. *J Perinatol* 2007; 27: 297-302.

Baergen RN. The Placenta as a Witness. *Clin Perinatol* 2007; 34: 393-407.

Baud O, d'Allest A-M, Lacaze-Masmonteil T, Zupan V, Nedelcoux H, Boithias C, Delaveauecoupet J, Dehan M. The early diagnosis of periventricular leukomalacia in premature infants with positive rolandic sharp waves on serial electroencephalography. *J Pediatr* 1998; 132: 813-7.

Bhutani VK, Donn SM, Johnson LH. Risk management of severe neonatal hyperbilirubinemia to prevent kernicterus. *Clin Perinatol* 2005; 32(1):125-39.

Blickstein I, Green T. Umbilical Cord Blood Gases. *Clin Perinatol* 2007; 34: 451-459.

Bloom SL, Leveno KJ, Spong CY, Gilbert S, Hauth JC, Landon MB et al. Decision-to-incision times and maternal and infant outcomes. *Obstet Gynecol* 2006; 108: 6-11.

Bullard J, Trajanowski M. Simulation and training. eNeonatal Review Newsletter 2011; 8(9):1-11.

Buonocore G, Perrone S. Biomarkers of hypoxic brain injury in the neonate. *Clin Perinatol* 2004; 31: 107-116.

Byard RW, Bourne AJ, Moore L, Little KE. Sudden death in early infancy due to delayed cardiac tamponade complicating central venous line insertion and cardiac catheterization. *Arch Pathol Lab Med* 1992; 116(6): 654-656.

Carroll AE, Buddenbaum JL. Malpractice claims involving pediatricians: epidemiology and etiology. Pediatrics 2007; 120(1):10-17.

Chauhan SP, Chauhan VB, Cowan BD, Hendrix NW, Magann EF, Morrison JC. Professional liability claims and Central Association of Obstetricians and Gynecologists members: Myth versus reality. *AJOG* 2005; 192:1820-8.

Chauhan SP, Hendrix NW, Magann EF, Sanderson M, Bofill JA, Briery CM et al. Neonatal organ dysfunction among newborns at gestational age 34 weeks and umbilical arterial pH < 7.00. *J Matern Fetal Neonatal Med* 2005; 17: 261-268.

Chauhan SP, Magann EF, Scott JR, Scardo JA, Hendrix NW, Martin JN Jr. Emergency cesarean delivery for nonreassuring fetal heart rate tracings: compliance with ACOG guidelines. *J Reprod Med* 2003; 48(12): 975-81.

Chow LC, Wright KW, Sola A, CSMC Oxygen Administration Study Group. Can changes in clinical practice decrease the incidence of severe retinopathy of prematurity in very low birth weight infants? *Pediatrics* 2003; 111(2):339-345.

Chuo J, Hicks RW. Computer-related medication errors in neonatal intensive care units. *Clin Perinatol* 2008; 35(1):119-39.

Cifuentes J, Bronstein J, Phibbs CS, Phibbs RH, Schmitt SK, Carlo WA. Mortality in low birth weight infants according to level of neonatal care at hospital of birth. *Pediatrics* 2002; 109(5):745-751.

Clark SJ, Belfort MA, Byrun SL et al. Improved Outcomes, Fewer Cesarean Deliveries, and Reduced Litigation: Results of a new paradigm in patient safety. *Am J Obstet Gynecol* 2008; 199: 105 e1-7.

Clark SL, Belfort MA, Dildy GA, Meyers JA. Reducing obstetric litigation through alterations in practice patterns. *Obstet Gynecol* 2008; 112: 1279-83.

Clark SL, Hankins GD. Temporal and demographic trends in cerebral palsy - fact and fiction. *Am J Obstet Gynecol* 2003; 188: 628-33.

Cornette L. Fetal and neonatal inflammatory response and adverse outcome. *Seminars in Fetal & Neonatal Medicine* 2000; (9)459-470.

Darling JC, Newell SJ, Mohamdee O, Uzun O, Cullinane CJ, Dear PR. Central venous catheter tip in the right atrium: a risk factor for neonatal cardiac tamponade. *J Perinatol* 2001; 21(7):461-464.

Donn SM, Faix RG, Roloff DW, Goldman EB. Medico-legal consultation: an expanded role of the tertiary neonatologist. *J Perinatol* 1987; 7(3):238-241.

Donn SM. Medicolegal issues get short shrift in pediatric residency training. *AAP News* 2006; 27(7):16.

Donn SM. Take steps to minimize risk when consulting with another physician. *AAP News* 2005; 26(12):24.

Early Treatment For Retinopathy Of Prematurity Cooperative Group. Revised indications for the treatment of retinopathy of prematurity: results of the early treatment for retinopathy of prematurity randomized trial. *Arch Ophthalmol* 2003; 121(12):1684-1694.

Falck AJ, Escobedo MB, Baillargeon JG, Villard LG, Gunkel JH. Proficiency of pediatric residents in performing neonatal endotracheal intubation. *Pediatrics* 2003; 112(6):1242-1247.

Ferriero DM. Neonatal brain injury. *N Engl J Med* 2004; 351: 1985-95.

Finer NN, Robertson CM, Richards RT, Pinnell LE, Peters KL. Hypoxic-ischemic encephalopathy in term neonates: perinatal factors and outcome. *J Pediatr* 1981; 98: 112-7.

Freeman RK. Medical and legal implications for necessary requirements to diagnose damaging hypoxic-ischemic encephalopathy leading to later cerebral palsy. *Am J Obstet Gynecol* 2008; 199:585-586.

Gaies MG, Morris SA, Hafler JP, et al. Reforming procedural skills training for pediatric residents: a randomized, interventional trial. *Pediatrics* 2009; 124(2): 610-619.

Gelfand SL, Fanaroff JM, Walsh MC. Controversies in the treatment of meconium aspiration syndrome. *Clin Perinatol* 2004; 31: 445-452.

Geva R, Eshel R, Leiner Y, Valevski AF, Harel S. Neuropsychological outcome of children with intrauterine growth restriction: a 9-year prospective study. *Pediatrics* 2006; 118: 91-100; www.pediatrics.org/cgi/dol/10.1542/peds.1005-2343.

Glass HC, Glidden D, Jeremy RJ, Barkovich AJ, Ferriero DM, Miller SP. Clinical neonatal seizures are independently associated with outcome in infants at risk for hypoxic-ischemic brain injury. *J Pediatr* 2009; 155(3):318-323.

Goldaber KG, Gilstrap LC III, Leveno KJ, Dax JS, McIntire DD. Pathologic fetal academia. *Obstet Gynecol* 1991; 78: 1103-7.

Goodwin TM, Milner-Masterson L, Paul RH. Elimination of fetal scalp blood sampling on a large clinical service. *Obstet Gynecol* 1994; 83:971-974.

Graham EM, Ruis KA, Hartman AL, Northington FJ, Fox HE. A systematic review of the role of intrapartum hypoxia-ischemia in the causation of neonatal encephalopathy. *Am J Obstet Gynecol* 2008; 199(6): 587-595.

Grether JK, Nelson KB. Maternal infection and cerebral palsy in infants of normal birth weight. *JAMA* 1997; 278: 207-211.

Guidelines for expert witness testimony in medical malpractice litigation. Committee on Medical Liability. American Academy of Pediatrics. *Pediatrics* 2002; 109(5):974-979.

Hankins GDV, MacLennan AH, Speer ME, Strunk A, Nelson K. Obstetric litigation is asphyxiating our maternity services. *Obstet Gynecol* 2006; 107: 1382-5.

Hayakawa F, Okumura A, Kato T, Kuno K, Watanabe K. Determination of timing of brain injury in preterm infants with periventricular leukomalacia with serial neonatal electroencephalography. *Pediatrics* 1999; 104: 1077-1081.

Hermansen MC, Hermansen MG. Perinatal infections and cerebral palsy. *Clin Perinatol* 2006; 33:315-333.

Hermansen MC, Hermansen MG. Pitfalls in neonatal resuscitation. *Clin Perinatol* 2005; 32(1):77-95

Hickson GB, Clayton EW, Githens PB, Sloan FA. Factors that prompted families to file medical malpractice claims following perinatal injuries. *JAMA* 1992; 267(10):1359-1363.

Hoffman MA, Johnson CL, Moore T, Pearl RH. Management of catastrophic neonatal midgut volvulus with a silo and second-look laparotomy. *J Pediatr Surg* 1992; 27(10):1336-1339.

Johnston MV, Donn SM. Hypoxic-ischemic encephalopathy and traumatic intracranial injuries. In: Donn SM, Fisher CW, eds. *Risk Management Techniques in Perinatal and Neonatal Practice.* Futura Publishing Company, Inc.: New York, 1996, p 453.

Kain ZN, Caldwell-Andrews AA. What pediatricians should know about child-related malpractice payments in the United States. *Pediatrics* 2006; 118(2):464-468.

Kirton A, deVeber G. Cerebral palsy secondary to perinatal ischemic stroke. *Clin Perinatol* 2006; 33:367-386.

Korst LM, Phelan JP, Ahn MO, Martin GI. Nucleated red blood cells: an update on the marker for fetal asphyxia. *Am J Obstet Gynecol* 1996; 175: 843-6.

Korst LM, Phelan JP, Wang YM, Ahn MO. Neonatal platelet counts in fetal brain injury. *Am J Perinatol* 1999; 16: 79-83.

Kuzniewicz MW, Escobar GJ, Newman TB. Impact of universal bilirubin screening on severe hyperbilirubinemia and phototherapy use. *Pediatrics* 2009; 124(4):1031-1039.

Larroque B, Bertrais S, Czernichow P, Leger J. School difficulties in 20-year-olds who were born small for gestational age at term in a regional cohort study. *Pediatrics* 2001; 108: 111-115.

Lee HC, Chitkana R, Halamek C, Hintz S. A national survey of pediatric residents and delivery room training experience. *J Pediatr* 2010; 157:158-6.

Lehmann CU, Kim GR. Prevention of medication errors. *Clin Perinatol* 2005; 32(1):107-23.

Leone TA, Rich W, Finer NN. Neonatal intubation: success of pediatric trainees. *J Pediatr* 2005; 146(5):638-641.

Levene MI, Sinha SK. Clinical management of the asphyxiated newborn. In: Donn SM, Sunil K. Sinha SK, Malcolm L. Chiswick ML, eds. *Birth Asphyxia and the Brain*: Basic Science and Clinical Implications. Armonk, NY: Futura Publishing; 2002:297-298.

Levine MI, Chervenak FA, Whittle M. Congenital structural defects of the brain. In: Bennett MF, Punt J (eds). *Fetal and Neonatal Neurology and Neurosurgery* 3rd Edition. Harcourt: London, 2001, pp 211-212.

Li AM, Chau V, Poskitt KJ, Sargent MA, Lupton BA, Hill A, et al. White matter injury in term newborns with neonatal encephalopathy. *Pediatr Res* 2009; 65: 85-89.

MacLennan A, Nelson KB, Hankins G, Speer M. Who will deliver our grandchildren? Implications of Cerebral Palsy Litigation. *JAMA* 2005; 294(13): 1688-1690.

Macones GA, Hankins GDV, Spong CY, Hauth J. The 2008 National Institute of Child Health and Human Development Workshop Report on Electronic Fetal Monitoring. *Obstet Gynecol* 2008; 112: 661-6.

Maisels MJ, Bhutani VK, Bogen D, Newman TB, Stark AR, Watchko JF. Hyperbilirubinemia in the newborn infant ≥ 35 weeks' gestation: an update with clarifications. *Pediatrics* 2009; 124(4):1193-1198.

Mangurten HH, Angst DB, See C, Boyle D, Beckman S. Professional liability in a neonatal intensive care unit: a review of 20 years' experience. *J Perinatol* 2000; 20(40):244-248.

Maung M, Saing H. Intestinal volvulus: an experience in a developing country. *J Pediatr Surg* 1995; 30(5):679-681.

McAbee G. Pediatrics among specialties with highest payments for closed malpractice claims in 1985-2005. *AAP News* 2006; 27(8):18.

Meadow W, Mendez D, Hipps R, Vakharia T, Husein G, Lantos J. The relationship between physician behaviors and blood gas values in the first hours of life--implications for "standards" of medical care for infants with respiratory distress. *Am J Perinatol* 1996; 13(8):457-464.

Mello MM, Studdert DM, Brennan TA. The new medical malpractice crisis. *N Engl J Med* 2003; 348(23):2281-2284.

Mendelson RA. Careful communication, charting can head off malpractice suits. AAP News 2009; 30(2):16.

Miller JD, Carlo WA. Pulmonary complications of mechanical ventilation in neonates. *Clin Perinatol* 2008; 35(1):273-81.

Miller SP, Ramaswamy V, Michelson D, Barkovich J, Holshouser B, Wycliffe N et al. Patterns of brain injury in term neonatal encephalopathy. *J Pediatr* 2005; 146: 453-60.

Muraskas JK, Morrison JC. A proposed evidence-based neonatal work-up to confirm or refute allegations of intrapartum asphyxia. *Obstet/Gynecol* 2010;116:261-8.

Nadroo AM, Glass RB, Lin J, Green RS, Holzman IR. Changes in upper extremity position cause migration of peripherally inserted central catheters in neonates. *Pediatrics* 2002; 110(1):131-136.

Naeye RL, Shaffer ML. Postnatal laboratory timers of antenatal hypoxemic-ischemic brain damage. *J Perinatol* 2005; 25: 664-668.

Nelson KB, Ellenberg JH. Apgar scores as predictors of chronic neurologic disability. *Pediatrics* 1981; 2:181-8.

Neonatal Seizures. In: Volpe J. *Neurology of the Newborn*, 5th ed. Philadelphia, PA: Elsevier Science; 2002:203-244.

Neufeld MD, Frigon C, Graham AS, Nueller BA. Maternal infection and risk of cerebral palsy in term and preterm infants. *J Perinatol* 2005; 25:108-113; doi:10.1038/sj.jp.7211219.

Newman TB, Liljestrand P, Jeremy RJ, et al. Outcomes among newborns with total serum bilirubin levels of 25 mg per deciliter or more. *N Engl J Med* 2006; 354(18):1889-1900.

Okerafor A, Allsop J, Counsell SJ, Fitzpatrick J, Azzopardi D, Rutherford MA, Cowan FM. Patterns of brain injury in neonates exposed to perinatal sentinel events. *Pediatrics* 2008; 121: 906-915.

Papoff P. Use of Hematologic Data to Evaluate Infections in Neonates. In: Christensen, (ed). *Hematologic Problems of the Neonate.* W.B. Saunders: Philadelphia, 2000, pp 389-404.

Pasternak JF, Gorey MT. The syndrome of acute near-total intrauterine asphyxia in the term infant. *Pediatr Neurol* 1998; 18: 391-398.

Perlman J. Intrapartum Asphyxia and Cerebral Palsy: Is There a Link? *Clin Perinatal* 2006; 33:335-353.

Phelan JP, Korst LM, Ahn MO, Martin GI. Neonatal nucleated red blood cell and lymphocyte counts in fetal brain injury. *Obstet Gynecol* 1998; 91: 485-489.

Phelan JP, Martin GI, Korst LM. Birth asphyxia and cerebral palsy. *Clin Perinatol* 2005; 32: 61-76.

Phibbs CS, Baker LC, Caughey AB, Danielsen B, Schmitt SK, Phibbs RH. Level and volume of neonatal intensive care and mortality in very-low-birth-weight infants. *N Engl J Med* 2007; 356(21):2165-2175.

Practical Neonatal Respiratory Care. In: RL Schreiner, JA Kisling (eds). Raven Press: New York, 1982, p 246.

Practical Neonatal Respiratory Care. In: RL Schreiner, JA Kisling (eds). Raven Press: New York, 1982, p 248.

Ramachandrappa A, Jain L. Iatrogenic disorders in modern neonatology: a focus on safety and quality of care. *Clin Perinatol* 2008; 35(1):1-34.

Ramasethu J. Complications of vascular catheters in the neonatal intensive care unit. *Clin Perinatol* 2008; 35(1):199-222.

Raval NC, Gonzalez E, Bhat AM, Pearlman SA, Stefano JL. Umbilical venous catheters: evaluation of radiographs to determine position and associated complications of malpositioned umbilical venous catheters. *Am J Perinatol* 1995; 12(3):201-204.

Riley RJ, Johnson JWC. Collecting and analyzing cord blood gases. *Clin Obstet Gynecol* 1993; 36: 13-23.

Rodger MA, Paidas M, McLintock C, Middeldorp S, Kahn S, Martinelli I et al. Inherited thrombophilia and pregnancy complications revisited. *Obstet Gynecol* 2008;112: 320-4.

Rutherford M, Counsell S, Allsop J, Boardman J, Kapellou O, Larkman D et al. Diffusion-weighted magnetic resonance imaging in term perinatal brain injury: a comparison with site of lesion and time from birth. *Pediatrics* 2004; 114: 1004-1014.

Rutherford M. Neuroimaging. In: Donn SM, Sinha SK, Chiswick ML (eds). In: *Birth Asphyxia and the Brain: Basic Science and Clinical Implications.* Futura Publishing Company, Inc.: New York, 2002, pp 320-321.

Rutherford MA. The asphyxiated term infant. In: Rutherford MA (ed). *MRI of the Neonatal Brain.* W.B. Saunders: London, 2002, p 101.

Sarnat HB, Sarnat MS. Neonatal encephalopathy following fetal distress: a clinical and electroencephalographic study. *Arch Neurol* 1976; 33: 696-705.

Sasidharan P, Billman D, Heimler R, Nelin L. Cardiac arrest in an extremely low birth weight infant: complication of percutaneous central venous catheter hyperalimentation. *J Perinatol* 1996; 16(2):123-126.

Shah DK, Zempel J, Barton T, Lukas K, Inder TE. Electrographic seizures in preterm infants during the first week of life are associated with cerebral injury. *Pediatr Res* 2010; 67(1):102-106.

Shah P, Perlman M. Time courses of intrapartum asphyxia: neonatal characteristics and outcomes. *Am J Perinat* 2009; 26(1): 39-44.

Shah PS, Shah V, Qiu Z, Ohlsson A, Lee SK, Canadian Neonatal Network. Improved outcomes of outborn preterm infants if admitted to perinatal centers versus free standing pediatric hospitals. *J Pediatr* 2005; 146(5):626-631.

Shalak LF, Laptook AR, Jafri HS, Ramilo O, Perlman JM. Clinical Chorioamnionitis, elevated cytokines, and brain injury in term infants. *Pediatrics* 2002;110: 673-680.

Stavroudis TA, Miller MR, Lehmann CU. Medication errors in neonates. *Clin Perinatol* 2008; 35(1):141-61.

Steinman KJ, Gorno-Tempini ML, Glidden DV, Kramer JH, Miller SP, Barkovich AJ, Ferriero DM. Neonatal watershed brain injury on magnetic resonance imaging correlates with verbal IQ at 4 years. *Pediatrics* 2009; 123: 1025-1030.

Strauss RS. Adult functional outcome of those born small for gestational age: twenty-six-year Follow-up of the 1970 British birth cohort. *JAMA* 2000; 283: 625-632.

Subhani M, Combs A, Weber P, Gerontis C, DeCristofaro JD. Screening guidelines for retinopathy of prematurity: the need for revision in extremely low birth weight infants. *Pediatrics* 2001; 107(4):656-659

Tawil KA, Eldemerdash A, Hathlol KA, Laimoun BA. Peripherally inserted central venous catheters in newborn infants: malpositioning and spontaneous correction of catheter tips. *Am J Perinatol* 2006; 23(1):37-40

The American College of Obstetricians and Gynecologists and American Academy of Pediatrics. *Neonatal encephalopathy and cerebral palsy*: defining the pathogenesis and pathophysiology. The American College of Obstetricians and Gynecologists, American Academy of Pediatrics: Washington, DC, 2003.

Thomson TL, Levine M, Muraskas JK, El-Zein C. Pericardial effusion in a preterm infant resulting from umbilical venous catheter placement. *Pediatr Cardiol* 2010; 31(2):287-290

Vargas JE, Allred EN, Leviton A, Holmes LB. Congenital microcephaly: phenotypic features in a consecutive sample of newborn infants. *J Pediatr* 2001; 139: 210-4.

Volpe J. Hypoxic-ischemic encephalopathy: clinical aspects. In: *Neurology of the Newborn*, 5th Edition. W. B. Saunders: Philadelphia, 2008, pp 400-480.

Walker MW, Shoemaker M, Riddle K, Crane MM, Clark R. Clinical process improvement: reduction of pneumothorax and mortality in high-risk preterm infants. *J Perinatol 2002*; 22(8):641-645

Wall SN, Handler AS, Park CG. Hospital factors and nontransfer of small babies: a marker of deregionalized perinatal care? *J Perinatol* 2004; 24(6):351-359

Warner B, Musial MJ, Chenier T, Donovan E. The effect of birth hospital type on the outcome of very low birth weight infants. *Pediatrics* 2004; 113(1):35-41

Westgate J, Garibaldi JM, Greene KR. Umbilical cord blood gas analysis at delivery: a time for quality data. *Br J Obstet Gynaecol* 1994; 101:1054-63.

Wirrell EC, Pelausa EO, Allen AC, Stinson DA, Hanna BD. Massive pericardial effusion as a cause for sudden deterioration of a very low birthweight infant. *Am J Perinatol* 1993; 10(6): 419-423

Wu YW, Escobar GJ, Grether JK, Croen LA, Greene JD, Newman TB. Chorioamnionitis and cerebral palsy in term and near-term infants. *JAMA* 2003; 290: 2677-2684.

Part 6

Frequently Used Medications Guide

16

Administration and Dose of the Most Frequently Used Drugs in Paediatrics

Şenay Çetinkaya
Pediatric Nursing,
Adana School of Health,
Çukurova University,
Turkey

1. Introduction

Though the main aim of modern medicine is the prevention of healthy people, the most of the medical service for treatment today is applied as medical treatment of patients. One of the very important reasons of the service of medical treatment is choice of wrong drugs, and the other is not be able to use the planned treatment truly. The patients may not take the drugs that clinicians suggested themselves. This situation is known to be closely related to the presence of social health organization of patients. The patients may misuse a true treatment. Also the clinicians may cause the problem of drug misuse, especially the antibiotics. Whatever the reason is, the drug misuse causes the public health to deteriorate and economical loses and, this is inevitable. Moreover, some of the drug misuses, like of antibiotics, may imbalance the ecology and cause the problem to convey to next generations (Gokalp & Mollaoglu, 2003).

World Health Organization has defined the use of rational medication as "providing medication to individuals easily, at the lowest prices, and for the most suitable dosages and periods according to clinical findings and personal characteristics of individuals" (Baytemur, 2005; Cetinkaya et al, 2010; Ozdemir, 2010). Antibiotics are among the most important discoveries of the past century (Çetinkaya et al, 2010; Karabay, 2009).

Antibiotic use among the infants at newborn intensive care units is gradually increasing. In a study conducted over 29 newborns in USA, it was determined that 43% of the patients used antimicrobial during their stay. Undergoing microbial application poses a risk in terms of resistance. To avoid the use of antibiotics, in this sense, there have been training programs developed by the American Society of Infection (Patel & Saiman, 2010).

Antibiotics sits atop in the list of most frequently used medication in all countries. Similarly in Turkey, antibiotics are placed on the top in terms of the average per capita medication with a ratio of 17-19% (Çetinkaya et al, 2010; Özdemir, 2010; Ozgunes, 2005). The frequency of antibiotics usage in Turkey for in-patients is over 30%. This ratio increases over 50% for intensive care units (Çetinkaya et al, 2010; Sardan, 2005). While the consumption costs of antibiotics in USA exceed 7 million dollars per year, such medications establish the 30% of the total medication budgets of all hospitals. Nearly half of the antibiotics usage is still not appropriate despite strict control programs and such effort (Akan, 2006; Çetinkaya et al, 2010). In Turkey, antibiotic treatment is prescribed too frequently (Bal, 2005; Celen et al, 2005; Çetinkaya et al, 2010; Özgüneş, 2005;). In a study it is stated that antibiotics are being prescribed to significant portion of the patients who apply to clinics (15-48%) and only 2-2.5% of those prescribed medication was based on culture results (Çetinkaya et al, 2010; Özgüneş, 2005).

Since the prevalence of drug errors are high, it is that imperative that nurses understand the factors leading to errors, and avoid them to the best of their ability (Dinc, 2011).

Without considering by whom it was prescribed, nurses are responsible for the every each medication that is administered personally on legal grounds, moral grounds, and ethical grounds (Dinç, 2011).

All professional nurses should take these issues seriously. Safe and correct medication is one of the principal responsibilities of a nurse during patient care. For a nurse to make free decisions over right medication, correct administration, and providing appropriate means for measurement and monitoring is important for the assessment of the side effects of medication and the patient reactions against it. Reliable medication requires knowledge synthesis, experience, critical approach and intellectual norms (Dinç, 2011).

Comparing to that on an adult, medication administration greatly differs on children, while bringing along responsibilities. It is of the physician's responsibility to write down the doses into drug master file. Nurse, on the other hand, is responsible for administering the medication at the correct amount and on the correct time. Nurse has to know when this medication would start to be effective, for how long it would be effective, what side-effects it might cause, any toxic indications, and counter-measures in respect thereof (Kavakli et al, 1998).

In a study carried out to analyze the knowledge and behavior of pediatricians regarding to the rational use of antibiotics, as well as the socio-demographic factors that might be affecting, 89.8% of the participants reported that, when prescribing antibiotics, they need to see the patient first, whereas, 78.1% indicated that they were prescribing antibiotics according to the patient's clinical condition, 71.1% reported that they had paid attention to the appropriateness of the symptoms, and 67.2% told that they were going to take microbiological culture samples for examination. As for the question '*who should give education about antibiotics*' 32.1% replied as the physician who had prescribed the medication, 23.4% said the junior doctors, 21.9% said pharmacists, 17.2% said the pediatric nurse, 9.4% said nurses (Çetinkaya et al, 2010).

The pediatrics nurses auditing the medication use, evaluation by them if the importance of regular use of the medication is understood or not, to obtain the suitable feedback from the patent and the patient's family by the prescribing physician, adverse effects and what they should do under such circumstances etc., providing training and consultancy on all these are among their duties (Çetinkaya et al, 2010; Çetinkaya &Tengir, 2006).

2. Pharmacological concepts

If taken by a living organism, drug is an agent that brings changes in body functions. Administration of drugs is of the principal practices in nursing. Safety of the patient is the basis in preparation of medication, and during their administration. Along with the nurse's skill in administering drugs, he / she has to possess adequate information about the drug (Gorgulu & Ulusoy, 1996).

2.1 Sources of drugs

These are the basic sources of drugs:

- **Natural sources:** Minerals (like Iron), animals (such as insulin), and plants (such as opium)
- **The synthetics** (*chemical agents manufactured in laboratories*): Synthetic drugs have the same chemical composition with the natural ones, and they are obtained much cheaper; just not every drug could be acquired in this way, though (Görgülü & Ulusoy, 1996).

2.2 Drug nomenclature

Drugs have multiple names:

- *"Chemical Name"* shows its chemical composition.
- *"Generic Name"* (family, registry name) describes the common name of the drug, given by its first manufacturer. This name is given after its chemical name.
- *"Official Name"* is the name for the official publications that would certificate the drug
- *"Trade Name"* or sometimes "Brand Name" is given by the drug's authenticated manufacturer. There can be more than one trade names.

Nurses can recognize the drugs they used frequently by their generic names and trade names (Çavuşoğlu, 2000; Dinç, 2011; Görgülü & Ulusoy, 1996). Because nurses happen to be facing the drugs under good deal of different names, they need to be careful about the name before its administration (Dinç, 2011).

2.3 Classification of drugs

Drugs are classified in various ways. As some could be classified by the body systems, such as "affecting respiratory system", "affecting cardiovascular system", some could be grouped by the syndromes they eliminate (Dinç, 2011; Görgülü & Ulusoy, 1996). Any drug may belong to more than one categories, as in the aspirin, which is an analgesic, antipyretic and anti-inflammatory drug (Dinç, 2011).

2.4 Pharmaceutical type of drugs

A pharmaceutical drug or medicine refers to the final state of medical substances, intended or ready for use in medical applications. The active element of the drug is processed to become useable with other solids or liquids. Drugs are available in different forms so they could be easily taken according to varying needs and conditions:

1. Solid Pharmaceutical Types: powder, cachet, package, capsules, tablet, pastille, pilular, sugar-coated pill, extracts.
2. Semi-liquid semi-solid Pharmaceutical Types: Suppository, ovular, ointments.
3. Liquid Pharmaceutical Types: Solutions, solution for injections, syrup, potion, elixirs, lotions, enema (Çavuşoğlu, 2000; Yüncü, 1994).

2.5 Drug effects

Nurse should be aware of the curing, thus, desired effect of a drug before administering it. Since drugs are chemical compounds they may result in more than one effect, therefore, they may not react the same way for every patient (Dinç, 2011).

2.5.1 Curing effects

These are the desired physiological effects of a drug. Every drug has an intended curing purpose. Aspirin can be used to wear off a pain, reduce fever, help inflammations over edema. It is important for a nurse to know about the curing effects of prescribed medicines. By this way, nurse can properly brief the patient and assess the desired effects of medicine. (Dinç, 2011).

2.5.2 Side effects / adverse effects

Drugs can result in undesired, and sometimes, unexplained reactions in the body. No drug is completely safe. The side-effects can be predictable; these effects can show up even if drug is taken at the appropriate doses. Should the severity of side-effects start exceeding the desired effects, this medication should be abandoned by whom it was prescribed (Dinç, 2011).

Adverse drug reactions are undesired, and, most often, unpredictable effects. They may result in anomalies which would incapacitate the patient. Some of them may show up at short notice, some may take even months (Dinç, 2011).Side effects are those which surface as an unsettling effect to the patient although the dose was appropriate. These may result from the preservatives and other ingredients, or even the drug itself (Çetinkaya &Tengir, 2006).

Nurses should be alarmed for any side effects especially when dealing with new drugs. A nurse should be aware of the fact that even mildly occurring adverse effects may result in severe allergic reactions with high toxicity. Early detection of adverse effects may prevent the patient from getting harmed (Dinç, 2011).

2.5.2.1 Toxic effects

Toxicity determines the level of toxication a substance can cause. The toxicity occurs with the accumulation of drug in the blood due to either high dosage, or oral administration and digestion of an non-oral medication, or failure in metabolism and excretion mechanism. Depending on the drug activity, toxic effects can be deadly (Dinç, 2011).

2.5.2.2 Idiosyncratic reactions

These are unusual reactions in which the patient shows either excessive or too little reaction against a medication. These are unpredictable and it is not possible to determine which patient might develop an idiosyncratic reaction (Dinç, 2011).

2.5.2.3 Allergic reactions

Drug reaction, according to the UN World Health Organization, is defined as "unexpected and harmful reactions that a medicine provided with appropriate doses for the intent of diagnosis, treatment, or preservation is causing" (Çetinkaya et al, 2008; Sin, 2005). Allergic reactions constitute only one part of undesired drug reactions (Çetinkaya et al, 2008; Sin,

2005). Due to lack of feedback, the frequency of reactions on the patients obtaining their medication at outpatient services cannot be determined (Çetinkaya et al, 2008; 2005; Sin, 2005; Tomaç & Üstündağ). As for the hospitalized incidents, the observation rate for drug reactions is 15 - 30% (Çetinkaya et al, 2008; Sin, 2005).

Allergic reactions can be mild as well as they could be serious. Allergic symptoms vary according to patient and medication. With respect to different drug types, antibiotics have the highest incidence rate for allergic reactions (Dinç, 2011).

Allergic medicine reactions, to get her with the most common form of skin reactions constitute 5-10% of the medicine side effects. It is presumed that the hospital expenses due to medicine reactions are 7000 per unit bed year and morbidity and mortality costs are presumed to be more than 136 million dollars only in USA (Çetinkaya & Tengir, 2008).

Antibiotics like Vancomycin, Cephalosporins, and Penicillins, besides, anticonvulsant drugs, narcotic analgesics, and anti-emetics are of the examples to the drugs that cause undesired effects on children. Because most of these effects proceed mildly, the situation can be brought under control easily. However, every three out of ten reactions last longer and require hospitalization. An example to such most serious reactions is "respiratory arrest" which is caused by anaphylaxis, or application of benzodiazepine - narcotic analgesic combination, following a Cephalosporin antibiotic treatment (Pala & Baktir, 2011).

Penicillin was found by Fleming in 1928. Penicillin group of drugs are the most frequently prescribed antibiotic, and they usually are the most common reasons of medicine allergy (Çetinkaya & Tengir, 2008).

Indeed, penicillin allergy is one of the most encountered problems (Çetinkaya et al, 2008; Tomaç & Üstündağ, 2005). It was determined in a study that three out of five antibiotics prescribed in the world in 1999 were derivatives of penicillin. For this reason, penicillin, among all drugs, constitutes the most researched antibiotic group for their allergic reactions (Çetinkaya et al, 2008; Mungan, 2005).

It is estimated that the chance for an allergic reaction to occur following penicillin is 2% for every treatment cure (Çetinkaya et al, 2008; Mungan, 2005). Among children, rate for penicillin allergy is not determined (Cetinkaya & Cag, 2004; Çetinkaya et al, 2008). For the children having medical history of their parents with penicillin allergy, the rate of allergy development by the age of 16 is 26%. The 39% of children who were hospitalized due to drug reactions later showed life-threatening incidents (Çetinkaya et al, 2008; Park & James, 2005).

A research to analyze the knowledge and application of nurses in Penicillin Allergy Test and the factors underlying has been conducted; a total of 161 nurses and midwifes working in twenty-two healthcare centers located in Konya, Turkey has participated. The 83.5% of the participants told that penicillin should be administered at the healthcare centers, 92.1% opted for a nearby medical facility in case of an emergency, and 91.3% of them told that a doctor, at least, should be present at the site of administration for the same reasons. In the end, it was suggested that nurses and midwifes should acquire knowledge about the penicillin test before any penicillin treatment was placed in order, so as precautionary actions could be taken during the application (Çetinkaya et al, 2008).

Patients should definitely be given adequate written material. They should be asked to carry special id cards indicating what drugs they had allergic reaction against. On these allergy cards, name of the active agent, drug's trade name, severity of the reactions that was observed, assessment tests (history, skin test, IgE test, IPT), suggested alternative drug and its doses should be indicated (Çetinkaya et al, 2008; Dursun & Bavbek, 2005).Administration method, the treatment and its length may affect allergic reactions' development. This is what all healthcare personnel should adequately know about. Physicians should monitor these reactions very carefully, because it will be decisive in respect to patient's future drug regime; and if ignored, the treatment will become more and more complicated, effectively requiring much higher costs (Çetinkaya & Tengir, 2008).

2.5.2.4 Drug tolerance and addiction

Any decrease in physiological response following the repeated use of medication or chemical compounds is called "drug tolerance". This tolerance is discovered when the patient starts requiring new doses after steady use of lower doses for a long period. For acute cases, this is not often the case, and tolerance does not develop. The time period required to observe such development can be one month, or even more. Moreover, "cross tolerance" may develop should any drug tolerance occurred initially, and caused other drugs of the similar pharmaceutical properties fail over the same receptor area (Dinç, 2011).

Drug tolerance is not drug addiction. There are two types of drug addictions: psychological and physical. In psychological addiction patient requires the medication not for its desired effects, but for other benefits (Dinç, 2011).

Opioid resistance develops among the long-time opioid users. Despite the increasing doses it gets never enough, and patient gradually starts showing abstinence syndrome (Anand, 2007).

2.5.2.5 Drug interactions

If a drug alters the effect of another drug, the matter at hand is a drug interaction. The occurrence of such is frequent among the people taking multiple medicines at once. Any drug can increase or decrease the effectiveness of another drug, can affect the metabolism and alter the rate of absorption and / or excretion (Dinç, 2011).

If the combined effects of two drugs equal to the sum of the effect of each drugs individually, drug accumulation takes place (Dinç, 2011).

Synergistic effect is told when two drugs are taken simultaneously. By this effect, the physiological effectiveness is increased comparing to that if taken one by one (Dinç, 2011).

2.6 Dose responses of drugs

The differences in people's drug responses are called polymorphism. Factors contributing to this can be environmental, genetic or cultural ones (Dinç, 2011).

The reason for treatment with medicine is to prevent diseases, decrease the effect of a disease or keep that under control. To this end, sufficient amount of medicine should be delivered to the targeted tissues without causing intoxication. Pharmacokinetics studies the period of time a medicine is absorbed, distributed inside, metabolized, and egested from the body. This period involves a steady and dynamic interaction between the human bodies and drugs (Çetinkaya &Tengir, 2006).

The term "bio-availability" is used for the part of the dose that reaches to the circulatory system. The dose interval between the beneficial part of a drug and that causing side effects is called "therapeutic index". The time it takes for drug concentration in blood serum to be halved is called "half-life". Half-life is affected by other drugs, tissue perfusion and organ functions. Determination of the blood level is easier than that of a tissue, in most of the cases. Volume of distribution is a parameter, used to determine the relation between the applied dose and blood concentration of a drug. Volume of distribution is affected by the chemical properties of the drug and patient's physiological condition. "Stable drug level" indicates the egested amount of drug matching the amount of drug which was taken. Usually in clinical practices, stable drug level is attained following 4-5 half-lives.

"Clearance" is the term showing the excretion rate of a drug. Clearance of any drug depends on the volume of distribution, half-life, and patient's physiology, blood circulation of organs, the organ functions, and drug's chemical properties. In clinical terms, clearance is studied in two types: linear (first degree) and nonlinear (zero degree). A drug showing linear pharmacokinetics results in proportional increase to blood and tissue concentrations as the dose increases. Most of the drugs used in newborns (amino glycosides, Vancomycin, Phenobarbital, caffeine, catecholamine) are egested this way. As for the drugs showing nonlinear pharmacokinetic properties, there will be a sharp increase in blood concentration even if there is a mild change in the dose level. Such an unpredictable change is related to enzyme saturation levels in the liver. Therefore, almost all of the drugs egested from liver have nonlinear pharmacokinetics. These drugs, on the other hand, tend to show linear excretion properties if given in therapeutic doses. Approaching to the toxicity levels, this relation becomes nonlinear. Phenytoin is a good example to such drugs (Ovali, 2008).

In order to measure the effects of some drugs, checking blood levels may be required. In the use of amino glycosides, the measurement of both the lowest and the highest concentrations in the blood might be useful. Should the lowest concentration be observed above expected, an excretion problem can be considered, thus, dose intervals are extended (or narrowed when the concentration was lower). Deviations in the maximum values, on the other hand, require changes in the dose amount, not in the interval. Because those inspections require considerable amount of blood taking, for the infants, it is a better idea to make with clinical overview instead of following the routine, unless the drug levels are required in case of necessity (Ovalı, 2008).

Factors related to the growth and development of a child may affect the drug effect and its excretion. Maturation lag or natal disorders do affect the drug absorption, its effect and excretion (Kavaklı et al, 1998).

Comparing to adults, newborns exhibit great differences physiologically, anatomically, and pharmacologically. Renal functions in the newborn are reduced since the glomerular and tubular functions are infrequent, and blood circulation at the kidneys is low. Glomerular filtration and tubular functions reach to their mature levels after 20 weeks from delivery, whereas, this is 2 years for renal functions. Newborn's ability for water-retention and excretion of solutes are insufficient. All of these reasons cause extended half-lives. On a full-term infant the liver is immature. Enzymes playing role in drug mechanisms are not sufficient. Only through the infant's growth, the blood circulation in liver increases, and the enzyme maturation is completed. Glycogen stores are minimal at the liver of premature infants; they cannot stockpile large protein molecules. The albumin and other proteins which are involved in drug metabolism are kept in minimum amounts; subsequently, the free fractionation of drugs increases (Ozcengiz, 2011).

Drug response in infants varies according to the body's muscle - fat - water distribution, protein binding, body temperature, the cardiac outflow, physiological maturation of heart, maturation of blood - brain barrier, efficiency of the liver and kidneys, and whether a congenital malformation exists or not. Total body water is higher in premature newborns comparing to a newborn, and in newborns in comparing to a 2 years old. The rate of fat and muscle increases with the age, a significant characteristic for the clinical applications of newborn. Water-soluble drugs have higher volume-distribution. Thus, starting doses are greater to attain desired blood-levels. Because the fat-rate is lower in newborns, drugs redistributed to the fatty tissues, as well as those redistributed to muscle-tissues have longer effects. There are also other factors affecting a newborn's drug-response. Since the volume-distribution is wider, the excretion is delayed. Liver and kidney functions are insufficient; the rate of protein binding is low. Moreover, the presence of prematurity, sepsis, congestive cardiac failure, increased intra-abdominal pressure, controlled ventilation, and insufficient nutrition do affect the drug response adversely. Ultimately, reviewing the drug pharmacokinetics and pharmacodynamics are required for each and every newborn (Özcengiz, 2011).

For a drug to be used in the body, first, it should be absorbed (should pass to the blood from its entry point), be distributed (its delivery through circulation to the impact area) and be transformed to its active state. Later on, it is broken up with the metabolism, and egested from body as a drug metabolite. This mechanism prevents the toxicity of regular medication due to accumulation in body. For infants and children, absorption, distribution, metabolism, and excretion mechanisms differ from those in adults due to the immaturity of their body systems (Çetinkaya &Tengir, 2006).

3. Drug pharmacokinetics

The term *pharmacokinetics refers to the way a drug is handled by the body. Pharmacokinetic* measures, such as area under the curve (AUC) and concentration at the maximum (Cmax) and parameters calculated from those measures, such as clearance, half-life, and volume of distribution, reflect the absorption (A), distribution (D), and elimination (E) of a drug from the body. A drug can be eliminated by both metabolism (M) to one or more active and inactive metabolites and excretion of the unchanged drug. The overall set of processes is often referred to as ADME, which ultimately controls systemic exposure to a drug and its metabolites after drug administration (Buxton & Benet, 2011).

This systemic exposure, reflected in plasma drug and/or metabolite concentrations, is generally used to relate dose to both beneficial and adverse effects. All drugs show inter- and intra-individual variance in pharmacokinetic measures and/or parameters (Buxton & Benet, 2011). Variances can sometimes be substantial. In the pediatric population, growth and developmental changes in factors influencing ADME also lead to changes in pharmacokinetic measures and/or parameters. To achieve AUC and Cmax values in children similar to values associated with effectiveness and safety in adults, it may be important to evaluate the pharmacokinetics of a drug over the entire pediatric age range in which the drug will be used. Where growth and development are rapid, adjustment in dose within a single patient over time may be important to maintain a stable systemic exposure.

Developmental changes in the pediatric population that can affect absorption include effects on gastric acidity, rates of gastric and intestinal emptying, surface area of the absorption site, and gastrointestinal enzyme systems for drugs that are actively transported across the gastrointestinal mucosa, gastrointestinal permeability, and biliary function.

3.1 Absorption

Absorption is the period of a drug to pass into body-liquids and to be brought to its receptor zone (Çetinkaya &Tengir, 2006).

Similarly, developmental changes in skin, muscle, and fat, including changes in water content and degree of vascularization, can affect absorption patterns of drugs delivered via intramuscular, subcutaneous, or percutaneous absorption (Buxton & Benet, 2011).

Drugs are delivered through intravascular (*intravenous*) or extravascular (*intramuscular, oral, sublingual, subcutaneous, or rectal*) routes. A drug administered via extravascular route should be absorbed in order to reach its receptor zone (Çetinkaya &Tengir, 2006).

The absorption of most drugs at the gastrointestinal system is through passive diffusion. Absorption is affected by the delivery route, drug density, medium's acidity, and the local circulation. For newborns and infants, the drugs given orally usually have a belated absorption (Çetinkaya &Tengir, 2006).

A drug to pass from cell-membrane shouldn't be ionized. Acidic drugs ionize at alkaline medium. Since these drugs do not ionize at the acidic medium they are absorbed well. The stomach pH of a newborn is acidic (1-3); by the 4th month the acidity approaches to that of an adult's 50%, and around the age of 3 it gets near-adult-values (0.9-1.5) (Çetinkaya &Tengir, 2006).

Decreasing stomach activity for newborns and infants affect the drug absorption, too. For newborns, stomach is empties in 6-8 hours; this number reaches to adult values of 2 hours at the age of 6-8 months. Irregular peristaltic movements until the 8th month cause this procrastination, also delaying drug's blood-levels. Furthermore, newborns do not exhibit efficient absorption since their intestinal enzyme developments were delayed (Çetinkaya &Tengir, 2006).

Absorption of intramuscular or subcutaneous drugs depends on the tissue perfusion at the primer application zone. Since the circulation at muscles and various tissues are less than sufficient, the absorption of intramuscular or subcutaneous drugs is decreased (Çetinkaya &Tengir, 2006).

Slow blood circulation can also affect the drug absorption in newborns. Drug distribution can be limited for the infants carrying cardiovascular disease (Çetinkaya &Tengir, 2006).

Oral use: Although oral use is the most frequent drug administration type, this is not preferred for newborns. Stomach acids secretion in newborns and infants is low; their digestive juice is close to neutral. The bioavailability of basic drugs is decreased, whereas that of acidic ones (*Ampicillin*) is increased. Moreover, gastro-intestinal motilities are irregular; these are slower in newborn and infants, while they are faster than adults in children (Pala & Baktır, 2011).

Rectal use: It is an alternative route when oral use is not applied due to nausea, vomiting, or other reasons. Some analgesic - antipyretic drugs, valproic acid, Diazepam, Phenobarbital, and some corticosteroids can be administered this way. Absorption of the drugs that are applied as a suppository in the rectum is neither regular, nor exact (Pala & Baktır, 2011).

Intramuscular use (IM): it is weak and irregular for newborns and infants. This is caused by the irregularities in blood circulation and vasomotor functions (Pala & Baktır, 2011).

Percutaneous use: With the stratum corneum layer too thin, skin hydration is excessive in newborns. Therefore, locally applied drugs are absorbed more than that in the adults, making undesired toxicity quite possible. Especially, topical preparations containing corticosteroid require significant attention (Pala & Baktır, 2011).

3.2 Distribution

Distribution of a drug may be affected by changes in body composition, such as changes in total body water and adipose tissue, which are not necessarily proportional to changes in total body weight. Plasma protein binding and tissue binding changes arising from changes in body composition with growth and development may also influence distribution (Buxton & Benet, 2011).

Prior to the absorption, drug is carried to organs and tissues through blood-circulation. Composition of body liquids and the drug's level of protein-binding affect the distribution level. Plasma albumin is a primer binding-place for drugs. This binding phenomenon delimits the amount of free drug in circulation, hence, preventing drug to attain at toxic levels (Çetinkaya &Tengir, 2006).

The amount of binding to plasma protein differs from one drug to another. Therefore, density and the amount of the drug that reached to the receptor zone are not proportional to dose. Neonatal albumin has lower binding capacity to some drugs (*Phenytoin*).

Should the active free drugs remain at high levels in blood, the chances for toxic effects to surface become more likely. The water amount in body is a significant parameter used to determine the highest attained drug density. The total water amount of premature infants constitutes the 80-85% of their total weight, whereas this ratio is 75% for interm infants, and it is at adult-like levels (50-60%) by the end of age two. Given the amount of total weight to adjust proportional dose levels, administering drugs that are water-soluble results in insufficient drug density in blood-plasma; thus, more appropriate doses are used for infants (Çetinkaya &Tengir, 2006).

The ability to metabolize drugs in newborns (especially premature infants) is quite limited due to physiological immaturity (Çetinkaya &Tengir, 2006).

Once metabolized, drugs transform into water-soluble compositions for excretion at kidneys. Most of this bio-transfer takes places in the liver. Two-to-three weeks from delivery, liver enzymes begins to maturate; at about the 4th week liver functions are fully developed and the excess drugs can be metabolized. If this period is not taken into account, the non-metabolized drugs begin to accumulate at toxic levels (Çetinkaya &Tengir, 2006).

Because the metabolism rate of an infant (and small child) is faster than an adult, certain drugs can be metabolized also faster. Another factor is the change in liver size. Fetal liver is the 4% of total weight in infants, while this is 2% for adults. This alone explains why many drugs are disposed more quickly, and, accordingly, why the children require medication in higher-doses (Çetinkaya &Tengir, 2006).

The volume of body liquids vary comparing to adults. Comparing to total weight, body liquids in children are more than they are in adults (Pala & Baktır, 2011).

The relative mass of fatty tissues and skeleton muscle tissues are less than those at adults. Especially fat-soluble drugs have greater distribution volume; they should be used in lower doses (Pala & Baktır, 2011).

The rate of drugs' protein binding is lower since the total protein concentration is lower than that in adults. Since the free drug concentration in the blood is higher, so is for the toxicity risk (Pala & Baktır, 2011).

The blood-brain barrier isn't fully developed. There is a risk for hypersensitivity against the drugs affecting the central (Pala & Baktır, 2011).

3.3 Metabollsm

Drug metabolism usually occurs in the liver, but may also occur in the blood, gastrointestinal wall, kidney, lung, and skin. Developmental changes in metabolizing capacity can affect both absorption and elimination, depending on the degree to which intestinal and hepatic metabolic processes are involved. Although developmental changes are recognized, information on drug metabolism of specific drugs in newborns, infants, and children is limited. In general, it can be assumed that children will form the same metabolites as adults via pathways such as oxidation, reduction, hydrolysis, and conjugation, but rates of metabolite formation can be different (Buxton & Benet, 2011).

There are qualitative and quantitative differences in biotransformation between a newborn and other age groups. (Pala & Baktır, 2011).

The metabolism capacity of most drugs is rudimental in newborns; on the contrary, various metabolism pathways show significant development during the first one year (Pala & Baktır, 2011).

In some cases, the dominant metabolic route differs at the infants and children. Caffeine synthesis due to the methylation of teophylline is developed well at infants (Pala & Baktır, 2011).

Glucuronidation at infants is insufficient (Pala & Baktır, 2011).

Sulfide conjugation is developed at infants. Paracetamol absorption is similar to adults (Pala & Baktır, 2011).

3.4 Protein binding

Protein binding may change with age and concomitant illness. In certain circumstances, an understanding of protein binding may be needed to interpret the data from a blood level measurement and to determine appropriate dose adjustments. In vitro plasma protein binding studies can determine the extent of binding of the parent and the major active metabolite(s) and identify specific binding proteins, such as albumin and alpha-1 acid glycoprotein. Optimal estimates of the degree to which protein binding is linear may be obtained by testing maximumand minimum observed concentrations (Buxton & Benet, 2011).

The main reason that age affects drug action is that drug elimination is less efficent in newborn babies and in old people, so that drugs commonly produce greater and more prolonged effects at the extremes of life. Other age-related factors, such as variation in pharmacodynamic sensitivity, are also important with some drugs.

3.5 Excretion

Drug excretion by the kidney is controlled by glomerular filtration, tubular secretion, and tubular re-absorption (Buxton & Benet, 2011). Because these processes mature at different rates in the pediatric population, age can affect systemic exposure for drugs where renal excretion is a dominant pathway of elimination. Consideration should also be given to the maturation of other excretory pathways, including biliary and pulmonary routes of excretion. Glomerular filtration rate (GFR) in the newborn, normalized to body surface area, is only about 20% of the adult value, and tubular function is also reduced. Accordingly, plasma elimination half-lives of renal eliminated drugs are longer in neonates than in adults. In babies born at term, renal function increases to values similar to those in young adults in less than a week, and indeed continues to increase to a maximum of approximately twice the adult value at 6 months of age. The increase in renal function occurs more slowly in premature infants. Renal immaturity in premature infants can have a very large effect on drug elimination. For example, in premature newborn babies the antibiotic Gentamicin has a plasma half-life of 18 hours or greater, compared with 1-4 hours for adults, and approximately 10 hours for babies born at term. It is, therefore, necessary to reduce and/or space out doses to avoid toxicity in premature babies.

Drugs and their metabolites are excreted through sweat, urine, stools, or enzymes. By the time kidney functions develop, disposing drugs via urinary system is limited. The glomerular filtration speed and the circulation in kidneys are 30-40% of adults; this ratio is even smaller for infants delivered before 34 weeks. Following the first two weeks, the glomerular filtration speed is doubled, eventually reaches to adult-levels in 2.5 - 5 months (Çetinkaya &Tengir, 2006). Glomerular filtration speed meets adult levels in 6 - 12 months (Pala & Baktır, 2011). The half-lives of drugs also change (Pala & Baktır, 2011).

4. Pharmacodynamic changes in children

Results obtained from clinical trials and experimentation with the animals show that receptor development leads to changes in drug response. Serotonin is a neurotransmitter paying important role in the behavioral and psychiatric disorders. Serotonin at the brain steadily decreases with the increasing age. The pharmacodynamic response of Dopamine, also an important neurotransmitter, varies largely in the newborn and adult test animals. Many neurological, psychiatric and behavioral disorders are related to the dopamine at SSS. Among the pharmacodynamic responses of the drugs which are being used against this type of disorders may show significant differences during infancy and childhood.

Major factors affecting the newborn's response to a treatment: Gestation age, chronological age, weight, development phase, liquid-electrolyte balance, disorder level at the organ systems and functions, presence of co-existing diseases, accompanying other medication (Ovalı, 2008).

5. Principles of pharmacotherapy for the pediatric patients

- Assessment of clinical / laboratory findings regarding to the drugs used,
- Confirmation of patient's age, body weight, and dose regime; making out the discrepancies in drug absorption, distribution, metabolism and excretion between the infants and children,
- Choosing the most suitable dose type and regime,
- Preparation of a stabile and suitable dose form if no commercial package is available,
- Using the most affective, safest, and fine tasted economic drugs by use of comparative tests,
- Monitoring adverse effects and drug reactions, recognizing the undesired outcomes on children,
- Applying changes in the drugs, dose, or dose intervals when necessary,
- Regular communication with the patient and patient relatives during the treatment (Pala & Baktır, 2011).

5.1 Major problems of pediatric patients related to drug use

- They have inadequate prospectus knowledge
- Dose forms are insufficient for the pediatric population
- Pharmacokinetics, effectiveness, and reliability data through clinical tests are either insufficient or completely absent
- The parameters regarding primary activity for each age groups should be determined
- Duration of disease, age groups, and maturation period should be considered
- Oral suspensions should be developed
- Tablets and capsule sizes should be at appropriate sizes for pediatric patients
- Appropriate dose types should be improved for individual use (Pala & Baktır, 2011).

The drug manufacturers design drugs according to adult population. With the increasing doses on pediatric patients, the drugs used in adults generally cause trouble (Schultheis et al, 2006). Although most drugs in the market are steadily used on pediatric patients today, only one fourth of these drugs have actually been approved by the FDA (Food and Drug Administration) for their use on infants (Pala & Baktır, 2011). FDA has a website in order to give assistance for who might be willing to carry out clinical tests on pediatric patients (Schultheis et al, 2006).

5.1.1 Dose forms

Regarding new products in the market, drug manufacturers generally take little interest in the production of liquid forms that are to be used on infants and children. Among the reasons, likely obligations, limited sources, and the little market share of pediatric drugs can be told. Not having been approved, most of the products are kept being used on the infants and children. Formulation of these medications may not be appropriate for pediatric patients just because they are fit for adults. Liquid forms are preferred for oral use on infants. Infants have difficulty in swallowing capsules and tablets. Besides they are too sized for them, their active ingredients are equally too much. Measuring the appropriate dose becomes, therefore, difficult. Most drugs do not dissolve in the water entirely. To make use of some drugs on the infants orally, suspensions should be formed. Carboxymethylcellulose and methylcellulose are used to achieve this. Most of the intravenous drugs used in adults are very concentrated. Therefore, their use on infants and children are quite difficult. Due to difficulties in dosing, toxic reactions are reported related to digoxin and morphine use on infants. The parenteral drugs to be used on infants, but are used in adults, are diluted in injection water or in 0.9% NaCl. The stability of these drugs should be tested for their active components and sterilities. The excipient components used in drug production are often inert matters, some of which might result in undesired effects. The benzyl alcohol used as preservative show serious toxic properties on infants; sorbitol used in high volumes as excipient may result in diarrhea. In addition, the propylene glycol used in preparations such as Phenytoin, Phenobarbital, digoxin, diazepam, vitamin D, and hydralzine, leads to hyperosmolarity on infants (Pala & Baktır, 2011).

5.1.2 Dosing in children

Calculation according to body weight is a preferred way of measuring the infant dose, especially using the Clark formula (Pala & Baktır, 2011).

Clark Formula:

Infant dose = Infant weight (kg)/ 72 x adult dose

Many clinic experiments show that the dose calculations according to the surface area (m^2) are more suitable than those using body weights for their least erroneous, thus, preferred aspect. Respiration metabolism, blood volume, extracellular liquid amount, glomerular filtration speed, and renal blood circulation are among the physiological parameters showing strong correlation with the body surface. Most of these functions have a direct affect on drug elimination (Pala & Baktır, 2011).

Since the metabolism is faster in children, infant doses (per kg. weight) can be greater than that of adults (Pala & Baktır, 2011).

Among the drugs given to infants in greater amount (per kg.) are as follow: Phenytoin, Diazepam, Imipramine, Phenobarbital, Teophylin, Chlomypramin, Carbamazepine, Enprophylin, Haloperidol, Ethosuximide, Digoxin, Chlorpromazine, Clonazepam, some anti-cancerogenic drugs (Pala & Baktır, 2011).

With the lower renal and hepatic functions, infants require longer drug intervals comparing to children and adults. For children to get appropriate doses, thorough clinical tests and drug's blood level studies are required. Due to certain ethical reasons, carrying out clinical studies over the children is difficult. In addition to the outstanding ethical reasons, too little size of the samples resulting in inefficiency in determination, insufficient experimental equipment specific to children, other varying parameters on a long-term study, contribute to such difficulties (Pala & Baktır, 2011).

6. Drugs

6.1 Antibacterial drugs

Antibacterial (chemical agents which cease the reproduction of microorganisms or kill them) agents are the most frequently used group of pediatric drugs. These drugs are to be influential as bactericide or bacteriostatic corrupting the structure or the functions of the microbial cell (Eroğlu, 2002; Ovalı, 2002).

6.1.1 Penicillin

Penicillin influences the gram-positive coccus, some gram-negative microorganisms and spirochetes. They are used in order to provide prophylaxis in streptococcus, pneumococcus, staphylococcus, salmonella, shigella infections, venereal diseases and also in rheumatic fever (Kavaklı et al, 1998).

6.1.1.1 Oral preparations

Penicillin G has a variable absorption level as it is acid-labile. *Penicillin V* is acid-resistant and absorbed better (Eroğlu, 2002).

400.000 U=250 mg penicillin, 25.000-50.000 U/kg/day rheumatic fever prophylaxis; 400.000 U/day (every 12 hours) (Eroğlu, 2002).

6.1.1.2 Parenteral preparations

6.1.1.2.1 Benzyl penicillin (crystallized penicillin G)

The antibacterial spectrum is limited. It cannot be administered by oral route as it is decomposed in gastric acid and is not well-absorbed by digestive tract (Rang et al, 1998; Dökmeci 2000).

Newborn: IV 15-30 min. 6 dose/day every 4 hours established optimal treatment.
Newborn: <2000g: 50.000 U/kg/day (every 12 hours)
In Meningitis: 100.000 U/kg/day (every 12 hours)
Newborn: >2000g: 75.000 U/kg/day (every 12 hours)
In Meningitis: 150.000 U/kg/day (every 12 hours)
Infant (I), child (C): 100.000-250.000 U/kg/day (every 4-6 hours)
In Serious Infections: 200-400.000 U/kg/day (every 4-6 hours)
Higher doses are required in B group streptococcal meningitis (Apak, 1996).
Side effects are as follows: allergy, shock, anaphylaxis, serum disease, rash, gastrointestinal system (GIS) (Eroğlu, 2002).

6.1.1.2.2 Procaine penicillin G

After IM injection it is a slowly absorbed, water-insoluble crystal salt of penicillin G. It is used in pneumococcus, streptococcus and meningococcal infections. Newborn: 50.000 U/kg/day IM (single dose); the others 25-50.000 U/kg/day IM (single dose) (Dökmeci, 2000).

Side effects: Allergy, shock (Apak, 1996).

6.1.1.2.3 Benzathine penicillin G

It is a salt of penicillin G which establishes quite low serum levels, which is water-insoluble and whose effect however remains for 3-4 weeks. In rheumatic fever prophylaxis, 600.000-1.200.000 U/dose IM (each month) is applied. Penadur LA, Deposilin are its derivatives. It does not cause shock (Apak, 1996; Dökmeci, 2000; Eroğlu, 2002).

Monitoring: Shall high doses be applied in patients with renal failure the serum sodium and potassium levels should be monitored. They should be monitored in terms of extravasation (Kanmaz, 2010).

Caution: The crystallized penicillin G should only be used IV. Procaine and benzathine penicillin G should only be used IM (Kanmaz, 2010).

Incompatible Drugs: Amphotericin B, aminophylline, aminoglycosides, metoclopramide (Kanmaz, 2010).

The things to be considered by nurse applying the drug: Nurse should know whether child is allergic to the drug or not (Kavaklı et al, 1998).

After the vial is diluted with sterile water the drug should be well dissolved before the desired dose is taken from the vial.

In case that high dose of Penicillin G is rapidly administered by IV route it can cause such electrolyte imbalances as potassium and sodium. So the drug should be administered very slowly. When administered by IM route, the injection area should be carefully selected; the drug should be administered deep and the area should be frequently changed (Kavaklı et al, 1998).

After the drug is administered by parenteral route the children should at least be monitored for an hour especially in terms of allergy and anaphylaxis. The presence of erythema and pallor in the injection area of IV and IM can be a sign of sensitivity. And also in case that the child is observed with anxiety, nausea, vomiting, dyspnea, tremor, instant febrility, and rash it should be considered that it might be an allergic reaction. Allergic reactions should immediately be notified to doctor. Drug, tools and equipment should all be available for an emergency (Kavaklı et al, 1998).

In case of an extravasation hyaluronidase can be used (Kanmaz, 2010).

Toxicity symptoms should be closely monitored in newborns, infants and people with renal failure. Bleeding time should be monitored (Kavaklı et al, 1998).

In oral route the best is to administer the drug with water pre-meals. Administering the drug 1 hour before, or 2 hours later than the meals decreases the effect of gastric acid or the possibility that foods delay the absorption of drugs. Child should be prevented from drinking acid beverages 1 hour before and after the administration of drug (Kavaklı et al, 1998).

Tablet drugs should be protected against light. Oral suspensions and syrups should be preserved in refrigerator. The infusion solutions of penicillin G can stay for 24 hours under room temperature (Kavaklı et al, 1998).

6.1.2 Penicillines resistant to penicillinase enzyme

This group of penicillin cannot hydrolyze with staphylococcal penicillinase. This antibiotic is preferred in staphylococcal infections resistant to penicillin (Eroğlu, 2002; Küçüködük, 1994).

6.1.2.1 Methicillin

In newborn,

IM, IV (15-30min.), <2000g <14 days: 50 mg/kg/day (every 12 hours),
<2000g >14 days: 75 mg/kg/day (every 8 hours),
>2000g <14 days: 75 mg/kg/day (every 8 hours),
>2000g >14 days: 100 mg/kg/day (every 6 hours),
For others: IV (15-30 min.), IM 100-200 mg/kg/day (every 4-6 hours), PO: 50-100 mg/kg/day (every 6 hours) (Eroğlu, 2002; Küçüködük 1994).
Side effects: It can cause interstitial nephritis. The dose should be adjusted in renal failure. Along with other penicillin it can produce cross allergic reaction (Apak, 1996).

6.1.2.2 Aminopenicillin

6.1.2.2.1 Amoxicillin

Even if administered with meals through GIS amoxicillin is absorbed faster and almost completely and has fewer side effects compared to ampicillin. It is an acid resistant ampicillin derivative and administered at a dose of PO; 25-50 mg/kg/day (every 8 hours) (Longo et al, 2002).

In a study where Feder and his friends (1999) compared the effects of Amoxicillin and Penicillin V it has been found out that amoxicillin does better than penicillin V in the treatment of angina caused by group a beta-hemolytic streptococcus (Feder et al, 1999).

6.1.2.2.2 Ampicillin

It covers the gram negative spectrum of penicillin. Newborn: IM, IV (15-30 min.), <7 days <2000 g: 50 mg/kg/day (every 12 hours), >2000 g: every 8 hours, >7 days <2000 g: 100 mg/kg/day, >2000 g: every 6 hours.

Infant, child: 50-100 mg/kg/day, PO (every 4-6 hours), Sepsis: 100-200 mg/kg/day IV (every 4 hours), Meningitis: 200-400 mg/kg/day IV (every 4 hours), in other infections: 100-200 mg/kg/day IV (every 4-6 hours) (Eroglu, 2002; Dokmeci, 2000; Kucukoduk, 1994).

Mode of Administration: IV slow
Preparation: Vials are prepared with 5-10 ml sterile water.
Miscible Serums: 5% Dex, SF
Drugs to be confronted at the end point: Fat emulsions, Acyclovir, Aminophylline, Calcium gluconate, Cefepime, Furosemide, Heparin, Insulin, Magnesium sulfate, Metronidazole, Potassium chloride, Vancomycin.
Incompatible Drugs: Dex/Amino acid, Amicasin, Dopamine, Epinephrine, Fluconazole, Gentamicin, Midazolam, Sodium bicarbonate.
Storage Conditions: Should be consumed in 1 hour.

6.1.2.2.3 Ampicillin sodium sulbactam

Dose: Dose is determined by your doctor. Typically, adults and children weighing over 30 kg - 375-750 mg 2 times daily for 5-14 days. Children under 30 kg body weight, have completed one year of age - 25 - 50 mg /kg body weight per day in two divided doses every 12 hours.

Uses: Broad-spectrum antibiotic useful against group *B. streptococcus, Listeria monocytogenes,* and suscetible *E coli* species

Adverse Effectes: Very large doses may results in CNS excitation or seizure activity. Moderate prolongation of bleeding times (by approximately 60 second) may occure after repeated doses. Hypersensitivity reaction (maculopapular rash, ulticarial rash, off fever) are rare in neonates (Young & Mangum, 2010).

6.1.3 Side effects of penicillin

6.1.3.1 Allergic reactions

Penicillin allergy can be diagnosed by taking a skin test. Acute allergic reactions can be such delayed reactions as anaphylaxis, angioneurotic edema and urticarial; and also be fever, eosinophilia, hemolytic anemia, serum disease, urticarial and maculopapular rash. The presence of rash is not indication to cease drug use (Eroğlu, 2002).

6.1.3.2 Dose-related effects

High doses can cause CNS toxicity, hypopotassemia and coagulation impairments (Apak, 1996; Eroğlu, 2002).

6.1.4 Cephalosporins

Their mechanisms of action resemble to penicillin. They are grouped in four generations. As the generation increases the activity against gram (-) also increases. The ones aside from cefuroxime and third-generation are not able to penetrate CNS. They cannot be used in bacterial meningitis treatment. Cephalosporins are commonly used because of their clinical utilities in the treatment of common infections (Rang et al, 1998; Zeph, 2002).

While maculopapular rash, drug-related fever and positive Coomb's test are the major side effects such reactions and anaphylaxis as urticarial and serum diseases are rarely seen (Rang et al, 1998; Zeph, 2002).

Cephalosporins cause allergic reactions in patients allergic to Penicillin. With the use of cephalosporin side effects are observed in 10% of the patients allergic to Penicillin (Puchner & Zacharisen, 2002).

6.1.4.1 First-generation cephalosporins

They are active against gram (+) cocci including staphylococcus aureus, and such gram (-) organisms as *E. coli* and *Klebsiella.* They are inactive against enterococci and H. influenzae. First-class cephalosporins cannot cross the blood-brain barrier and so are not effective in the treatment of central nervous system infections (Apak, 1996; Behrman & Kliegman, 2001; Dökmeci, 2000; Eroğlu, 2002).

6.1.4.1.1 Cephadroxil

Administered at the dose of 30 mg/kg/day (every 12 hours) PO, It has such side effects as hypersensitivity reactions, rarely renal toxicity, neuropathy, and eosinophilia (Apak, 1996; Behrman & Kliegman, 2001; Eroğlu, 2002).

6.1.4.1.2 Cephalothin

Newborn; IV (15-30 min.), IM <7 days; 40 mg/kg/day administered every 12 hours; >7 days; 60 mg/kg/day administered every 8 hours. The side effects are the same as in cephadroxil (Apak, 1996; Eroğlu, 2002).

6.1.4.1.3 Cefazolin sodium

Newborn; 40 mg/kg/day IM-IV administered every 6 hours. Cefazol, Cefamezin, Maksiporin, Cefozin are its derivatives. It rarely has such side effect as rash, positive Coomb's test, coagulopathy in uremic patients (Apak, 1996; Eroğlu, 2002).

6.1.4.2 Second-generation cephalosporins

They are used in gram (+) cocci, penicillinase producing and not producing H. influenzae, in *Klebsiella pneumonia* related bronchopulmonary infections, in E. Coli or proteus related nosocomial infections, in urinary infections caused by enterobacters and in the treatment of sinusitis and otitis media for the ones allergic to amoxicillin (Dökmeci, 2001).

Unlike others Cefuroxime is the only second-generation cephalosporin to cross blood-brain barrier. In case of an infection it is able to penetrate CNS. It is especially used in H. influenzae meningitis and sepsis treatment (Eroğlu, 2002).

6.1.4.2.1 Cefaclor

It is used in the treatment of upper and lower respiratory tract, urinary tract, skin and soft tissue infections as well as in otitis media and susceptible organisms. And it is administered every 8 hours at a dose of 20-40 mg/kg/day (Behrman & Kliegman, 2001; Eroğlu, 2002).

6.1.4.2.2 Cefoxitin

In children older than 3 months it is administered every 6-8 hours at a dose of 60-80 mg/kg/day either as IV or IM. It can cause thrombophlebitis, diarrhea and pseudomembranous colitis (Apak, 1996; Eroğlu, 2002).

6.1.4.3 Third-generation cephalosporins

Compared to first-generation cephalosporins they are less active against gram (+) cocci; however more active against most of the strains of gram (-) cocci. While they are moderately active against *Pseudomonas aeruginosa* they are more active against *H. influenza* and *N. gonorrhoeae*. They can easily penetrate into CNS from inflamed meninges. They are usually discharged from kidneys (Dökmeci, 2000).

6.1.4.3.1 Cefotaxime sodium

Treatment of neonatal meningitis and sepsis caused by susceptible gram-negative organisms (e.g. *E coli, H influenzae,* and *Klebsiella*), Treatment of disseminated gonococcal infections.

Dose: 50 mg/kg IV (Young & Mangum, 2010).

Newborn; < 7 days: (100 mg/kg/day) 12 hours interval, > 7 days; (150 mg/kg/days) IV-IM 8 hours interval, others; 100-200 mg/kg/days IV-IM 6-8 hours interval, for Meningitis; 200 mg/kg/days IV 6 hours interval (Apak, 1996; Eroğlu, 2002; Küçüködük, 1994).

Adverse Effects: neurotoxicity risk increases if used with Aminoglykosides. It may result in hypersensitivity for penicillin sensitive people (Apak, 1996; Eroğlu, 2002). Side effects are rare but include rash, phlebitis, diarrhea, leukopenia, granulocytopenia, and eosinophilia (Young & Mangum, 2010).

6.1.4.3.2 Ceftazidime

Treatment of neonatal meningitis and sepsis caused by susceptible gram-negative organisms (e.g. *E. coli, H. influenze, Neisseria, Klebsiella,* and *Proteus* species), especially *Pseudomonas aeruginosa*. Resistance among strains of *Serratia* and *Enterobacteriaceae* is increasing (Kanmaz, 2010; Young & Mangum, 2010).

Dose: 30 mg/kg per dose IV infusion by syringe pump over 30 minutes, or IM. To reduce pain at IM injectione site, ceftazimide may be mixed with 1% lidocaine without epinephrine (Kanmaz, 2010; Young & Mangum, 2010).Newborn; IM-IV <7 days and <2000 g; 100 mg/kg/days every 12 hours, >2000 g; 100 mg/kg/days every 8 hours, >7 days; 100-150 mg/kg/days every 8 hours, for others; 100-150 mg/kg/days (max 6 g) IV-IM every 8 hours (Apak, 1996; Eroğlu, 2002).

Adverse Effects: Reported adverse effects are uncommon but include rash, diarrhea, elevated hepatic transminases, eosynophilia, and positive Coombs' test (Kanmaz, 2010; Young & Mangum, 2010).

Administration and Storage Conditions: When the drug in powder gets diluted it can be stored for 24 hours under room temperature; and 7 days in refrigerator. It has not been approved to use preparations containing L-Arginine on children. As the forms administered to children contain sodium carbonate it releases carbon dioxide bubbles when diluted (Kanmaz, 2010).

Incompatible Drugs: Fluconazole, Midazolam, Vancomycin (Kanmaz, 2010).

6.1.4.4 Fourth-generation cephalosporins

6.1.4.4.1 Maxipime

Administered at a dose of 50-100 mg vial every 8 hours (Eroğlu, 2002).

6.1.5 Aminoglycosides

They inhibit the protein synthesis ribosomes. They have bactericidal effects on gram (-) enteric bacilli and *S. aureus*. And they are discharged from kidneys. Dose adjustment is important even in minor renal failures (Eroğlu, 2002).

6.1.5.1 Amicacin

Uses: Amicacin belongs to the aminoglycoside family of antibiotics. It has a very broad spectrum of activity. Bactericidal effect on bacteria of the strains of Gram-positive and Gram-negative and are resistant to certain enzymes produced by bacteria - betalactamase. Amicacin bacteria disrupts protein synthesis (Young & Mangum, 2010).

Newborn ; Gestation age $\leq 27 \rightarrow$ 18 mg/kg/dose every 48 hours
28-30 $\rightarrow$ 18 mg/kg/dose every 36 hours
31-33 $\rightarrow$ 16 mg/kg/dose every 36 hours
$\geq 34 \rightarrow$ 15 mg/kg/dose every 24 hours (Kanmaz, 2010).

Side Effects: Nephrotoxicity, ototoxicity, arthralgia, rash, eosinophil, neuromuscular block may develop (Apak, 1996).

> 1/100- Dizziness, sense of hearing and balance.

1/1000- Fever. Rash and itching. Disturbances in liver function. Changes in the blood picture.

<1/1000- Headache. Lowering blood pressure. Reducing the number of white blood cells, platelet count. Anemia. Tingling. Convulsions. Arthralgia (Young & Mangum, 2010).

Incompatibility: Lipid solution, Ampicillin, amphotericin B, phenytoin (Kanmaz, 2010).

6.1.5.2 Gentamicin

It is one of the most commonly used aminoglycosides (Kırdak & Kilicturgay, 1996; Rang et al, 1998).

Uses: Treatment of infections caused by aerobic gram-negative bacilli (e.g. *Pseudomonas, Klebsiella, E. coli*). Usually used on combination with a B-lactam antibiotic (Young & Mangum, 2010). High serum levels are required for bactericidal effect. Side effects are less seen with longer dose intervals. The volume of distribution increases in patients with PDA and clearance decreases. In premature and asphyxiated infants serum half-life prolongs (Kanmaz, 2010).

Gestation age $\leq$29 weeks$\rightarrow$ 0-14 mg/kg/dose every 72 hours
30-36 weeks $\rightarrow$0-14 mg/kg/dose every 48 hours
>14 mg/kg/dose every 24 hours
37-44 weeks$\rightarrow$ 0-7 mg/kg/dose every 48 hours
>7 mg/kg/dose every 24 hours
$\geq$45 weeks every 24 hours for all (Kanmaz, 2010).

Adverse Effects: The most frequently reported adverse reactions are occular burning and irritation upon drug instillation, non-specific conjunctivitis, conjunctival epithelial defects, and conjunctival hyperemia.

Other adverse reactions which have occurred rarely are allergic reactions, thrombocytopenic purpura, and hallucinations (Young & Mangum, 2010).

Garamycin, Genta, Gensif, Gentamicin, Gentrex are its derivatives. It has ototoxic and nephrotoxic side effects (Kırdak & Kılıçturgay, 1996; Rang et al, 1998). Temporary tubular dysfunction: loss of calcium, magnesium and sodium via the urinary system. Vestibular and auditory toxicity. When used with patients using pancuronium neuromuscular blockage may increase. In the event that extravasation develops hyaluronidase can be used. Other concomitant ototoxic and nephrotoxic drugs increase the toxicity (Kanmaz, 2010).

Incompatible Drugs: Amphotericin B, Ampicillin, Furosemide, Heparin (>1 U/ml), Imipenem/Cilastatin, Indomethacin, Methicillin, Mezlocillin, Nafcillin, Oxacillin, Penicillin G, Propofol, Cefepime, Ticarcillin/Clavulanate (Kanmaz, 2010).

6.1.5.3 Streptomycin sulfate

It is an antibiotic and anti-tuberculostatic drug. It affects some gram negative and positive microorganisms (Kavaklı et al, 1998). It is used with Isoniazid and other tuberculosis drugs in tuberculosis meningitis and progressive tuberculosis. In tuberculosis meningitis it is administered by IM route every 12 hours 20-40 mg/kg/day. The maximum dose is 1 g/day. The length of treatment period is usually 2-3 months. Higher doses and/or more prolonged therapy may result to destruction in 8th cranial nerve (Eroğlu, 2002).

Side effects: Myocarditis, Ataxia, nuisance, vomiting, ototoxicity, nephrotoxicity and hypersensitivity can be seen (Kavaklı et al, 1998).

6.1.5.4 tobramycin

It is more active against P. Aeruginosa than gentamycin. Newborn; IV (30-60 min.) , IM; <7 days <34 weeks <1500g; 3 mg/kg every 24 hours, >1500g; 2.5 mg/kg every 18 hours, >34 weeks >1500g; 2.5 mg/kg every 12 hours, >after 7 days; 5 mg/kg every 12 hours, for older people; 5-7.5 mg/kg/day IM, IV every 6-8 hours (Eroğlu, 2002; Küçüködük, 1994).

6.1.5.5 Netilmicin

Treatment of infections caused by aerobic gram-negative bacilli (Young & Mangum, 2010). It is antimicrobial effective and indicated for the treatment of sepsis caused by susceptible E. *coli, Klebsiella, Enterobacter, Pseudomonas, H. influenza, Salmonella, Shigella, Staphylococci* and of respiratory tract and surgical infections. And it is used in the treatment of complicated urinary system infections, sepsis, skin and skin joint infections, lower respiratory infections and intra-abdominal infections (Köksal & Mangum, 2010).

Uses: Serious life-threatening infections with bacteria sensitive to Netromycin (sepsis, endocarditis) (Young & Mangum, 2010).

Dose: The dose to be used in the first week ≤29 gestational weeks 5 mg/kg/dose every 48

The dose to be used in the first week	≤29 gestational weeks 5 mg/kg/dose every 48 hours
	30-33 weeks 4.5 mg/kg/dose every 48 hours
	34-37 weeks 4 mg/kg/dose every 36 hours
	≥38 weeks 4 mg/kg/dose every 24 hours

After the first week 4 mg/kg is administered as first dose. After 12-24 hours following the end of infusion the dose interval is calculated on the basis of serum concentration (Kanmaz, 2010).

Side Effects: 1/100- Rash, pruritus. Protein in the urine, an increase of uric acid in urine. Dizziness and balance disorders. The deterioration of hearing. 1/1000- Changes in blood picture. Urticaria. Changes in the liver. <1/1000- Headache. Anemia. Lowering blood pressure. Kidney damage (Young & Mangum, 2010).

Administration and Storage Conditions: Ampoules should be diluted before use. The drug diluted with SF can be stored for 3 days in refrigerator (Kanmaz, 2010).

Incompatible Drugs: Amphotericin B, Ampicillin, Furosemide, Heparin, Methicillin, Mezlocillin, Nafcillin, Oxacillin, Penicillin G, Propofol, Ticarcillin/Clavulanate (Kanmaz, 2010).

6.1.6 Macrolides

6.1.6.1 Erythromycin

It inhibits the protein synthesis by binding to ribosome. It can be used with sulphonamide for otitis media treatment (Eroğlu, 2002; Gallardo & Thomas, 1999).

Uses: Erythromycin is used alternatively instead of penicillin to treat bacterial infections, especially in patients allergic to penicillin. The drug is effective in the treatment of diphtheria treatment of whooping cough, pneumonia caused by Mycoplasma pneumonia (including infants), Legionnaires' disease, the treatment of Chlamydia, Gonorrhea, Syphilis, endocarditis, urinary tract inflammation, conjunctivitis (Young & Mangum, 2010).

Dose: 10 mg/kg PO (Young & Mangum, 2010). While erythromycin estolate should be administered every 3 hours; ethylsuccinate one should be administered every 6 hours with food. In chlamydia treatments: Estolate form 12.5 mg/kg/dose every 6 hours for 14 days. In serious infections 5-10 mg/kg/dose every 6 hours with a slow infusion for 60 min. or 10 mg/kg/dose PO. In ophthalmia neonatorum treatment: 0.5% cream for each conjunctiva (Kanmaz, 2010).

Side effects: It is accepted as one of the most dependable antibiotics. The side effects are rarely seen and usually light and limited to skin. However in several occasions angioedema and urticarial have been observed to develop (Gallardo & Thomas, 1999).

Drug Interaction: The plasma clearance of midazolam decreases by 50%. Theophylline and carbamazepine serum concentration may increase. When used together with sisapride, it causes serious dysrhythmias (Kanmaz, 2010).

Monitor: Heart rate and blood level should be monitored during IV use. Liver function tests should be carried out. Hemogram can be used for eosinophilia (Kanmaz, 2010).

6.1.6.2 tetracyclines

It inhibits bacteria protein synthesis. It has wide-spectrums active against gram (+) and gram (-) bacteria (Behrman & Kliegman, 2001; Eroğlu, 2002). Its use is limited in infants and children because of the side effects. Tetracycline prevents growth accumulating in bones and teeth. It should be used on ones older than 8 years old. It may increase intracranial pressure in infants (Eroğlu, 2002).

6.1.6.2.1 Chlortetracycline hydrochloride

PO: administered every 6 hours at a dose of 25-50 mg/kg/day (Köksal & Reisli, 2002).

6.1.6.2.2 Oxytetracycline

Child; PO: 25-50 mg/kg/day every 8 hours, IM: 15-20 mg/kg/day every 8-12 hours, IV: 10-20 mg/kg/day every 12 hours (Eroğlu, 2002).

6.1.7 Other antimicrobial drugs

6.1.7.1 Clindamycin

It is a derivative of lincomycin. It inhibits protein synthesis. It is active against gram (+) cocci and anaerobes (Köksal & Reisli, 2002). Its metabolism in premature is highly variable (Kanmaz, 2010).

Dose: 5-7.5 mg/kg/dose IV slow infusion for 30 min. or PO (Kanmaz, 2010).

Newborn; (IM/IV), <7 days <2000g: 10 mg/kg/day every 12 hours >2000g: 15 mg/kg/day every 8 hours, >7 days <2000g: 15 mg/kg/day every 8 hours, >2000g: 20 mg/kg/day every 4 hours, infant and children; 10-25 mg/kg/day (PO) every 6-8 hours or 25-40 mg/kg/day IV, IM every 6-8 hours (Eroğlu, 2002).

Side effects: Such gastrointestinal symptoms as nausea, vomiting, nuisance, and diarrhea are frequent (Apak, 1996; Eroğlu, 2002). Pseudomembranous enterocolitis may develop. Given fast by infusion it may cause syncope and respiratory arrest. Cleocin, Clindan, Klinoksin are its derivatives (Eroğlu, 2002).

6.1.7.2 Chloramphenicol

It inhibits protein synthesis. It has wide spectrum. It is bacteriostatic for many organisms in low concentrations. Newborn; <14 days 25 mg/kg/day PO, IV, every 12 hours >14 days <2000g: 25 mg/kg/day PO, IV, every 4 hours, >2000g: 50 mg/kg/day PO, IV every 4 hours, infant and children; 50-100 mg/kg/day PO, every 6 hours IV 100 mg/kg/day every 4 hours (Eroğlu, 2002; Dökmeci, 2001).

Side effects: Non dose-related aplastic anemia is a rarely seen; but a serious complication. Dose-related bone marrow suppression is frequently seen and reversible (Eroğlu, 2002).

6.1.7.3 Rifampicin

It is an antimicrobial and antibacterial agent. It is used with at least one more antituberculosis agent in tuberculosis treatment. And administered as single dose 10-20 mg/kg/day PO (Dökmeci, 2001).

6.1.7.4 Vancomycin

It inhibits cell wall synthesis in gram (+) bacteria (Dökmeci, 2001).

Uses: Drug of choice for serious infections caused by Methicillin-Resistant Staphylococcus (e.g. S. Aureus and S. Epidermidis) and Penicillin-Resistant Pneumococci (Dökmeci, 2001; Young & Mangum, 2010). Dose restriction is required in case of a renal failure. It cannot be administered by oral route as it cannot be absorbed well enough. IM administration causes tissue necrosis. It is administered only by IV route in systemic infection treatments (Dökmeci, 2001).

Dose: IV infusion by syringe pump over 60 minute. Meningitis: 15 mg/kg per dose. Bacteremia: 10 mg/kg per dose (Young & Mangum, 2010). Newborn; IV, <7 days <1200g; 15 mg/kg/day every 24 hours, >1200g; 30-45 mg/kg/day every 12 hours, >7 days <1200g; 15 mg/kg/day every 24 hours, >7 days >1200g; 30-45 mg/kg/day every 8-12 hours. For others; 45-60 mg/kg/day every 6-8 hours (Dökmeci, 2001; Ekenel et al, 2001; Eroğlu, 2002).

Adverse Effects: Nephrotoxity and ototoxity: Enhanced by aminoglycoside therapy. Rash and hypotension (red man syndrome): Appears rapidly and resolves within minutes to hours. Lengthening infusion time usually eliminates risk for subsequently doses. Neutropenia: Reported after prolonged administration (more than 3 weeks). Phlebitis: May be minimized by slow infusion and dilution of the drug. (Eroğlu, 2002; (Young & Mangum, 2010).

Preparation: The maximum concentration should be 5 mg/ml.

Miscible Serums: 5% Dex, 10% Dex, SF

Drugs to be confronted at the end point: Dex/Amino acid mixture, Lipid solution, Acyclovir, Aminophylline, Ampicillin, Amicasin, Fluconazole, Heparin (concentration ≤1 U/ml), Calcium gluconate, Meropenem, Midazolom, Potassium chloride, Ranitidine, Sodium bicarbonate.

Incompatibility: Cefazolin, Cefepime, Cefotaxime, Ceftazidime, Ceftriaxone, Dekort, Heparin (concentration >1 U/ml)

Storage Conditions: The solution diluted with sterile water as 50 mg/ml can be stored for 14 days in refrigerator.

6.1.7.5 Sulphonamide

The main indications are non-complicated urinary infections. Erythromycin-sulphonamide combination is effective in the treatment of otitis media. It is used in acute rheumatic fever prophylaxis. However it is not effective in group A streptococcus infection. Such drug-related reactions as fever and rash may develop (Dökmeci, 2001).

6.2 Antiviral drugs

6.2.1 Acyclovir

Acyclovir is one of the most commonly used antiviral drugs (Kavaklı et al, 1998). Treatment of neonatal herpes simplex infections varicella zoster infections with CNS and pulmonary involvement, and herpes simplex encephalitis (Kavaklı et al, 1998; Young & Mangum, 2010).

It can be used for the treatment of herpes simplex virus infections of newborn, varicella infections of children taking immunosuppressive and of immunodeficient children (Kavaklı et al, 1998).

Dose: 20 mg/kg per dose Q8 hours IV by syringe pump over 1 hour. Prolong the dosing interval in prematures infant <34 weeks PMA, or in patients with significant renal impairment or hepatic failure. Treat localized herpes simplex infections for 14 days, disseminated or CNS infections for 21 days (Young & Mangum, 2010).As this drug's intestinal absorption is not that good it should be taken by oral route at high doses. The drug reaches its peak after 1.5-2 hours following being administered by oral route. Almost 30-90% of it is discharged by urinary system (Kavaklı et al, 1998).

Adverse Effects: The most common side effects are nausea, vomiting, diarrhea and headache. Other reported side effects include agitation, confusion, rash, anemia, and muscle pain. Hypersensitivity reactions, seizures, agitation, confusion, anemia, hepatitis, and muscle pain have also been reported (Apak, 1996; Kavaklı et al, 1998; Young & Mangum, 2010).

The things to be considered by nurse applying the drug: In application by IV route a vial of 500 mg is diluted with 10 ml sterile water. The vial is shaken until the drug is fully dissolved. The desired dose is taken into syringe. In order to decrease concentration a single dose should be administered every 1 hour with infusion solution and if possible with infusion pump. Fast application may result in phlebitis and kidney destruction. The infusion area should be changed in order to avoid thrombophlebitis. The prepared solution should be used within 12 hours.

As the drug gets discharged from urinary system the child should be provided with adequate hydration pre-application and during application. The nephrotoxicity risk decreases after 2 hours following infusion application.

Nurse should attentively observe the observable side effects of the drug and should notify doctor if any is observed. If necessary, drug use should be ceased at once (Kavaklı et al, 1998).

6.2.2 Gansklovir

It is an antiviral drug used for the prevention of hearing loss in infants with symptomatic congenital CMV infection (Dökmeci, 2001; Kanmaz, 2010).

Children; first line treatment, 10 mg/kg/day IV (1 hour, slow) every 8-12 hours, 14-21 days; Maintenance, 5-6 mg/kg/day IV every 12-24 hours for 5 days in a week (Dökmeci, 2001). The dose should be halved in case of a serious neutropenia (<500/mm3) (Kanmaz, 2010).

Side Effects: Granulocytopenia, anemia, thrombocytopenia (Kanmaz, 2010).

Incompatible Drugs: Enalaprilat, Fluconazole, Linezolid, Propofol, Remifentanil, Aztreonam, Cefepime, Piperacillin-Tazobactam (Kanmaz, 2010).

6.2.3 Interferons

These composites produced by body cells against viral infections can be synthesized via recombinant DNA technology in our day. The activities of these substances in the treatment of virus infections are a matter of research (Biçer, 2008).

6.3 Antifungal drugs

6.3.1 Amphotericin B liposome

It destroys the cell membrane permeability. It is used in progressive and fatal infections as a result of toxicity (Apak, 1996; Dökmeci, 2001; Eroğlu, 2002).

Uses: Treatment of systemic fungal infections resistant to conventional amphotericin B therapy or in patients with renal or hepatic dysfunction (Young & Mangum, 2010).Dose: 5 to 7 mg/kg dose Q24 hours IV infusion by syringe pump over 2 hours (Young & Mangum, 2010).

It is administered by IV route every 2-6 hours in a 5% dextrose solution. It is started with 0.25 mg/kg/day and increased by 0.25 mg/kg/day in 1-2 days and can be advanced up to 1-1.5 mg/kg/day (Apak, 1996; Dökmeci, 2001; Eroğlu, 2002).

Side Effects: Anemia, thrombocytopenia, hypokalemia, nausea/vomiting, and fever/chills (Young & Mangum, 2010).

6.3.2 Fluconazole

It is active against oropharynx, esophagus, urinary and systemic candidiasis. It is orally well- absorbed. It interacts with Warfarin, Phenytoin, Cyclosporine and Rifampin (Eroğlu, 2002).

6.3.3 Nystatin

It is used in skin and mucosal candidiasis infections (Apak, 1996; Kanmaz, 2010). It resembles to Amphotericin B as structure. It cannot be absorbed via gastrointestinal channels, skin and mucosae. It may have fungicidal or fungistatic effect (Kanmaz, 2010).

Dose: Topical: cream or ointment can be used on the affected area every 6 hours. Therapy should be maintained even after symptoms disappear (Kanmaz, 2010).

PO: from 100.000 U/ml solution 2 ml for term infants, 1 ml for preterm ones every 6 hours for each side of mouth. Therapy should be maintained even after symptoms disappear (Kanmaz, 2010).

Side effects: Cream or ointment related rash (Kanmaz, 2010).

Administration Properties: Oral suspension must be shaken well before use. This suspension includes <1% alcohol, saccharin, 50% sucrose (Kanmaz, 2010).

6.4 Other drugs

6.4.1 Acetaminophen

It is a drug whose analgesic and antipyretic effect is almost equal to aspirin. However it does not resemble to aspirin in terms of gastric mucosa destruction and bleeding. It has no antirheumatic effect being only active against mild and moderate fever. It is used in cases of nuisance, muscle and joint pain, neuralgia and fever. It is also advised in situations where aspirin is contraindicated or not tolerated (Kavaklı et al, 1998).

The dose, route of administration, duration and discharge of drug:

Oral: loading dose 24 mg/kg, maintenance dose 12 mg/kg/dose
Rectal: loading dose 30 mg/kg, maintenance dose 20 mg/kg
Maintenance dose intervals
Preterm ≤32 weeks: 12 hours

>32 weeks: 8 hours
Term 6 hours (Kanmaz, 2010).

age-appropriate daily dose:
0-1 month→ 40 mg
4-11 months →80 mg
1-2 age →120 mg
2-3 age →160 mg
4-5 age →240 mg
6-8 age →320 mg
9-10 age→400 mg
11 years old and older→480 mg (Kavaklı et al, 1998).

The drug is administered every 4-6 hours. It should not exceed more than 5 doses within 24 hours. The drug can be in tablet, capsule, drop, suspension, syrup and suppository forms. The drug gets absorbed by gastrointestinal system, reaches the highest level in blood within half an hour-one hour and sustains its effect for almost 5 hours.

It is metabolized in liver and discharged from body via urinary system. It reaches fetus through placenta (Kavaklı et al, 1998).

Side effects of the drug: As a result of higher dose intake and more prolonged therapy vomiting, nausea, confusion, fever, coma, hepatic and renal tubular necrosis can be observed (Kavaklı et al, 1998). Liver toxicity occurs with excessive doses or after prolonged administration (>48 hours) of therapeutic doses. Rash, fever, thrombocytopenia, leupenia, and neutropenia have been reported in children (Young & Mangum, 2010).

The things to be considered by nurse applying the drug: Nurse should be warned not to exceed recommended dose. For children who have received higher doses and more prolonged therapy liver, kidney and hematopoietic functions should be analyzed.

In case of children with nutritional deficiency it may result in toxicity in liver even if higher doses are not administered.

If the drug is used to reduce fever it should not be forgotten that it can mask the serious disease condition.

The drug should be stored in tight-closed, light-proof bottles and kept away from the reach of children (Kavaklı et al, 1998).

6.4.2 Adenosine

Acute treatment of sustained paroxysmal supraventricular tachycardia. It may also be useful in establishing the cause of the SVT.

Dose: 50 mcg/kg rapid IV push (1 to 2 seconds). Increase dose in 50 mcg/kg increments Q2 minutes until return of sinus rhythm.

Adverse Effects: > 1 / 100 Pain in the chest. Shortness of breath. Dizziness and headache. The in flow of hot face. Speeding up heart rate. Tingling in the extremities. Nausea. 1/100-1/1000 Sweating. Lowering blood pressure. Anxiety. Seeing the fog. >1/1000 The attack of an asthma attack.

6.4.3 Adrenaline

As a bronchodilator in asthma attack it is administered 2 times at 20 minutes intervals by SC route at a dose of 0.01 mg/kg/dose. Higher dose Administration may result in arrhythmia and/or hypotension (Kartal, 2002).

Uses: The resuscitation - the cessation of the heart - together with other measures. Injections performed only by health services, which provides further information about the drug.

Dose: 0.0.1 to 0.03 mg/kg. IV push or SC (Young & Mangum, 2010).

6.4.4 Activated charcoal

It is used as absorbent in oral drug overdose treatment. The dose of 0.25-1 gr/kg can be administered by PO route every 4 hours if necessary (Eroğlu, 2002).

6.4.5 Albuterol

Albuterol is used as a bronchodilator in the treatment of bronchospasm developed in children with reversible respiratory tract disease. It affects the smooth muscles (Kavaklı et al, 1998).

The dose, route of administration, duration and discharge of drug:

The age-appropriate daily dose of albuterol:

2-6 age → 0.1-0.2 mg/kg/dose 3 times a day, 4 mg 3 times a day (the highest applicable dose)

6-12 age → 2 mg/dose 3 times a day, 24 mg/day (the highest applicable dose)

12 ages and older → 2-4 mg/dose 3-4 times a day, 8 mg 4 times a day (the highest applicable dose).

The drug is administered every 4-6 hours as 0.5% solution 0.01-0.05 ml/kg by inhalation via nebulizer. It can be administered more frequently on children with need.

Aerosol inhalation is administered on children above 12 at 90 µ/sprey and the drug reaches the highest level in blood after ½- 2 hours. It is metabolized in liver and discharged from body via urinary system (Kavaklı et al, 1998).

Side effects of the drug: Tachycardia, peripheral vasodilatation, tremor, nervousness, hyperactivity, hypokalemia, irritation in oropharynx are potential side effects (Kavaklı et al, 1998).

The things to be considered by nurse applying the drug: The drug should be well shaken before inhaler application. Mouth should be washed with water after each application in order to avoid mouth and throat dryness.

It should be administered with precaution in children with hyperthyroidism, diabetes, mellitus and heart disease. Addictiveness may develop in prolonged therapy and the usual dose may not be enough.

It has more effect when used with drugs decreasing congestion.

The serum potassium level, heart rate, respiration rate, blood gases of children should be closely monitored when the drug is administered (Kavaklı et al, 1998).

6.4.6 Aminophylline

Treatment of neonatal apnea, including post-extubation, post-anesthesia, and prostaglandin E1-inducted. Bronchodilator. May improve respiratory function (Kavaklı et al, 1998; Young & Mangum, 2010).

Dose: Loading dose: 8 mg/kg IV infusion over 30 minutes, or PO. Maintenance: 1.5 to 3 mg/kg per dose PO, or IV slow push Q8 to 12 hours. In preterms infants, changing from IV aminophylline to PO theophylline requires no dose adjustment (Young & Mangum, 2010).

The dose of 20 mg/kg/day should not be exceeded in rectal application. IM administration of drug is not advised as it causes long-term pains in the injection area (Kavaklı et al, 1998). When the drug is administered by IV route it reaches the highest level in blood within 30 minutes; by oral route it reaches within 1-2 hours.

The drug is metabolized in liver and discharged from body via urinary system. It reaches fetus through placenta in pregnancy period and is transmitted to child through natural nutrition in lactation period (Kavaklı et al, 1998).

Side Effects: An allergic reaction (difficulty breathing; closing of your throat; swelling of your lips, tongue, or face; or hives); seizures; increased or irregular heartbeats; or severe nausea or vomiting (Kavaklı et al, 1998; Young & Mangum, 2010).

The things to be considered by nurse applying the drug: The solution should be given in 20-30 minutes in IV administration. In infants younger than 6 months it should be slowly administered by infusion prepared in 5% dextrose. And it should not be mixed with other drugs.

In oral administration the drug should be administered with water half an hour or one hour before or 2 hours after meals as drug absorption is faster when child is hungry. Child should not break or chew the tablet; but swallow it as a whole. Tablet is not advised for children under the age of 12. Rectal route of administration is used for children who cannot take by oral route. If possible, drug use should be adjusted according to the excretion times of children as drug absorption is faster when rectum is empty. After the administration of drug child should be laid in supine position for 15-20 minutes. As the absorption via rectal route in children is way faster than adults the probability of toxicity is also higher. So nurse should be warned not to exceed recommended dose.

Vital signs and inputs/outputs are observed and recorded at frequent intervals. Instant and clear tachycardia is one of the symptoms of toxicity.

When side effect-related symptoms appear the drug should not be administered and doctor should be notified. In the event that the symptoms are light it can be administered with higher doses.

Such commonly consumed beverages as coffee, tea, coke can increase the reactions. While a diet rich in protein increases the output of drug; a diet rich in carbohydrate decreases the output of it. These conditions result in changes in the drug level in blood. So it may be required to readjust the dose.

The drug should be stored in refrigerator. Suppository forms should be stored either outside or in refrigerator according to the recommendation of the manufacturer (Kavaklı et al, 1998).

6.4.7 Acetylsalicylic acid

As an antipyretic and analgesic it is administered 4-6 times a day at a dose of 30-65 mg/kg/day via PO route in infants and children (Dökmeci, 2000).

6.4.8 Atropine

Reversal of severe sinus Bradycardia, particularly when parasympathetic influences on the heart predominate. Also used to reduce the muscarinic effects if neostigmine when reversing neuromuscular blockade.

Dose: IV: 0.01 to 0.03 mg/kg per dose IV over 1 minute, or IM. Dose can be repeated Q10 to 15 minutes to achieve desired effect, with a maximum total dose of 0.04 mg/kg (Young & Mangum, 2010).

Endotracheal: The same dose can be administered from ET tube. Right after ET tube, 1 ml SF should be given and PPV should be applied for homogenous distribution.

Oral: 0.02 mg-0.09 mg/kg/dose every 4-6 hours (Kanmaz, 2010).

Adverse Effects: Cardiac arrhythmias can occurs, particularly during the first 2 minutes following IV administration; usually a simple A-V dissociation more often caused by smaller rather than larger doses. Fever, especially in brain-damaged infants. Abdominal distention with decreased bowel activity. Esophageal reflux. Mydriasis and cyclopedia (Young & Mangum, 2010).

6.4.9 Calcium gluconate 10%

Uses: Treatment and prevention of hypocalcaemia, usually defined as a serum ionized calcium concentration less than approximately 4 mg/dL. Treatment of asymptotic infants is controversial.

Dose: Symptomatic hypocalcaemia - acute treatment: 100 to 200 mg/kg per dose. Maintenance treatment: 200 to 800 mg/kg per day (Young & Mangum, 2010).

The things to be considered by nurse applying the drug: The drug should be administered by IV route in a way not to exceed 0.5 ml per minute. Besides, 1000 ml serum, prepared in physiologic, can be administered every 12-24 hours. The temperature of solution should be close to the body temperature. The fast delivery of calcium to heart at higher concentrations may result in fatal cardiac arrest. So the drug should be administered very slowly when parenteral route is used. The heart rate should be checked and monitored. When the drug is administered by non-diluted IV route paresthesias, peripheral vasodilatation and hypotension can be observed. If the child is observed with any symptom drug administration should be ceased and the child should be ensured to rest for half an hour or one hour. It can cause extravasation (the process of exuding or passing out of a vessel into surrounding tissues) tissue irritation and necrosis. Nurse should closely monitor the injection area.

In order to ensure well absorption by oral route the drug should be administered 1-1.5 hours after meals. In order to promote intestinal absorption the use of milk and milk products should be decreased. As calcium gluconate increases the digital toxicity it should be attentively administered in patients receiving digital.

The effect of drug on tetany treatment is evaluated by neuromuscular recovery (Kavaklı et al, 1998).

Administration: It can be either slowly administered by IV route in 10-30 minutes or used as continuous infusion.

Miscible Serums: 5% Dex, 10% Dex, SF

Drugs to be confronted at the end point: Dex/Amino acid, Lipid solution, Aminophylline, Ampicillin, Amicasin, Dobutamine, Furosemide, Heparin, Midazolom, Meropenem, Potassium chloride, Vancomycin

Incompatibility: Amphotericin B, Fluconazole, Sodium bicarbonate

Side effects: Bradycardia, cardiac arrest, tissue necrosis, intestinal bleeding, diarrhea, gastric irritation. It should be used carefully in patients who receive digital treatment and has bradypnea.

6.4.10 Captopril

Uses: Treatment of moderate to severe hypertension. Afterload reduction in patients with congestive heart failure.

Dose: 0.01 to 0.05 mg/kg per dose PO Q8 to 12 hours. Adjust dose and interval based on response. Administer 1 hour before feeding.

Adverse Effects: Captopril produces the following side effects: Angioedema with involvement of the face, mouth, larynx, tongue, and glossitis, neutropenia, anemia and thrombocytopenia, proteinuria, acidosis, tachycardia, cardiac arrest, arrhythmias, rash and erythema multiform, exfoliate dermatitis, photosensitivity, elevated liver enzymes in serum, liver cell injury, cholestasis jaundice, gastric irritation, hepatitis, drowsiness, nervousness, depression, paresthesias of hands, confusion, ataxia, bronchitis, bronchospasm, pneumonia eosinophil, rhinitis (Young & Mangum, 2010).

6.4.11 Ceftriaxone

Uses: Treatment of neonatal sepsis and meningitis caused by susceptible gram-negative organisms (e.g. E coli, Pseudomonas, Klebsiella, H influenzae). Treatment of gonococcal infections.

Dose: Septis and disseminated gonococcal infection: 50mg/kg Q24 hours. Meningitis: 100 mg/kg loading dose, then 80 mg/kg Q24 hours. Uncomplicated gonococcal ophthalmia: 50 mg/kg (maximum 125 mg) single dose. (note: topical antibiotic therapy alone is inadequate and is unnecessary if systemic treatment is administered). IV administration: infusion by syringe pump over 30 minutes. Avoid administration of calcium-containing solution or products within 48 hours of the last administration. IM administration: to reduce pain at the injection site, reconstitute with 1% lidocaine without epinephrine.

Adverse Effects: Not recommended for use in neonatal with hyperbilirubinemia! Displaces bilirubin from albumin binding sites, resulting in higher free bilirubin serum concentration. Concurrent administration of ceftriaxone and calcium-containing solutions or products in neonates is contraindicated. Eosinophilia, Thrombocytosis, leukopenia. Increase in AST and ALT. Skin rash. Transient gallbladder precipitations occasionally associated with colicky abdominal pain, nausea, and vomiting (Young & Mangum, 2010).

6.4.12 Chloral hydrate

Uses: Sedative/hypnotic for short-term use only. Chloral hydrate has no analgesic after a feeding to reduce gastric irritation.

Dose: 25 to 75 mg/kg per dose PO. Oral preparation should be diluted or administered after feeding to reduce gastric irritation.

Adverse Effects: Chloral hydrate may lead to unpleasant side effects, including: drowsiness, nausea, vomiting, and diarrhea. Toxic doses (overdoses) can cause a marked drop in blood pressure and severely compromised respiration (breathing). Signs of an overdose of chloral hydrate can include: confusion, seizures, difficulty breathing, slurred speech, slow or irregular heartbeat, vomiting, weakness, and a lowered body temperature. Chronic use of chloral hydrate is also associated with a severe withdrawal syndrome and may induce liver damage (Young & Mangum, 2010).

6.4.13 Iron

Indication: The prevention and treatment of iron-deficiency induced anemia.

Pharmacology: Ferrous salts are preferred as they are absorbed 2-3 times better than ferric salts when administered by oral route. Ferrous sulfate, ferrous fumarate, ferrous gluconate can also be used. Absorption is better on an empty stomach. Half or one-third of it is absorbed when taken with food.

Dose: Premature infants: Elemental iron 2 mg/kg/dose PO, started after 4 weeks in doses divided into 2-3. For babies lighter than 1000 gr 4 mg/kg/day may be administered. For patients receiving EPO treatment: 6 mg/kg/day

Iron dextran: For ones who cannot take by oral route 0.4-1 mg/kg/day is administered as continuous infusion in D/AA.

Side effects: Iron treatment should not be launched as long as premature infants do not get adequate vitamin E. Hemolysis may increase in that case. Diarrhea and constipation, lethargy, hypotension, black-colored stool and erosion in gastric mucosa can be observed. It may be required to seek for occult blood in stool in suspicious cases (Kanmaz, 2010).

6.4.14 Dexamethasone

Uses: Dexamethasone is used primarily in the intensive and short-term treatment of severe allergic conditions such as asthma, also in rheumatic diseases, skin diseases, eye, blood and certain cancers.

Dose: 0.075 mg/kg per dose Q12 hours for 3 days, 0.05 mg/kg per dose Q12 hours for 3 days, 0.025 mg/kg per dose Q12 hours per 2 days, and 0.1 mg/kg per dose Q12 for 2 days IV or PO.

Adverse Effects: 1/100 Accumulation of fat around the body and face, growth retardation in children, susceptibility to infectious diseases, the activation of diabetes, muscle weakness, abnormal menstruation, body hair in women, akne. Most of these symptoms occurs as a result of long-term glucocorticoid therapy. 1/1000 Disturbances in water management, reducing the level of potassium in the body, accumulation of water in the body, raised blood pressure, heart failure, allergic reactions, accelerated blood clotting, gastrointestinal disorders, increased appetite, weight gain, damage the lining of the digestive tract, sagging skin, mental disorders manifested by extreme changes in mood, insomnia, headache, increased intraocular pressure in the eye lens opacity. If there are troublesome symptoms should seek medical attention.

6.4.15 Diazepam

It is effective as anxiolytic and muscle- relaxing agent. In treatment of status epilepticus 0.1-0.5 mg /kg/dose is administered 2 times at 5-15 minutes intervals by IV route in newborns-infants-children. Its effect by IM route is limited. To decrease anxiety: 4 times 0.2-0.3 mg/kg/day PO (Eroğlu, 2002).

6.4.16 Digoxin

Digoxin is an antiarrhythmic and cardiac glycoside drug (Kavaklı et al, 1998). It is a highly active cardiac glycoside with a half-life of 48 hours (Dökmeci, 2000; Küçüködük, 1994).

Uses: Treatment of heart failure caused by diminished myocardial contractility. Treatment of SVT, atrial flutter, and atrial fibrillation (Young & Mangum, 2010).

Dose:	*Old*	*Dose*	*Maintenance*	*Interval*
	29 <	*0.015 mg/kg*	*0.004 mcg/kg*	*24*
	30-36	*0.02 mg/kg*	*0.005 mg/kg*	*24*
	>37	*0.035 mg/kg*	*0.006 mg/kg*	*12 (Young & Mangum, 2010).*

Total digoxin dose; premature baby: 0.02 mg/kg PO, after birth of newborn; 0.01-0.03 mg/kg IM, IV / 0.04 mg/kg PO, infant; 0.03-0.04 mg/kg IM, IV / 0.05 mg/kg PO, children; 0.010-0.015 mg/kg IM, IV, PO. Higher doses result in fatal arrhythmias (Dökmeci, 2000; Küçüködük, 1994).

Adverse Effects: Toxic Cardiac Effects: PR interval prolongation, sinus bradycardia or SA block, trail or nodal ectopic beats, ventricular arrhythmias. Nontoxic Cardiac Effects: QTc interval shortening, ST segment sagging, T-wave amplitude dampening, heart rate slowing (Young & Mangum, 2010).

The things to be considered by nurse applying the drug: Before nurse administers Digoxin to a child he or she should very carefully obtain prior Digoxin use history. Serum digoxin, potassium, magnesium and calcium levels should be determined by laboratory investigations before digoxin administration. Nurse should measure radial heart rate for a minute before administrating the drug to child and if any abnormality presents he or she should check apical pulse and its rate, rhythm and properties and notify doctor. The drug can be administered by IV route either directly or via a solution including 5% dextrose or 9% sodium chloride. Absorption may delay if the drug is administered by oral route after meals. And absorption may also delay when administered with antacids. IM administration of drug is not advised especially for children with diabetics or mild tissue perfusion as it causes pain. When IM route is used the drug should be administered deep into a large muscle mass and then the area should be massaged after injection. No more than 5 mL should be administered in one area. In case that digoxin is administered with such drugs as diuretics which decrease potassium level and some antibiotics toxicity may develop. Besides, calcium should not be administered to digitalized children. It may have fatal consequences. If the drug is used for atrial fibrillation treatment purposes nurse should check heart rate and if it is below 60 or above 100 beats per minute then he or she should notify doctor. The drug should be administered with precaution and at fewer doses in children with hyperkalemia having kidney and hepatic impairment. The inputs/outputs of child should be followed, edema should be monitored and daily weight check should be ensured. Cardiac arrhythmia and anorexia in children are early symptoms of toxicity. Nurse should pay attention to those symptoms. If it is suspected of toxicity blood digoxin level should be measured and EGK should be performed. Nurse should store the drug in tight-closed and light-proof bottles. If any color change is observed the drug should not be used (Kavaklı et al, 1998).

6.4.17 Dobutamine

It is used in temporary treatment of heart failures related to the depression caused by cardiac rigidity. 0.0025-0.010 mg/kg/min is administered by IV infusion according to the patient's response (Eroğlu, 2002).

Dose: 2 to 20 mg/kg per minute continuous IV infusion. Begin at a low dose and titrate by monitoring effects. Use a large vein for IV (Kanmaz, 2010).

Side Effects: Volume replacement should be performed before drug use as it may cause hypotension in hypovolemic patients. Tachycardia may develop at higher doses. Arrhythmia, hypertension and vasodilatation in skin may also develop. If it exudes or passes out of a vessel it causes tissue ischemia (Kanmaz, 2010).

Administration and Storage Conditions: Diluted drug can be stored for 6 hours under room temperature and 48 hours in refrigerator. Slight color change does not mean that the drug is spoiled (Kanmaz, 2010).

6.4.18 Dopamine

It is indicated for all kinds of hypotension, heart failure and circulatory impairments. To increase cardiac output and to improve organ perfusion it is started to be administered by IV infusion at a dose of 0.002-0.005 mg/kg/min (100 mg dopamine in 250 ml 5% dextrose) as 0.400 mg/ml solution. It can be advanced up to 0.020 mg/kg/min (Apak, 1996).

Uses: Treatment or hypotension

Dose: 2 to 20 mcg/kg per minute continuous IV infusion. Begin at a low dose and titrate by monitoring effects. Use a large vein for IV.

Adverse Effects: > 1/100 Headache. Additional heartbeat, increased heart rate. Pain in the chest. Nausea and vomiting. Shortness of breath. 1/1000 Heart arhythmia. Changes in the ECG. Lowering blood pressure. Allergic reactions. Pulmonary edema (Young & Mangum, 2010).

Monitor: Heart rate and intra-arterial blood pressure should continuously be monitored. Urinary output and peripheral perfusion should be observed. A large vein is recommended to use. Extra care should be shown in terms of extravasation. Pallor may be observed through the subject vein. If it exudes or passes out of a vessel it causes necrosis, in which case 1 mg/ml phentolamine should be injected around lesion (Kanmaz, 2010).

Administration and Storage Conditions: The opened ampoule should be stored in refrigerator and consumed within 24 hours. Ampoules with color change should not be used (Kanmaz, 2010).

Miscible Serums: 5% DX, 5% DSF, SF, D/AA, fat emulsions (Kanmaz, 2010).

Incompatible Drugs: Amphotericin B, Acyclovir, Furosemide, Indomethacin, Insulin, Sodium bicarbonate (Kanmaz, 2010).

6.4.19 Fentanyl

Uses: Anelgesia, sedation, anesthesia.

Dose: Sedation and analgesia: 0.5 to 4 mcg/kg per dose IV slow push. Repeat as require (usually Q2 to 4 hours).

Infusion rate: 1 to 5 mcg/kg per hours. Tolerance may develop rapidly following constant infusion.

Anesthesia: 5 to 50 mcg/kg per dose (Young & Mangum, 2010).

Neonatal dose: IV slow 0.3-2 mcg/kg/dose
IV infusion dose: 0.3-5 mcg/kg/hour (Anand, 2007).

Adverse Effects: Respiratory depression, Sometimes nausea, Vomiting, Bradycardia, Hypotension, Extremely bronchospasm. At high doses observed in a small chest muscle stiffness, which may hamper rescue breathing (Young & Mangum, 2010).

Preparation: 1 ml fentanyl from 50 mcg/ml ampoules gets diluted with 4 ml SF.

Miscible Serums: 5% DX, 10% DX, SF

Drugs to be confronted at the end point: Dex/Amino acid mixture, Dekort, Dobutamine, Dopamine, Furosemide, Heparin, Midazolam, Potassium Chloride.

Incompatible Drugs: Phenytoin, Azithromycin.

Storage Conditions: It should be protected against light. Diluted ampoules can be stored for 24 hours in refrigerator.

6.4.20 Furosemidum

Uses: Diuretic that may also improve pulmonary function. It is used in pulmonary edema, in heart failures and for increasing urinary discharge

Dose: 1 mg/kg IV slow push, IM or PO. May increase to a maximum of 2 mg/kg per dose IV or 6 mg/kg per dose PO.

Adverse Effects: > 1 /100 Decreased blood potassium levels, which implies a weakening of the muscles. Decreased levels of magnesium, calcium and sodium. Increasing levels of uric acid in the blood. Reduce the volume of blood in case of longer treatment. 1/1000 Digestive disorders. <1/1000 Phlebitis. Changes in the blood picture. Allergic reactions. If you get a rash you should immediately contact your doctor and stop taking the drug. Dizziness and tinnitus. Increased blood sugar levels (Young & Mangum, 2010).

It develops hypotension, hyponatremia, hypokalemia, alkalosis and hypercalciuria. It is highly ototoxic especially when administered fast.

Administration and Storage Conditions: The ampoules should be protected against light.

Compatible: SF and sterile water.

Incompatible: Dopamine, Dobutamine, Erythromycin, Fluconazole, Midazolam.

6.4.21 Glucagon

Uses: It is used in patients with diabetes in decline due to excessively low blood sugar. This condition usually occurs as a result of too much insulin.

Dose: 200 mcg/kg per dose IV, IM, SC

Adverse Effects: 1 /100 Nausea and vomiting. 1/1000- <1/1000 Allergic reactions (Young & Mangum, 2010)

6.4.22 Heparin

Uses: Preventing blood clots, the risk of their formation is increased, e.g. after surgical procedures in acute myocardial infarction. Heparin is also used to treat blood clots in the legs and lungs in congestion of the arteries. The use of heparin also gives good results in the treatment of frostbite and burns (Young & Mangum, 2010). Prevention of peripheral and central catheters from congestion. Its use in renal vein thrombosis is still a matter of discussion (Kanmaz, 2010).

Dose: IV for each ml of liquid 0.5-1 Unit

For thrombosis treatment 70 Unit/kg bolus in 10 minutes, 28 Unit/kg/hour continuous infusion (Young & Mangum, 2010). 75 units/kg bolus over 19 minutes.

Adverse Effects: Side effects in the form of bleeding occurs in approximately 10% of patients. >1/100 Bleeding. A decline in platelet count. Changes in the functions of the liver. <1/1000 Allergic reactions, allergic shock. Disturbances in the function of the adrenal cortex. Hair loss (Young & Mangum, 2010).

Preparation: Added onto the solution as half of the total.

Miscible Serums: SF, 5% DX, 10% DX

Drugs to be confronted at the end point: Dex/Amino acid mixture, Acyclovir, Amphotericin B, Ampicillin, Calcium gluconate, Cefazolin, Cefepime, Cefotaxime, Ceftazidime, Ceftriaxone,

Dekort, Dobutamine, Dopamine, Fentanyl, Fluconazole, Furosemide, Insulin, Meropenem, Midazolom, Penicillin G, Potassium chloride, Sodium bicarbonate, Bactrim (Young & Mangum, 2010).

Incompatible Drugs: Amicasin (if concentration is intense), Diazem, Gentamicin (if concentration is intense), Phenytoin, Vancomycin (Kanmaz, 2010).

Storage Conditions: It should be stored at room temperature under 25°C in its package (Young & Mangum, 2010).

6.4.23 Hydroxyzine hydrochloride

Uses: Sedative/hypnotic. Anesthesia induction. Treatment of refractory seizures.

Dose: IV: 0.05 to 0.15 mg/kg over at least 5 minutes. Repeat as required, usually Q2 to 4 hours. May also be given IM. Dosage requirements are decreased by incurrent use of narcotics.

Adverse Effects: Pediatric patients: desaturation 4.6%, apnea 2.8%, hypotension 2.7%, paradoxical reactions 2.0%, hiccough 1.2%, seizure like activity 1.1% and nystagmus 1.1%. The majority of airway-related events occurred in patients receiving other CNS depressing medications and in patients where midazolam was not used as a single sedating agent (Young & Mangum, 2010).

6.4.24 Ibuprofen

It is a non-steroidal anti-inflammatory agent with analgesic and antipyretic effect. As an analgesic and antipyretic it is administered at a dose of 10-15 mg/kg/dose every 4-6 hours by PO route and 40-60 mg/kg/day at maximum (Dökmeci, 2000).

Uses: Rheumatic Diseases. Menstrual pain. Pain of different origins.

Dose:

3-6 months > 5 kg 50 mg 3-4 times a day

6-12 months 50 mg 3 times a day

1-4 ages 100 mg 3-4 times a day

The maximum dose for children and newborns is:

3 months- 4 age 30 mkg 3-4 times a day (Pursell, 2010).

Adverse Effects: >1/100 Abdominal pain, burning sensation in the throat, nausea, diarrhea. Fatigue.
Headache. Rash. 1/1000 Allergic reactions. Symptoms of allergy may be asthma, rhinitis, and rash. Bleeding from the gastrointestinal tract. Gastric ulcer. Blurred vision. The deterioration of hearing. Anxiety. Insomnia (Young & Mangum, 2010).

6.4.25 Indomethacin

Uses: Closure of ducts arteriosus. Prevention of intraventricular hemorrhage.

Dose:(mg/kg)

Age at 1st dose	1st	2nd	3rd
<48	0.2	0.1	0.1
2 to 7 d	0.2	0.2	0.2
>7 d	0.2	0.25	0.25

Adverse Effects: The most common side effects are nausea, vomiting, diarrhea, stomach discomfort, heartburn, rash, headache, dizziness and drowsiness (Young & Mangum, 2010).

6.4.26 Imipenem

Uses: Restricted to treatment of no-CNS infections caused by bacteria, primarily Enterobacteriaceae and anaerobes, resistant to other antibiotics (Kanmaz, 2010; Young & Mangum, 2010).

Dose: 20 to 25 mg/kg per dose Q12 hours IV infusion over 30 minutes

Adverse Effects: Seizures occur frequently in patients with meningitis, preexisting CNS pathology, and severe renal dysfunction. Local reaction at the infection and increased platelet counts are the most frequent adverse effects. Other including eosinophilia, elevated hepatic transaminases, and diarrhea also occur in more than 5% of patients (Young & Mangum, 2010).

Incompatible Drugs: Amicasin, Fluconazole, Gentamycin, Clonazepam, Sodium bicarbonate, Tobramycin (Kanmaz, 2010).

6.4.27 Insulin

Indication: For adjuvant treatment in hypoglycemia and hyperpotassemia.

Pharmacology: It ensures intracellular glucose transmission. It converts glucose into glycogen, ensures amino acid intake and transmission of K into muscle tissue and cell. It increases fat synthesis. It inhibits lipolysis and the conversion of protein to glucose. It is decomposed in liver and kidneys. Serum half-life is 9 minutes for adults.

Dose: Intermittent dose: 0.1-0.2 U/kg, every 6-12 hours SC

Continuous infusion: 0.01-0.1 U/kg/hour

Only regular insulin can be given IV. The dose is adjusted according to blood sugar.

Side effects: Hypoglycemia and increase in insulin resistance. It can cause normoglycemic hyperinsulinemia and metabolic acidosis.

Monitor: Blood sugar should be monitored at 15-30 min. intervals after infusion and dose adjustment.

Administration and Storage Conditions: A solution of 1 U/ml concentration should be prepared by diluting with sterile water or SF. Should wait for 20 minutes to give time for connection of plastic to IV catheters before continuous infusion. It should be stored in refrigerator.

Incompatible Drugs: Aminophylline, Dopamine, Phenytoin, Phenobarbital, Pentobarbital (Kanmaz, 2010).

6.4.28 intralipid

Uses: Parental nutrition source of calories and essential fat acids.

Adverse Effects: 1/100- 1 / 1000 Fever. Chills. Nausea. Redness of the skin. <1/1000 Allergic shock. Changes in the blood picture, which occur most frequently in infants. Increase or decrease in blood pressure. Rash. Changes in liver function. Shortness of breath. Long-term painful erection (Young & Mangum, 2010).

6.4.29 Caffein

It is MSS stimulator and vasoconstrictor of cerebral vessels. It is used for vascular headache and as analeptic. Neonatal apnea loading dose: 10 mg/kg, maintenance 5-10 mg/kg/day (Biçer, 2008).

6.4.30 Ketamine

General anesthetic, sedative, hypnotic, analgesic and amnestic. IV, IM. It protects cardiovascular functions. It improves lung compliance, has bronchodilator effect. As ketamine favorably alters the heart and respiratory functions it can be used as a sedative agent in patients who receive mechanical ventilation and have myocardial depression induced by benzodiazepines and opiates. It can be used in cases where spontaneous ventilation is requested while sedation is provided (Biçer, 2008).

Neonatal Dose:

IV slow	0.5-2 mg/kg/dose
IV Inf. Dose	0.5-1 mg/kg/h
IM, SC	2 mg/kg/dose
Oral	5-8 mg/kg/dose (Anand, 2007).

Sedation: 0.5-2 mg/kg/dose IV, can be repeatedly administered at doses of 0.5 mg/kg/dose at 2-5 min. intervals or with 1-2 mg/kg/hour infusion until adequate sedation is achieved (Max. 5 mg/kg). 4-5 mg/kg/dose IM (if adequate sedation is not achieved within 10 minutes), one more dose of 2 mg/kg/dose can be administered. Rapid sequential intubation: 0.5-2 mg/kg/dose IV or 3-7 mg/kg/dose IM (1 dose). Caution: It acts fast; but slow. Aspiration and laryngospasm can be observed in patients who ventilate spontaneously in the unprotected airway. Atropine and glycopyrronium bromide are advised to use before ketamine as it increases saliva and bronchial secretions. It should not be administered in cases of increase in intracranial pressure, suspected head trauma and in convulsions whose etiology is unknown and where intracranial pressure may have increased. It can cause such reactions as hallucination and delirium and these phenomena increase by age and dose. The administration of benzodiazepines 5 minutes before ketamine is active against these phenomena (Biçer, 2008).

Side Effects: Laryngospasm, out-of-anesthesia reaction, tachycardia, hypertension, increase in intracranial pressure (Biçer, 2008).

6.4.31 Levothyroxine

Uses: Treatment of hypothyroidism

Dose: PO: 10 to 14 mcg/kg. IV 5 to 8 mcg/kg

Adverse Effects: Prolonged over treatment can produce premature craniosynostosis and acceleration of bone age (Young & Mangum, 2010).

6.4.32 Magnesium sulfate

Uses: Postpartum eclampsia. Tetanus.

Warning: Injection should not be administered in renal failure. Injections should be done slowly by controlling the breath of the patient (Young & Mangum, 2010).

6.4.33 Meropenem

Uses: Limited to treatment of pneumococcal meningitis and other serious infections caused by susceptible gram-negative organisms resistant to other antibiotics, especially extended-spectrum beta-lactamase producing *Klebsiella pneumonia* (Young & Mangum, 2010).

Dose: 20 mg/kg per dose IV

Less than 32 weeks GA, less than or equal to 14 days PNA: administered Q12 hours; after 14 days PNA: administered Q8 hours. 32 weeks and older GA, less than or equal to 7 days PNA: administered Q12 hours; after 7 days PNA: administered Q8 hours. Meningitis and infections caused by Pseudomonas species, all ages: 40mg/kg per dose Q8 hours. Give as an IV infusion over 30 minutes. Longer infusion times (up to 4 hours) may be associated with improved therapeutic efficacy (Young & Mangum, 2010).

Adverse Effects: Diarrhea (4%), nausea/vomiting (1%) and rash (2%). May cause inflammation at the injection site. The use of carbapenem antibiotics can result in the development of cephalosporin resistance in *Enterobacter, Pseudomonas, Serration, Proteus, Citrobacter,* and *Acinetobacte*r species. The risk of pseudomembranous colitis and fungal infections are also increased (Young & Mangum, 2010).

Administration: IV 30 min. infusion

Preparation: 500 mg meropenem is diluted with 10 ml proper solution. 50 mg/ml concentration is obtained.

Miscible Serums: 5% Dex, 10% Dex, SF

Drugs to be confronted at the end point: Dex/Amino acid, Lipid solution, Acyclovir, Aminophylline, Dopamine, Dobutamine, Fluconazole, Gentamicin, Heparin, Sodium bicarbonate, Vancomycin.

Incompatibility: Amphotericin B, Metronidazole, Acyclovir, Calcium gluconate, Diazepam, Zidovudine.

Storage Conditions: Diluted with sterile distilled water it can be stored for 2 hours under room temperature, 12 hours in refrigerator; diluted with SF for 2 hours under room temperature, 18 hours in refrigerator; diluted with 5% Dex for 1 hour under room temperature, 8 hours in refrigerator. These periods of time are valid for 50 mg/ml concentration (Kanmaz, 2010).

6.4.34 Metronidazole

Uses: Reserved for treatment of meningitis, ventriculitis, and endocarditis caused by Bacteroides fragilis and other anaerobes resistant to penicillin; treatment of serious intra-abdominal infections; and treatment of infections caused by Trichomonas vaginalis. Treatment of C. difficile colitis.

Dose: Loading dose: 15 mg/kg PO or IV infusion by syringe pump over 60 minutes Maintenance dose: 7.5 mg/kg per dose PO or IV infusion over 60 minutes. Begin one dosing interval after initial dose. Adverse Effects: Seizures and sensory polyneuropathy have been reported in a few adult patients receiving high doses over a prolonged period. Drug metabolites may cause brownish discoloration of the urine (Young & Mangum, 2010).

6.4.35 Phenobarbital

It is a long-term effective MSS depressant. For sedation: infants and children; 2-3 mg/kg/day PO every 8-12 hours. For sleep: infants and children; 2-3 mg/kg/dose PO, if IM required it is repeated after 12-24 hours (Eroğlu, 2002).

Dose: 20 mg/kg IV, given slowly over 10 to 15 minutes. Refractory seizures: Additional 5 mg/kg doses, up to a total of 40 mg/kg.

Neonatal Abstinence Syndrome: 16 mg'kg PO on day 1.

Uses: Epilepsy, seizures primarily large, so called and grand mal seizures, which cover only part of the brain. Seizures in newborns.

Adverse Effects: Respiration and respiratory depression (Kanmaz, 2010). > 1 / 100 Drowsiness. Disturbances in attention. Irritability, especially in young children. The difficulty of concentration of vision. The difficulty in coordinating movements. Changes in the blood picture. Rash. Confusion, especially in older patients. 1/1000 The risk of mucous membrane of the mouth and teeth, especially during prolonged treatment. <1/1000 - Anemia (Young & Mangum, 2010).

Follow: The therapeutic concentration is 15-30 mcg/ml. Respiratory depression is observed in concentration exceeding 60 mcg/ml. The serum half-life is longer in the first 1-2 weeks. The serum half-life differs in patients taking phenytoin and valproate (Kanmaz, 2010).

Administration and Storage Conditions: The ampoules should be used within 30 minutes after opening (Kanmaz, 2010).

Incompatible Drugs: Fat emulsions, Hydralazine, Hydrocortisone, Insulin, Clindamycin, Methadone, Midazolam, Morphine, Pancuronium, Ranitidine, Vancomycin (Kanmaz, 2010).

6.4.36 Phenytoin

Uses: Anticonvulsant often used to treat seizures refractory to phenobarbital.

Dose: 15 to 20 mg/kg IV infusion over at least 30 minutes, after that 4 to 8 mg/kg Q24 hours IV or PO. Max 0.5 mg/kg/minute.

Adverse Effects: Due to the central nervous system: Nystagmus, slurred speech, impaired motor coordination, may rarely occur: dizziness, insomnia, irritability, involuntary muscle spasms, headache, in very rare cases you may experience dyskinesia.

Due to the gastrointestinal tract: most - nausea, vomiting, constipation, in rare cases can lead to hepatotoxicity.

On the part of the skin: various forms of skin rashes, systemic lupus erythematous, Stevens - Johnson syndrome, toxic epidermolysis.

On the part of the hematopoietic system: in rare cases there may be abnormal blood cell production - thrombocytopenia, leukopenia, granulocytopenia, and anemia Megaloblastic makrocytosis (equivalent of treatment with folic acid) (Young & Mangum, 2010).

Administration Type: Loading dose IV 30 minutes infusion, Maintenance dose IV slow.

Preparation: The maximum concentration should be 10 mg/ml when it is diluted with SF. 5 mg/ml concentration is obtained diluting 50 mg/ml with 9 ml SF.

Miscible Serums: SF. Stability is ruined with most of the IV liquids.

Drugs to be confronted at the end point: Fluconazole, Sodium bicarbonate

Incompatible Drugs: 5% Dex, 5% with Dextrose, Dex/Amino acid, Lipid emulsions, Aminophylline, Amicasin, Dobutamine, Fentanyl, Heparin, Potassium chloride, Vitamin K1.

Storage Conditions: Unopened ampoules should be protected against light under room temperature. Opened ampoules should not be delayed.

6.4.37 Potassium chloride

Uses: Potassium deficiency. Prevention of excessive potassium smothering as a result of taking diuretics, diabetes, long-term diarrhea.

Dose: 0.5 to 1 mEq/kg per day divided an administered with feedings. 1g KCl = 13.4 mEq K+

Adverse Effects: Confusion, anxiety, feeling like you might pass out; uneven heartbeat; extreme thirst, increased urination; leg discomfort; muscle weakness or limp feeling; numbness or tingly feeling in your hands or feet, or around your mouth; severe stomach pain, ongoing diarrhea or vomiting; black, bloody, or tarry stools; or coughing up blood or vomit that looks like coffee grounds (Young & Mangum, 2010).

Administration: IV infusion

Preparation: Maximum concentration via peripheral line is 40 mEq/L. and 80 mEq/L. through central vein. The desired amount is added to total solution.

Miscible Serums: Compatible with all standard IV solutions.

Incompatibility: Amphotericin B, Diazepam, Phenytoin.

6.4.38 Sodium bicarbonicum 8.4%

Uses: Treatment of normal anion gap metabolic acidosis caused by renal or GI losses. Sodium bicarbonate is not a recommended therapy in neonatal resuscitation guidelines. Administration during brief CPR may be determinal.

Dose: 1 to 2 mEq/kg IV over at least 30 minutes

Adverse Effects: Excess sodium in the body, which can manifest itself in the body of water retention, swelling, weakness, anxiety, swollen tongue, dizziness and headaches, fever, decrease in saliva and urine, pressure drop, rapid heart rate, apnea (Young & Mangum, 2010).

6.4.39 Ranitidine

Dose: PO: 2 mg/kg per dose Q8 hours. IV: 1.5 mg/kg per dose Q8 hours.

Uses: Prevention and treatment of stress ulcers and GI hemorrhage aggravated by gastric acid secretion.

Adverse Effects: 1/100 Fatigue. Diarrhea, rash, dizziness. 1/1000 Allergic reactions such as swelling of the skin rash, fever, seizures or asthma. Changes in the blood picture and liver function. Jaundice. Depression, hallucinations, disorientation, especially in debilitated and elderly patients. Seeing the fog. Pain in muscles and joints (Young & Mangum, 2010).

6.4.40 Steroids

Steroids are used as anti-inflammatory, immunosuppressive or in rheumatic diseases in order to increase sensitivity against beta adrenergic, chronic ulcerative colitis, nephrotic syndrome, tuberculosis meningitis and asthma.

Dose:

Hydrocortisone	10-20 IV, IM, Oral
Methylprednisolone	0.4-2 IV, IM, Oral
Prednisone	1-2 Oral

The drug can be administered 1-2 times a day by oral route. Hydrocortisone should be administered deeply IM and delta frame should not be performed. Steroids should be administered by SC route as they cause sterile abscess and pseudoatrophy. The duration of therapy may differ from 3-5 days to weeks or months depending on the diagnosis of child. The drug is metabolized in liver and discharged from body via urinary system.

Side Effects: Edema, hypertension, headache, convulsion, acne, skin atrophy, hypokalemia, alkalosis, Cushing syndrome, hyperglycemia, peptic ulcer, nausea, vomiting, cataract, glaucoma and muscle weakness are observed side effects (Kavaklı et al, 1998).

The things to be considered by nurse applying the drug: The recommendation of manufacturer on the route of administration should be taken into consideration. Nurse should administer the drug slowly by IV route. In oral administration it should be administered at meal intervals or after meals to decrease gastric irritation of drug. Salt is limited in foods. If possible diets rich in potassium and protein are prepared. The blood pressure and other vital signs, input-output, sleeping condition and daily weight check of child is observed in recorded. Oral and hygienic care is provided at frequent intervals. Steroid can cause hyperkalemia when used with certain diuretics. Phenobarbiturates decrease the effect of steroids. Urinary and blood glucose investigations should be carried out especially in children with diabetics. It may be necessary to increase insulin dose. As it is a drug decreasing hypophyseal stimulation for a long-term it may cause adrenal insufficiency, in which cases such symptoms as loss of appetite, nausea, anorexia, pain, fever and painful urination may appear in children. The drug should be administered carefully in patients with previous psychological problems. The behaviors, emotional status, sleeping order and psychomotor activity changes of child should be monitored and notified to doctor especially on long-term treatments. The treatment should be ceased by gradually decreasing dose. Long-term applications should be avoided in that it has many side effects. Unless otherwise stated by manufacturer nurse should protect drug against light and frost (Kavaklı et al, 1998).

6.4.41 Surfactant

Uses: Prophylaxis of infants at high risk for RDS (those < 29 weeks gestation).

Mode of Action: Preparation obtained from the lungs of beef. Lowers the surface tension of pulmonary alveoli, allowing easy opening of the alveoli and facilitates the process of respiration (Young & Mangum, 2010).

6.4.42 Tracutil

Administration: It is added to TPN solution in order to meet daily trace element need. IV infusion: Infusion should not be less than 6 and less than 24 hours. Contains Iron, Zinc, Manganese, Copper and Selenium.

Dose: 0.2 cc/kg in first week and then 0.5 cc/kg

Preparation: It can be used by being added to parenteral nutrition solutions.

Miscible Serums: 5% Dex, 10% Dex, SF, Ringer lactate, Amino acid solution.

Incompatibility: Sodium bicarbonate

Storing Conditions: Unopened ampoules are stored at room temperature under 25°C.

6.4.43 Vecuronium

Uses: Loosening the muscles before surgery.

Dose: 0.1. Mg/kg IV

Adverse Effects: The preparation is generally well tolerated. <1/1000- Allergic reactions. Allergic shock. Irritation at the injection site (Young & Mangum, 2010).

6.4.44 Vitamin K

Uses: Prophylaxis and therapy on hemorrhagic disease of the newborn. Treatment of hypoprothrombinemia secondary to factors limiting absorption or synthesis of vitamin K.

Dose: Preterm infants, 32 weeks gestation: BW > 1000 grams: 0.5 mg/kg IM. BW < 1000 grams: 0.3 mg/kg IM (Young & Mangum, 2010).

7. Drug management in pediatric nursing

Many drugs can be stored under room temperature (5-25°C). And some drugs need to be protected against sunlight. The list of drugs to be stored and not to be stored in refrigerator should be attached on the refrigerator in service. No IV drug including the diluted ones with more than 24-hour preservation period should be kept more than 24 hours. Preservation period for oral drugs explicitly written at the prospectuses are acceptable. If there is no period stated they are discharged after 30 days. That is why the first opening and discharge dates are always noted on the oral drugs (Çavuşoğlu, 2000).

Vital signs and clinical findings should be carefully evaluated. Therapeutic and toxic drug effects should be closely monitored. Kidney functions should be evaluated by monitoring the input-output liquid. The track of serum levels on drugs with limited therapeutic boundary should be ensured. The volume of the administered drug should be continuously monitored. With drugs requiring special safety measures those measures should be followed to the letter. The drugs which are not risky to administer on infants should be tagged with catchy titles and be kept away from the preparation area. One should be careful against potential side effects of the drugs which are underutilized and have limited reported experience on infants (Çetinkaya &Tengir, 2006). In terms of dose, some drugs are readjusted for infants by breaking the tablet, opening capsules, mixing with different liquids, or weighing the raw drug. Whether the drug was given at desired dose or if its bio-availability and microbial stabilities were variable cannot be determined when this method is used. Therefore, it is recommended not to resort to these methods unless otherwise is strictly required (Young & Mangum, 2010).

When a drug is administered the aim is to get the desired effects while keeping undesired ones at minimum. Pediatric nurse evaluates the response of the infant to drug and is the one to interfere if necessary. The knowledge of medication principles for newborns ensures a reliable drug administration (Çetinkaya &Tengir, 2006).

The following information should be obtained from parents before administering any drugs:

- Is the newborn allergic to any drugs?
- How does the newborn response to drug treatment?
- What are the names, doses, schedules and taking reasons of previously administered drugs?
- If newborn is breastfed, it should be found that whether the mother uses any drug or not.
- Does the infant or family know the reason why the drug has been prescribed or what are its desired effects (as well as potential side effects)?

Drug effectiveness and the tolerance of infants can be determined by the help of these questions. Besides, infant's development level, the needle size and suitable gauge for injection, how and when infants should be prepared can also be found out.

To avoid mistakes and to ensure safe, reliable drug administration, the principle called "*eight corrects*" is of a significant importance:

1. *Correct Drug:* The nurse should know the name and commercial name of the drug given by its first manufacturer. Name and dose should be checked three times before the use (Çavuşoğlu, 2000; Çetinkaya &Tengir, 2006).
2. *Correct Dose:* The dose should be calculated according to the body weight (kg) and its surface area (m^2). It is highly important to measure all the drugs properly (Çavuşoğlu, 2000; Çetinkaya &Tengir, 2006; Ovalı 2002).
3. *Correct Route:* The recommended route is checked along with the availability of that route and the condition of infant for that route (Çetinkaya &Tengir, 2006; Eroğlu 2002).
4. *Correct Patient (infant):* Each hospital has its own way of patient identification and recognition. There may be ID cards attached to the wrists or ankles for these purposes. Name of the child should be double-checked to avoid any confusion (Çavuşoğlu, 2000; Çetinkaya &Tengir, 2006).
5. *Correct Timing:* It takes longer time to administer drug to infants than administering it to adult patients. In this sense, timing of the previous administration should be checked carefully; and if it was not timely made, a new time-schedule should be arranged accordingly (Çetinkaya &Tengir, 2006; McKinney et al, 2000).
6. *Correct Approach:* During drug administration to infants, their fears, weaknesses and their ways for dealing with them are taken into account with regards to their development levels (Çavuşoğlu, 2000; Çetinkaya &Tengir, 2006).
7. *Correct Information:* The child and family should be informed about the purpose and duration of the drug treatment along with its desired effects and potential side effects. By this way, the recommended drugs can be used more safely (Çavuşoğlu, 2000; Çetinkaya &Tengir, 2006).
8. *Correct Record:* Prior to administration the nurse writes down the name of the drug, its dose, administration hour, and administration route on the observation form. The nurse performing this administration signs up the observation form with his / her name (Çetinkaya &Tengir, 2006; McKinney et al, 2000).

Pediatric drug doses are calculated according to body weight and body surface. Body surface area of the infants in proportion to their weight is much larger than that of the children and adults. This is why the dose for infants calculated with body surface is much higher than that calculated with body weight. Therefore, during the premature term and infancy periods body surface area is not used for dose calculation purposes (Çetinkaya &Tengir, 2006).

Generally, pediatric drug doses are described as gram or milligram per kilogram of body weight. Safe dose amounts differ according to infant's age and his/her ability to metabolize the drug. Before any drug is administered the recommended dose is checked and rechecked whether it should have been calculated properly. So there should be a drug guide in each pediatric unit (Çetinkaya &Tengir, 2006).

Since the pediatric doses are relatively fewer than adult ones, any mistake in the amount may have serious consequences. The biggest responsibility in drug administration falls onto nurses. The nurse should be well aware of the pharmacokinetic and pharmacodynamic effects of the drugs in order to assess the clinical effects and risky conditions (Çetinkaya &Tengir, 2006).

For premature infants, newborns and early infants the immatureness of their body systems affects the drug administration. Among the factors accompanying toxicity of drugs are an immature enzyme system in the liver, decrease of the protein fields that drugs bind, and immature kidney system. Likewise, drugs leading to acid-base imbalance also affect toxicity. For example, overdose of salicylates can easily lead to metabolic acidosis in infants. The drug level in serum, its side effects and urinary excretion should be evaluated to avoid drug toxicity (Çetinkaya &Tengir, 2006).

The electrolyte - fluid balance is closely monitored during drug treatment. Newborns have limited ability to concentrate urine, so they should be provided with adequate liquid to discharge both drugs and metabolites. Dehydration may increase the drug toxicity risk. An immature blood - brain barrier also serves for drug toxicity. The immature myelination of the central nervous system increases the permeability of blood - brain barrier. The myelination forming this barrier is not fully mature until the infant is 2 years old. As the permeability of blood - brain barrier increases during the diseases like meningitis and brain tumor, side effects of the drugs administered into central nervous system should be monitored closely (Çetinkaya &Tengir, 2006).

The skin absorption rate of the topical drugs is significant. Infants have a thin layer of dermis and epidermis, hence their absorption rate would be greater compared to adults. Besides, greater body surface in proportion to weight is an important factor when drug is administered on wide skin surface. Infants, therefore, should be monitored for their sensitiveness to the drugs applied on skin surface (Çetinkaya &Tengir, 2006).

If the patients taking numerous drugs together yield different findings than the anticipated results in the light of laboratory findings, drug interactions should be taken into consideration. Some drugs affect the absorption of other drugs through the gastrointestinal system (GIS). This interaction or behavior results from changes in pH, changes in flora, and drug binding to intestine lumen. For example, antacids do not only cause intestinal pH to change; but also inactivate the drugs by binding to them (Çetinkaya &Tengir, 2006).

The period of drug use differs from 1 week to 5 weeks before any symptom appears; following the next dose the symptoms reappear instantly. Redness, fever, joint pain and inflammation, lymphadenopathy, eosinophilic leukopathy can be observed (Çetinkaya &Tengir, 2006).

Drug Mistakes Caused by Nurse: Administration of drugs prior to a non-official request, administration of drugs without a physician's request, administration of wrong drug because of misspelling or resemblance in appearance, miscalculation of drug dose or administration at wrong dose, inattention to information provided on the drug container or package, forgetting the administration (Çetinkaya &Tengir, 2006).

Medical mistakes have a potential of becoming 8 times more harmful at the newborn intensive care units. One of those mistakes is the administration of the similar drugs at different concentrations given in different doses, whereas other mistakes could be system-related.

These are the most common mistakes made on newborns regarding drug administration:

- Administration of wrong dose because of the resemblance between Adult Vitamin K (10 mg/ml) and Neonatal Vitamin K (1 mg/0.5 ml) ampoules
- To confuse Vancomycin and Heparin vials
- Though not exactly a drug administration, vaccination at wrong doses through mistaking adult and infant versions of Diphtheria-Tetanus vaccine. Moreover, the administration of DTaP and Hib combination vaccine on inappropriate age groups in terms of their effectiveness on infants (although pentaxim or infanrix can be received under 1 year of age, combination vaccines, in general, has low effectiveness on such infants).
- To confuse Vecuronium (1mg/ml) (preparation: 0.25 mg/0.25 ml) and Cisatracurium (2 mg/ml) (preparation: 0.5 mg/0.25 ml (Used for avoiding muscle paralysis. Sedation effective) (Sauberan et al, 2010).

In this sense, the physician requests should be re-checked, any questions in mind should be asked to physician and be well understood, and the medication should be carried out on time and be recorded appropriately; by this way, any medical or legal danger caused by the drug mistakes either by nurses or physicians can be avoided. Since the pediatric doses are relatively fewer than those for adults, any quantitative mistake may lead to serious consequences (Çetinkaya &Tengir, 2006).

The factors leading to inadequate adaptation to prescribed drugs:

- Not obtaining the prescription, or not having it at the pharmacy
- Unclearness of the purpose regarding drug use
- Surmising the ineffectiveness of the drug
- Occurrence of actual side effect, or the thought of side effects appearing
- Unclearness of the instructions regarding drug intake
- Physical difficulty during the administration (handling small tablets, or unpacking drug container)
- Repelling formulations (e.g. unpleasant taste) (Kayaalp, 2001).

It is noteworthy again that the pediatric nurse to administer drug on patients should find out first that if the dose and route of the administration asked by physician is appropriate or not. The nurse should be careful for potential drug interactions. Infant's developmental characteristics affect the techniques and approaches used in drug administration. The infant and parents should be prepared besides with the drug. Attentive observation should be performed in and after the process. Observations about administration should be recorded. Patient should be kept well-monitored against undesired effects prior to administration. It is important to provide information and consultation services to the patient and/or family about drugs.

In conclusion, any mistake in drug amount for infants may have serious consequences. Nurse should be well informed about the preparation and administration of the drugs. Nurse should know about his/her legal responsibilities that might require in the process, and the pharmacologic properties of drugs. Nurse should also know about the generic and commercial names of drugs, and remain utmost careful during the administration. Pediatric nurses, in particular, should always update their knowledge about drugs.

	Ampicilline	Cefotaxime	Ceftazidime	Gentamicin	Vancomycin	Naphthalene	Penicillin	Impenem	Ciprofloxacin	Amphotericin	Acyclovir	Dobutamine	Dopamine	Fentanyl	Morphine	Heparin	Insulin	Lipid	Sodium Bicarbonate	Calcium	Potassium	Sodium Chloride	%5 dex	%10 dex	Ranitidine	PGEI	Propanadol	Epinephrine	Pentoxifylline
Pentoxifylline																						c	c	c					
Epinephrine	x											c	c			c			x		c	c	c	c		c			
Propanadol																c						c	c						
PGEI				c								c	c		c	c					c	c	c	x	c			c	
Ranitidine				c	c					x	c	c	c	c	c	c		c				c	c	c		c			x
%10 dex	c	c	c	c	c	c	c	c	c	c	c	c	c	c	c	c	c	c	c		c	c	c		c	x		c	
%5 dex	c	c	c	c	c	c	c	c	c	c	c	c	c	c	c	c	c	c	c	c	c	c		c	c	c	c	c	c
Sodium Chloride	c	c	c		c	c				x	c	c	c	c	c	c	c	c	c		c		c	c		c	c	c	c
Potassium	c	c	c		c	c				x	c	c	c	c	c	c	c	c	c			c	c	c		c	c	c	c
Calcium																			x			c	c	c					
Sodium Bicarbonate	x	x	c		c	c				c	c	x	c	c	c	c	x	c		x		c	c	c				x	
Lipid	x			c									c			c	c		c		c	c	c	c	c				
Insulin	c			c	c	x						c			c	c		c	x		c		c	c					
Heparin	c	c	c	x	c	c				c	c	c	c	c	c		c	c	c		c	c	c	c	c	c	c	c	
Morphine	c	c	c	c	c	c					c	c	c	c		c	c		c		c	c	c	c	c	c	c		
Fentanyl						c									c	c			c		c	c	c	c	c				
Dopamine	c			c						x	x	c			c	c		c	x		c	c	c	c	c	c		c	
Dobutamine											x		c		c	c	c		x		x	c	c	c	c	c	c	c	
Acyclovir	c	c	c	c	c	c						x	x		c	c			c		c	c	c	c	c				
Amphotericin				x				x					x			c			c		x	x	c	c	x				
Ciprofloxacin								x																					
Impenem	x	x	x		x	x	x		x	x												c	c	c					
Penicillin				x				x														c	c	c					
Naphthalene				x				x			c			c	c	c	x		c		c	c	c	c					
Vancomycin								x			c				c	c	c		c			c	c	c	c				
Gentamicin	x					x	x	x		x	c		c		c	x	c	c				c	c	c	c	c			
Ceftazidime								x			c				c	c			c		c	c	c	?					
Cefotaxime								x			c				c	c			x		c	c	c	c					
Ampicilline				x				x			c	c	c		c	c	c	x	x		c	c	c	c				x	

c : Compatible (can be given together or can be mixed)
x : Incompatible (cannot be mixed, cannot be administered consecutively through the same path)
? : Unknown

Table 1. Compatibility Chart of Some of the Most Frequently Used Drugs in Pediatrics (Katzung, 1998; Loeb, 1990; Trissel, 1992; Wong et al, 1992; Young & Magnum, 2008).

8. References

Akan, H. (2006). Akılcı Antibiyotik Kullanımı ve Türk Hematoloji Derneği. [*The rational use of antibiotics and the Turkish Hematology Association*]. ANKEM Derg 20(1):65-67.

Anand, K.J. (2007). Pharmacological Approaches to the management of Pain in the Neonatal İntensive Care Unit. Journal of Perinatology. ss. 4 -11.

Apak, H. (1996). Drugs used in paediatrics. In: Onat, T. Çocuk Sağlığı ve Hastalıkları. 1. Baskı. 2. Cilt. Eksen Yayınları. ss: 1140-1160.

Bal, Ç. (2005). Etkene Yönelik Tedavide Antibiyogram Yorumu. [*Antibiogram interpretation at the agent-oriented treatment*]. Turkiye Klinikleri J Int Med Sci 1(11):39-49.

Baytemür, M. (2005). Akılcı Antibiyotik Kullanımında Birinci Basamakta Sorunlar. [*The Questions at Primary Healthcare Regarding to Rational Use of Antibiotics*]. ANKEM Derg 19 (Ek 2):182-184.

Behrman, R.E. & Kliegman, R.M. (2001). Drug doses. In: Tuzcu, S. (Çeviren). Essential of Pediatrics. 3. Baskı. Nobel Tıp Kitapevleri. ss: 783-807.

Biçer, S. (2008). Frequently used drugs at the infant intensive-care units. In: Karaböcüoğlu, M., Köroğlu, T.F. (Edt). Çocuk Yoğun Bakım Esaslar ve Uygulamalar. 1. Baskı. İstanbul: İstanbul Medikal Yayıncılık, OHAN Matbaa, ISBN: 978-9944-211-36-9. ss. 1143-1171.

Buxton, I. L. O. & Benet, L. Z. (2011). Pharmacokinetics: The Dynamics of Drug Absorption, Distribution, Metabilism, and Elimination. In: Brunton, L., Chabner., B, Knollman, B. (Edt). Goodman's & Gillman's The Pharmacological Basis of Therapeutics. United States: The McGraw-Hill Companies. ss. 17-41.

Canlı, H., Erdoğan, F. & Özşahin K. (2009). Birinci Basamakta Antibiyotik Kullanımı. [*The use of antibiotics at primary healthcare*]. STED.18 (5) :94-96.

Çavuşoğlu, H. (2000). Paediatric nursing. 4. Baskı. Cilt: 2. Ankara: Bizimbüro Basımevi. ISBN: 975-94996-3-0, 975-94996-5-7. ss: 247-264.

Çelen, M.K., Hoşoğlu, S., Geyik, M.F., Akalın, Ş. & Ayaz, C. (2005). Dicle Üniversitesi Hastanesi' ndeki Antibiyotik Tüketimi İndeksi ve Geliştirilen Kontrollü Antibiyotik Kullanımının Etkileri. [*The antibiotic consumption index and the effects of the controlled antibiotic use that was developed at the Dicle University Hospital*]. FLORA Dergisi 10(4):180-184.

Cetinkaya, F. & Cag, Y. (2004). Penicillin sensitivity among children without a positive history for penicilin allergy. Pediatr Allergy Immunol.15: 278-280.

Çetinkaya Ş, Karataş Y, Antmen A. B., Alhan E. (2010). Knowledge and behavior of the pediatricians on rational use of antibiotics. African Journal of Pharmacy and Pharmacology, November, Vol. 4(11). pp. 783-792.

Çetinkaya, S., Parlak, A. & Tengir, T. (2008). Nurses' and Midwifes' Knowledge and Application Associated with Penicillin Allergy Test in Konya Province Primary Health Care Services. Turkiye Klinikleri J Pediatr, 17:80-88.

Çetinkaya Ş, Tengir T (2006). Drug management in paediatric nursing. Atatürk Ü. Hemşirelik Yüksekokulu Dergisi, Cilt: 9, Sayı: 1, ss. 86-97.

Çetinkaya, Ş. & Tengir, T. (2008). Penicillin Allergy and Penicillin Allergy Test: ReviewTurkiye Klinikleri J Pediatr, 17:175-182

Dinç L (2011). Preparation for application of drugs. In: Klinik Uygulama Becerileri ve Yöntemleri. Editör: AG Perry, PA Potter. Clinical Nursing Skills&Techniques.

Klinik Uygulama Becerileri ve Yöntemleri. Türkinaz Atabek Aştı, Ayişe Karaadağ (Çev. Edt). Adana: Nobel Kitapevi. ss. 609-631.
Dursun, B. & Bavbek, S. (2005). In Vivo Diagnostics in drug allergies. In İlaç Alerjileri Sevim Bavbek, Zeynep Mısırlıgil (Edt). Ankara: Bilimsel Tıp Yayınevi, ss. 39-63.
Dökmeci, İ. (2000). Farmakoloji. Nobel Tıp Kitapevleri, Tayf Ofset. ss: 841-842, 861, 870-878.
Dökmeci, İ. (2001). Farmakoloji Dersleri ve Konularla İlgili Sorular. Nobel Tıp Kitapevleri, Tayf Ofset. ss: 56-61.
Eroğlu L. (2002). Paediatric pharmacology. In: Neyzi, O., Ertuğrul, T. (Ed). Pediatri. 3. Baskı, Nobel Tıp Kitabevleri, Tayf Ofset. ss. 571-591.
Feder, H.M., Gerber, M.A., Randiph, M.F., Stelmach, P.S. & Kaplan, E.L. (1999). Once-Daily Theraphy for Streptococcal Pharyngitis with Amoxicillin. Pediatrics. January, 103 (1): 47-51.
Gallardo, M.A. & Thomas, I. (1999). Hypersensivity Reaction to Eritromycin. Cutis. 64 (6): 375.
Gökalp, O. & Mollaoğlu, H. (2003). Inappropriate drug usage. Süleyman Demirel Üniversitesi Tıp Fakültesi Dergisi. 10 (2):17-20.
Görgülü, R.S. & Ulusoy, M.F. (1996). Temel Kuram Kavram İlke ve Yöntemler. Nursing basics. 2. Baskı. Cilt: 1. Ankara: TDFO Ltd Şti. ISBN: 975-96014-0-0. ss: 183-231.
Kanmaz, G. (2010). Frequently used drugs. In: Dilmen, U. (Edt). Yenidoğan Rehberi. Ankara: Sarıyıldız Ofset. ISBN: 978-605-88354-0-5. ss. 374-443.
Karabay, O. (2009). Türkiye'de Antibiyotik Kullanımı ve Direnç Nereye Gidiyor? [*Where are the use of antibitoics and antibitotic resistance going to in Turkey?*]. ANKEM Derg 23 (Ek 2):116-120.
Kartal, F.A. (2002). Pharmacokinetics in newborns and infants. In: Yücel, A., Özyalçın, N.S. (Edt) Pain at the infancy. Nobel tıp Kitabevleri. ss: 248-253.
Katzung, B.G. (1998). Clinical Pharmacology, Londan: Appleton & Lange.
Kavaklı, A., Pek, H. & Bahçecik, N (1998).Frequently used drugs in the infants, and normal serum values. In: Çocuk Hastalıkları Hemşireliği. Düzeltilmiş 2. Baskı. İstanbul: Çevik matbacılık. ss.459-511. ISBN: 975 411 100-6.
Kayaalp, O. (2001). Türkiye İlaç Kılavuzu 2001 Formülleri. İstanbul:Turgut Yayıncılık. ss: 1
Kırdak, T. & Kılıçturgay, S. (1996). Prophylactic antibiotics in surgery . Sendrom. 8 (3): 32-42.
Köksal, Y. & Reisli, İ. (2002). Acute Otitis Media in Children. Journal of Ankara Medical School. 24 (1): 19-25.
Küçüködük, Ş. (1994).Newborn pharmacology and illnesses. Yenidoğan ve Hastalıkları. Feryal Matbaa. ss: 629-653.
McKinney, E.S., Ashwill, J.W., Murray, S.S. James, S.R., Gorrie, T.M. & Droske, S.C. (2000). Maternal and Child Nursing. W.B. Saunders Company. pp: 991-1000.
Mungan, D. (2005). Allergy to Beta-lactam antibiotics. In İlaç Alerjileri Sevim Bavbek, Zeynep Mısırlıgil (Edt). Ankara: Bilimsel Tıp Yayınevi. ss. 85-99.
Loeb, S. (1990). Pediatric Drug Therapy. Pennsylvania, Springhouse Co.
Longo, G., Barbi, E. &Wald, E.R. (2002). Amoxicillin Dosage/in Reply. Pediatrics. 110 (1) 195.
Ovalı, F. (2002). Principles of medication for newborns. In: Dağoğlu, T., Görak, G. (Ed) Temel Neonatoloji ve Hemşirelik İlkeleri. Nobel Tıp Kitabevleri. ss: 186-188.

Ovalı, F. (2008). Principles of medication for newborns. In: Dağoğlu, T., Görak, G. (Ed) Temel Neonatoloji ve Hemşirelik İlkeleri. Nobel Tıp Kitabevleri. ss:743-755.

Özdemir, D. (2010). Çocuk Acil Serviste Akılcı Antibiyotik Seçimi. [*The rational choice of antibiotics at pediatric emergency services*]. Clinic Pediatri, Çocuk Acil Özel Sayısı, Ocak-Şubat 5(1):1-4.

Özgüneş, İ. (2005). Akılcı Antibiyotik Kullanımında Hastane Pratiğinde Sorunlar. [*Problems in the rational use of antibiotics related to hospital practice*]. ANKEM Derg 19 (Ek 2):185-189.

Özcengiz, D. (2011). Newborn physiology and pharmacology. http://lokman.cu.edu.tr/anestezi/anestezinot/ yeni_sayfa_4.htm Erişim Tarihi: 25.08.2011

Pala, Z. & Baktır, G. Drug use in children. http://www.teb.org.tr/images/upld2/ecza_ akademi/makale/20110113033750cocuklarda_ilac_kullanimi.pdf Erişim Tarihi: 22.08.2011.

Park, M.A. & James, T.C. (2005). Diagnosis and Management of Penicilin Allergy. Mayo Clinic Proceedings. Mar 80(3): 405-410.

Patel, S.J. & Saiman, L. (2010). Antibiotic Resistance in Neonatal İntensive Care Unit Pathogens: Mechanisms, Clinical İmpact, and Prevention İncluding Antibiotic Stewardship. Clin Perinatol. Sep;37(3):547-63.

Puchner, T.C. Jr., & Zacharisen, M.C. (2002). A Survey of Antibiotic Prescribing and Knowledge of Penicilin Allergy. Annals of Allergy, Asthma and Immunology, Palatine, 88 (1): 67.

Pursell, E. (2010). İbuprofen For Treatment of Fever in İnfants, Practice Nursing. Oct (21);10: 533-538.

Rang, H.P., Dale, M.M., Ritter, J.M. (1998). Pharmacology. Third Edition, Churchill Livingstone. pp: 729-735.

Sauberan, J.B., Dean, L.M., Fiedelak, J. & Abraham, J.A. (2010). Orgins of and Solution for Neonatal Medication-Dispensing Errors, Am J Health-Syst Pharm. Jan 1; 67 (1): 49-57.

Schultheis, L.W., Mathis, L.L., Roca, R.A.R., Simone, A. F. S., Hertz, S. H. & Rappaport, B. A. (2006). Pediatric Drug Development in Anesthesiology: An FDA Perspective. Anesthesia & Analgesia. July 103(1):49-51.

Sin, A. S. (2005). The immunopathogenicity of drug allergies. In İlaç Alerjileri Sevim Bavbek, Zeynep Mısırlıgil (Edt). Ankara: Bilimsel Tıp Yayınevi. ss. 21-38.

Şardan, Y.Ç. (2005) Akılcı Antibiyotik Kullanımı. [*The rational use of antibiotics*] Turkiye Klinikleri J Int Med Sci 1(11):27-31.

Tomaç, N. & Üstündağ, G. (2005). Epidemiology of drug allergies, risk factors, social and economical effects. In İlaç Alerjileri Sevim Bavbek, Zeynep Mısırlıgil (Edt). Ankara: Bilimsel Tıp Yayınevi. ss. 13-19.

Trissel, L.A. (1992). Handbook on Injectable Drugs. 7th Edition. American Society of Hospital Pharmacist, Inc.

Wong, A.,F., McCulloch, L.M. & Sola, A. (1992). Treatment of peripheral tissue ischemia with topical nitroglycerin oinment in neonates. J Pediatr. 121: 980-983.

Young, T.E. & Magnum, O.B. (2008). Neofax 2008. New Jersey: Thomson Reuters.

Young TE, Mangum B (2010). Neofax 2010. Twenty - Third Edition 2010, Thomson Reuters.
Yüncü F. (1994). Pharmacology course-book. Ankara: Yüncü Yayınları. ss: 2-19.
Zeph, B. (2002). Management of Patients with Cefalosporin Allergy. American Family Physician. 65 (6): 1196.